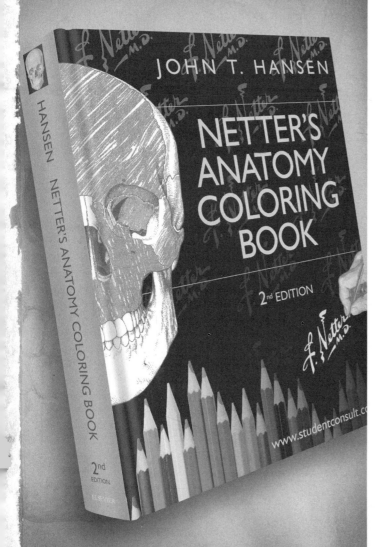
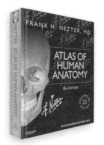
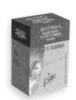
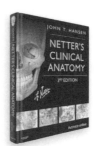
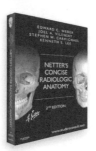

Netter's Anatomy **Coloring Book**

2nd Edition

John T. Hansen, PhD

Professor of Neurobiology and Anatomy
Associate Dean for Admissions
University of Rochester School of Medicine and Dentistry
Rochester, New York

ARTISTS

Art based on the works of the **Frank H. Netter, MD,** collection
www.netterimages.com

Modified for coloring by
Carlos A.G. Machado, MD
and
Dragonfly Media Group

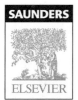

SAUNDERS

ELSEVIER

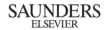

SAUNDERS
ELSEVIER

1600 John F. Kennedy Blvd.
Ste 1800
Philadelphia, PA 19103-2899

NETTER'S ANATOMY COLORING BOOK, SECOND EDITION   ISBN: 978-0-323-18798-5

ISBN: 978-0-323-18798-5

Senior Content Strategist: Elyse O'Grady
Senior Content Development Specialist: Marybeth Thiel
Publishing Services Manager: Patricia Tannian
Senior Project Manager: John Casey
Senior Book Designer: Lou Forgione

Printed in United States of America

Last digit is the print number: 9 8 7 6 5 4 3 2

For **Amy**, daughter, wife, mother, and physician, who colored her way through medical school and made me a believer...

For **Sean**, son, husband, father, and engineer, who colored outside the lines and showed me his creativity...

And, for **Paula**, wife, mother, grandmother, teacher, and soul mate, who understood the value of coloring and always gave us encouragement.

About the Artists

Frank H. Netter, MD

Frank H. Netter was born in 1906, in New York City. He studied art at the Art Student's League and the National Academy of Design before entering medical school at New York University, where he received his MD degree in 1931. During his student years, Dr. Netter's notebook sketches attracted the attention of the medical faculty and other physicians, allowing him to augment his income by illustrating articles and textbooks. He continued illustrating as a sideline after establishing a surgical practice in 1933, but he ultimately opted to give up his practice in favor of a full-time commitment to art. After service in the United States Army during World War II, Dr. Netter began his long collaboration with the CIBA Pharmaceutical Company (now Novartis Pharmaceuticals). This 45-year partnership resulted in the production of the extraordinary collection of medical art so familiar to physicians and other medical professionals worldwide.

In 2005, Elsevier, Inc. purchased the Netter Collection and all publications from Icon Learning Systems. There are now over 50 publications featuring the art of Dr. Netter available through Elsevier, Inc. (in the US: www.us.elsevierhealth.com/Netter; outside the US: www.elsevierhealth.com).

Dr. Netter's works are among the finest examples of the use of illustration in the teaching of medical concepts. The 13-book *Netter Collection of Medical Illustrations*, which includes the greater part of the more than 20,000 paintings created by Dr. Netter, became and remains one of the most famous medical works ever published. *The Netter Atlas of Human Anatomy*, first published in 1989, presents the anatomical paintings from the Netter Collection. Now translated into 16 languages, it is the anatomy atlas of choice among medical and health professions students the world over.

The Netter illustrations are appreciated not only for their aesthetic qualities, but, more important, for their intellectual content. As Dr. Netter wrote in 1949, "…clarification of a subject is the aim and goal of illustration. No matter how beautifully painted, how delicately and subtly rendered a subject may be, it is of little value as a *medical illustration* if it does not serve to make clear some medical point." Dr. Netter's planning, conception, point of view, and approach are what inform his paintings and what makes them so intellectually valuable.

Frank H. Netter, MD, physician and artist, died in 1991.

Learn more about the physician-artist whose work has inspired the Netter Reference collection:

http://www.netterimages.com/artist/netter.htm

Carlos A.G. Machado, MD

Carlos Machado was chosen by Novartis to be Dr. Netter's successor. He continues to be the main artist who contributes to the Netter collection of medical illustrations.

Self-taught in medical illustration, cardiologist Carlos Machado has contributed meticulous updates to some of Dr. Netter's original plates and has created many paintings of his own in the style of Netter as an extension of the Netter collection. Dr. Machado's photorealistic expertise and his keen insight into the physician/patient relationship inform his vivid and unforgettable visual style. His dedication to researching each topic and subject he paints places him among the premier medical illustrators at work today.

Learn more about his background and see more of his art at:

http://www.netterimages.com/artist/machado.htm

PREFACE: HOW TO USE THIS BOOK

Human anatomy is a fascinating and complex subject, and one that is interesting to virtually every one of us. Learning anatomy does not have to be difficult and can actually be enjoyable. Exploring human anatomy in a simple, systematic, and fun way is what the *Netter's Anatomy Coloring Book* is all about. This coloring book is for students of all ages; curiosity is the only prerequisite!

The images in *Netter's Anatomy Coloring Book* are based on the famous beautifully rendered medical illustrations of human anatomy by Frank H. Netter, MD, as compiled in his *Atlas of Human Anatomy*. This anatomy atlas is the most widely used anatomy atlas in the world and is translated into 16 different languages, and with good reason. The Netter illustrations have withstood the test of time and have illuminated human anatomy for millions of students around the world.

Why use an anatomy coloring book? The best reason, in my opinion, is because "active learning" always trumps passive learning. Seeing, doing, and learning go hand-in-hand; said another way, "eye to hand to mind to memory." This is how most of us learn best. Textbooks, flash cards, videos, and anatomy atlases all have their place in learning human anatomy, but those elements that engage us the most and allow us to participate in an active learning experience "cement" the material into our memory.

The *Netter's Anatomy Coloring Book* approaches human anatomy by body system. Footnotes to the illustrated pages refer to Dr. Netter's *Atlas of Human Anatomy* and *Netter's Clinical Anatomy*—the sources of the original full-color, fully labeled illustrations—for your further review and reference. In each coloring book plate, the most important structures are emphasized. The coloring exercises, labels, text, bullet points of essential material, and tables are provided to help you understand why the carefully chosen views of the human body are important both anatomically and functionally. I intentionally did not over-label each image because I want you to focus on the most important aspects of the anatomy; however, this is *your* coloring book! Feel free to color everything you wish; add your own labels as desired; cover structures to quiz yourself; in short, use each image as creatively as you wish to enhance your learning experience. In most cases, I let you choose the colors you want but would encourage you to color arteries bright red, veins blue, muscles reddish-brown, nerves yellow, and lymph nodes green, as these are common colors used in most color atlases of anatomy. Finally, I think you probably will find that colored pencils work best; but if crayons, colored pens, highlighters, or markers are your preferred medium, by all means use them! Most of all, have fun learning anatomy—after all, it is your anatomy too!

JOHN T. HANSEN, PHD

Contents

Contents

Chapter 1 **Orientation and Introduction**

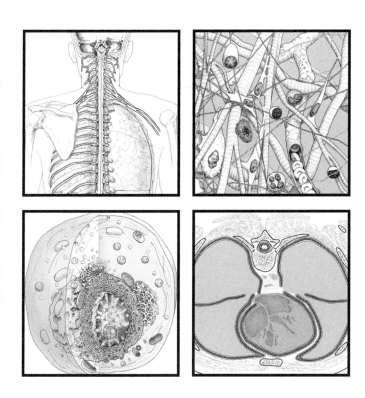

Anatomy requires a clinical vocabulary that defines position, movements, relationships, and planes of reference. By convention, anatomical descriptions of the human body are based on a person standing in the "**anatomical position.**" This position is defined as:

- Standing erect and facing forward
- Arms hanging at the sides, palms facing forward
- Legs placed together, feet slightly apart and directed forward

Regions of the body are defined by using the original Latin or Greek terms, although current usage in English-speaking countries uses more familiar terms. Regardless, some of the original terms are still used and seen in textbooks. The images on Plate 1-1 show some of the major regions and specific areas of the human body that are commonly used in anatomy and clinical settings.

COLOR the major regions, beginning with the head and working inferiorly to the lower limb, using a different color for each region:

1. Head (cephalon)
2. Neck (cervicis)
3. Thorax (chest)
4. Abdomen
5. Pelvis
6. Upper limb
7. Lower limb

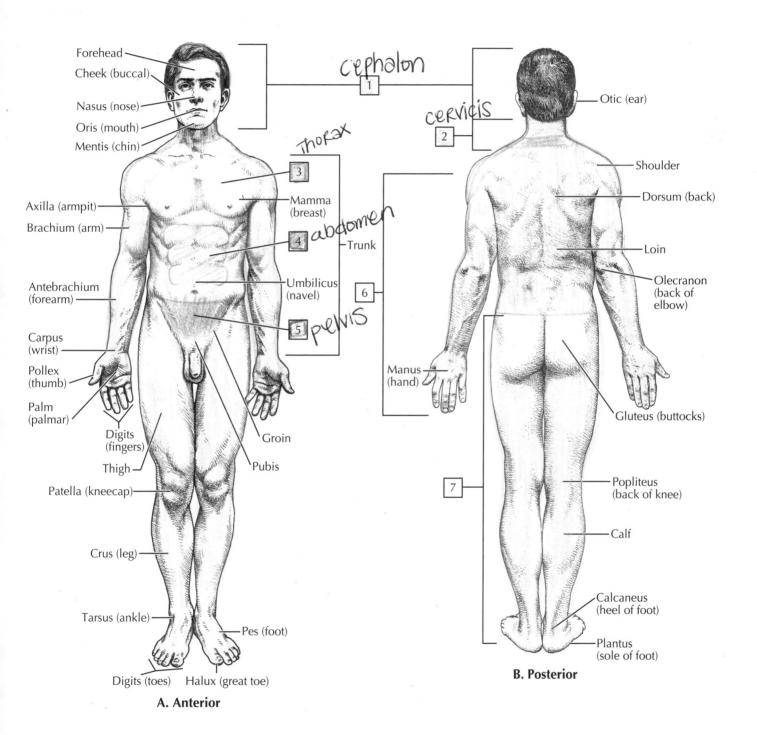

Forehead

Cheek (buccal)

Nasus (nose)

Oris (mouth)

Mentis (chin)

cephalon

1

cervicis

2

Otic (ear)

thorax

3

Shoulder

Mamma
(breast)

Dorsum (back)

Axilla (armpit)

Brachium (arm)

abdomen

4

Trunk

Loin

Umbilicus
(navel)

6

Olecranon
(back of
elbow)

Antebrachium
(forearm)

pelvis

5

Carpus
(wrist)

Pollex
(thumb)

Palm
(palmar)

Manus
(hand)

Digits
(fingers)

Groin

Gluteus (buttocks)

Thigh

Pubis

Patella (kneecap)

7

Popliteus
(back of knee)

Crus (leg)

Calf

Tarsus (ankle)

Pes (foot)

Calcaneus
(heel of foot)

Digits (toes)   Halux (great toe)

Plantus
(sole of foot)

A. Anterior

B. Posterior

Anatomical descriptions are referenced to one of four body planes that pass through the human body in anatomical position. The **four planes** include the following:

- The median plane, also known as the median sagittal or **midsagittal plane**, is a vertical plane that passes through the center of the body, dividing it into equal right and left halves.
- Sagittal planes, other than the median sagittal plane, are vertical planes that are parallel to the median sagittal plane and are often called **parasagittal planes**.
- Frontal planes, also known as the **coronal planes**, are vertical planes that pass through the body and divide it into anterior (front) and posterior (back) sections.
- Transverse planes, also known as cross sections, horizontal, or **axial planes**, are planes that are at right angles to the sagittal and frontal planes and divide the body into superior and inferior sections.

Also, when anatomists or physicians refer to right and left, it is always the person or patient's right and left side that we are referring to, NOT your right or left side.

COLOR the three planes shown on the figure using different colors.

1. **Median plane (median sagittal)**
2. **Frontal plane**
3. **Transverse plane**

TERM	DESCRIPTION
Anterior (ventral)	Nearer the front
Posterior (dorsal)	Nearer the back
Superior (cranial)	Upward or nearer the head
Inferior (caudal)	Downward or nearer the feet
Medial	Toward the midline or median plane
Lateral	Farther from the midline or median plane
Proximal	Near to a reference point
Distal	Away from a reference point
Superficial	Closer to the surface
Deep	Farther from the surface
Median plane	Divides body into equal right and left halves
Midsagittal plane	Median plane
Sagittal plane	Divides body into unequal right and left halves
Frontal (coronal) plane	Divides body into equal or unequal anterior and posterior parts
Transverse plane	Divides body into equal or unequal superior and inferior parts (cross sections or axial sections)

A. Body Planes

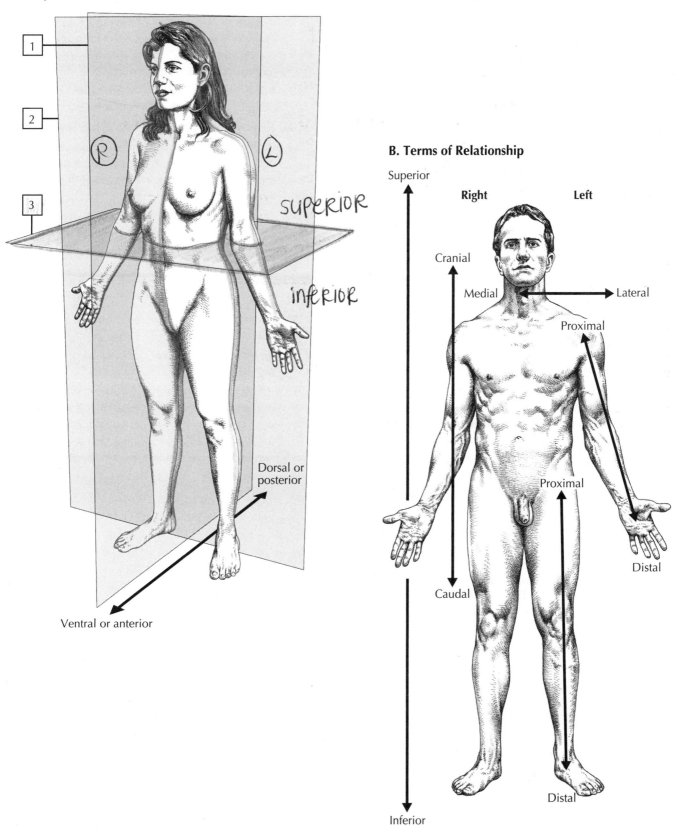

SUPERIOR

INFERIOR

1

2

3

Dorsal or posterior

Ventral or anterior

B. Terms of Relationship

Superior

Right   Left

Cranial

Medial   Lateral

Proximal

Proximal

Distal

Caudal

Distal

Inferior

Body movements occur at the joints, the points of articulation between two or more adjacent skeletal elements. Generally, when we refer to body movements we are focusing on movements about a joint that occur from the contraction (physical shortening) of skeletal muscle. These contractions result in the movement of a limb, the bending of the spine, the fine movements of our fingers, or the tensing of our vocal cords for speaking (phonation). Of course, many other types of movements also occur throughout the body, but the major movements about the joints are highlighted in the following list and illustrated.

COLOR the circle on the images corresponding to the numbered movement in the following list, using a different color for each movement. Note that the letter abbreviation of the movement (e.g., F = flexion) is shown in the circle and corresponds to the key in the list below.

1. **Abduction (AB): movement away from a central reference point**

1. **Adduction (AD): movement toward a central reference point; the opposite of abduction**

1. **Lateral rotation (L): turning a bone or limb around its long axis laterally or away from the midline**

1. **Medial rotation (M): opposite of lateral rotation; turning medially toward the midline**

2. **Flexion (F): usually a movement that decreases the joint's angle**

2. **Extension (E): usually a movement that increases the joint's angle; the opposite of flexion**

3. **Elevation (EL): lifting superiorly, as in shrugging your shoulders**

3. **Depression (D): a movement of a portion of the body inferiorly**

4. **Flexion (F) and extension (E) of the spine (as it relates to the spine, flexion decreases the angle between the vertebral bodies and extension increases this angle). When we bend forward we flex our spine, and when we bend backward to arch our back we are extending our spine.**

5. **Flexion (F) and extension (E) at the elbow**

6. **Flexion (F) and extension (E) at the wrist**

7. **Pronation (P): rotation of the radius about the ulna in the forearm causes the palm to face posteriorly (in anatomical position) or inferiorly (if hand held forward with the palm upward)**

7. **Supination (S): opposite of pronation; causes the palm to face anteriorly or superiorly**

8. **Flexion (F) and extension (E) at the knee joint**

9. **Circumduction (C): movement in space that circumscribes a circle or cone about a joint (circumduction of the lower limb at the hip joint is illustrated)**

10. **Dorsiflexion (DF): lifting the foot at the ankle joint (similar to extension at the wrist, but at the ankle it is referred to as dorsiflexion rather than extension)**

10. **Plantarflexion (PF): a downward movement or depression of the foot at the ankle (similar to wrist flexion)**

11. **Eversion (EV): movement of the sole of the foot laterally**

11. **Inversion (I): movement of the sole of the foot medially**

12. **Retraction (R): posterior displacement of a portion of the body without a change in angular movement**

12. **Protraction (PT): anterior displacement of a portion of the body without a change in angular movement**

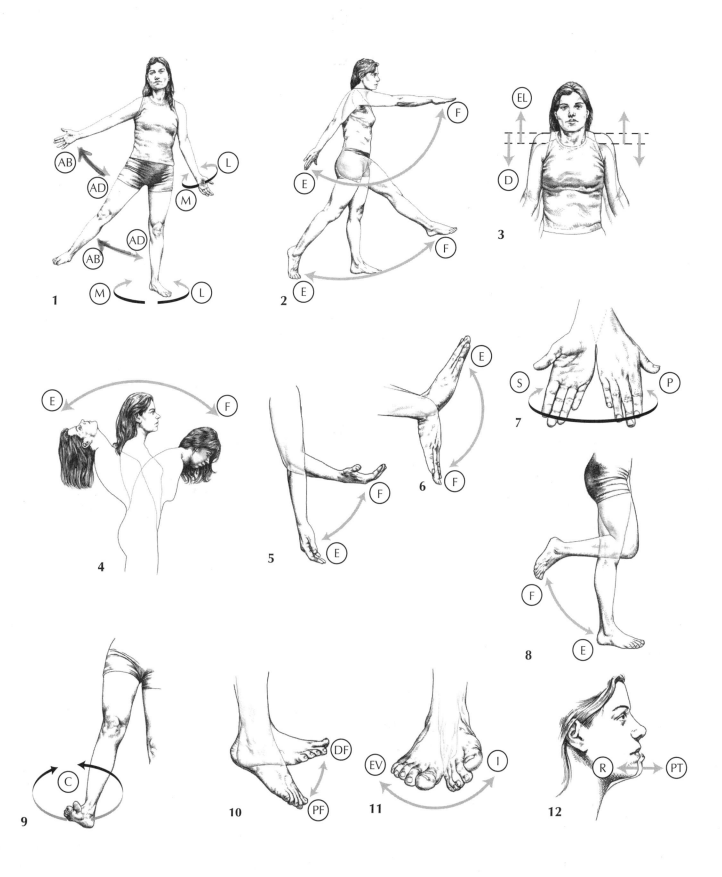

1 The Cell

The cell is the basic unit, structurally and functionally, of all of the body's tissues. Like people, cells come in many different varieties, but, also like people, almost all cells share many basic internal structures that we call **organelles**. Organelles function cooperatively in a variety of ways that allow the cell and tissues to perform their unique functions. Depending upon the type of cell, some will contain more of one type or another of an organelle or inclusion (unlike organelles, inclusions are not surrounded by a membrane).

COLOR each of these 13 cellular components, using different colors, noting their morphology and function as you do so.

 1. **Peroxisomes:** smaller vesicles containing enzymes that degrade hydrogen peroxide and fatty acids

 2. **Golgi apparatus:** flattened stacks of membranes that modify and package proteins and lipids for intracellular or extracellular use

 3. **Plasma membrane:** the "cell" membrane, composed of a lipid bilayer that functions in protection, secretion, uptake, sensitivity, adhesion, and support. The plasma membrane also can fuse with a secretory vesicle to release its contents, called exocytosis, or take up extracellular substances in a process called pinocytosis. The membrane also may possess specialized receptors along its surface.

 4. **Cytoplasm:** the aqueous matrix of the cell outside of the nucleus, containing inorganic ions, organic molecules, intermediate metabolites, carbohydrates, proteins, lipids, and RNA

 5. **Mitochondria:** produce ATP via oxidative phosphorylation for energy. Mitochondria possess an outer membrane and a folded inner membrane.

 6. **Lysosomes:** vesicles containing digestive enzymes

 7. **Endoplasmic reticulum:** membranous network in the cytoplasm, studded with ribosomes for protein synthesis (rough ER, 7A) or lacking ribosomes and involved with lipid and steroid synthesis (smooth ER, 7B)

 8. **Centrioles:** paired bundle-like inclusions essential for chromosome movement in cell division

 9. **Nucleolus:** condensation of RNA and proteins within the nucleus

 10. **Cell nucleus:** membrane-surrounded (inner and outer membranes) structure that contains chromosomes, enzymes, and RNA. The nuclear membrane, or envelope, is perforated by small nuclear pores.

 11. **Ribosomes:** RNA and proteins, both free and attached to rough ER. Ribosomes are involved in protein synthesis by translating the amino acid protein coding under the direction of mRNA.

 12. **Microfilaments:** inclusions that provide strength and support for the cell

 13. **Microtubules:** inclusions that comprise the cytoskeleton and assist in intracellular transport

Plate 1-4   **Orientation and Introduction**

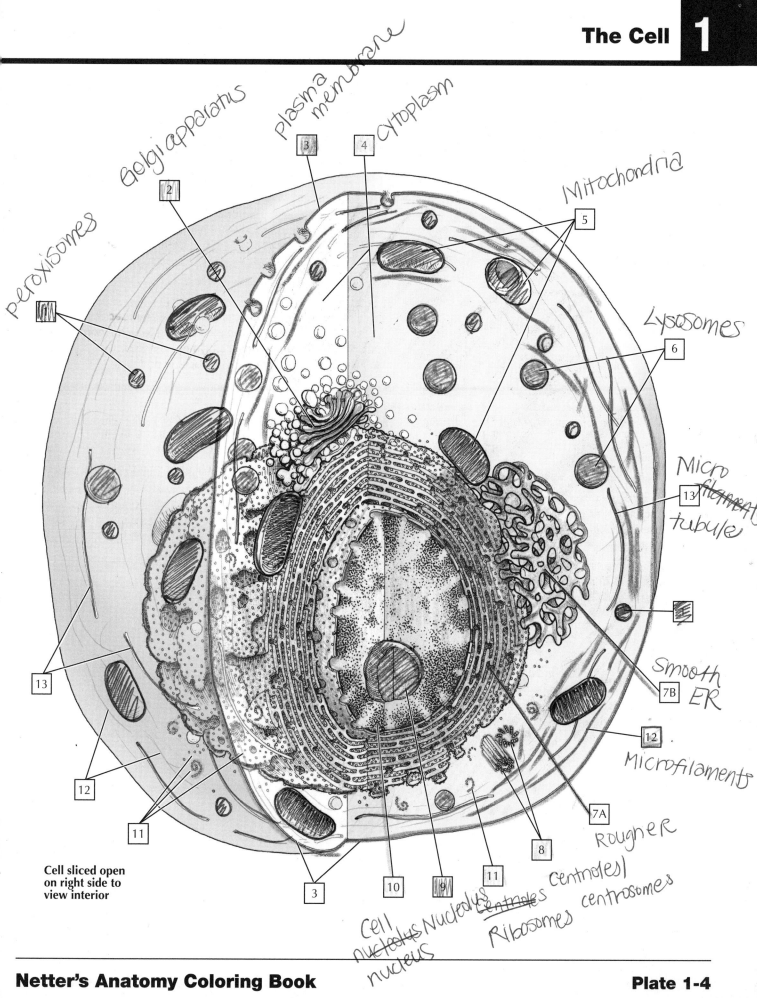

Peroxisomes

Golgi apparatus

plasma membrane

Cytoplasm

Mitochondria

Lysosomes

Micro filaments tubule

Smooth ER

Microfilaments

Rougher

Cell nucleus Nucleus nucleus

Centroles Centroles/ centrosomes

Ribosomes

Cell sliced open on right side to view interior

The epithelial cells form one of the four basic tissue types found in the human body (the other three are connective tissue, muscle tissue, and nervous tissue). The epithelium covers the body surfaces; lines the body cavities, the ducts of organs and glands, the vasculature, and organs; and forms the secretory portions of glands. Adjacent epithelial cells may form tight junctions between their cells and provide a barrier function; the cells may participate in absorption or secretion and/or possess the ability to distend and spread out along an expanded surface (the epithelium lining of the distended urinary bladder). The epithelium rests on a basement membrane.

Epithelium is classified based on the number of cell layers that comprise a tissue and includes:
• **Simple epithelium**: one cell layer in thickness
• **Stratified epithelium**: two or more cell layers in thickness

Additionally, epithelium is described based on the shape of the individual epithelial cells.

COLOR the three types of epithelium based on cell shape:

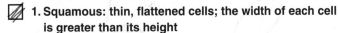 1. **Squamous: thin, flattened cells; the width of each cell is greater than its height**

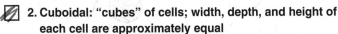 2. **Cuboidal: "cubes" of cells; width, depth, and height of each cell are approximately equal**

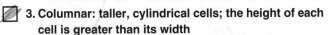 3. **Columnar: taller, cylindrical cells; the height of each cell is greater than its width**

The combination of cell layers and shapes combine to give six different kinds of epithelia, plus two specialized types called pseudostratified and transitional, for a total of eight types of epithelia.

Clinical Note:
In adults, the most common types of cancer (neoplasm) originate in epithelial cells, and are called carcinomas. Tumors may be benign or malignant and usually undergo a precancerous change described as dysplasia (abnormal development) or metaplasia (abnormal transformation).

COLOR examples of the eight types of epithelia typically seen in tissues and organs:

☐ 4. **Simple squamous: lines body cavities and vasculature, offering a barrier to transport or functioning as an exchange system, often by simple diffusion**

☐ 5. **Simple cuboidal: lines ducts of glands and kidney tubules, offering a passageway with or without the ability for absorption and secretion**

☐ 6. **Simple columnar: lines much of the gastrointestinal system, offering a surface for absorption and secretion**

☐ 7. **Pseudostratified: trachea, bronchi of the lungs, and ductus deferens, offering a passageway with or without barrier or secretory functions**

☐ 8. **Stratified squamous: the skin, oral cavity, esophagus and vagina, offering a protective surface; the skin may have a protective layer of keratin overlying the epithelium**

☐ 9. **Stratified cuboidal: ducts of sweat glands and other large exocrine glands, offering a conduit and/or a barrier to transport**

☐ 10. **Stratified columnar: large ducts of exocrine glands, offering a conduit and barrier**

☐ 11. **Transitional: lines the urinary system, offering a conduit and the ability to distend**

Plate 1-5 **Orientation and Introduction**

BM: Basement membrane
CT: Connective tissue

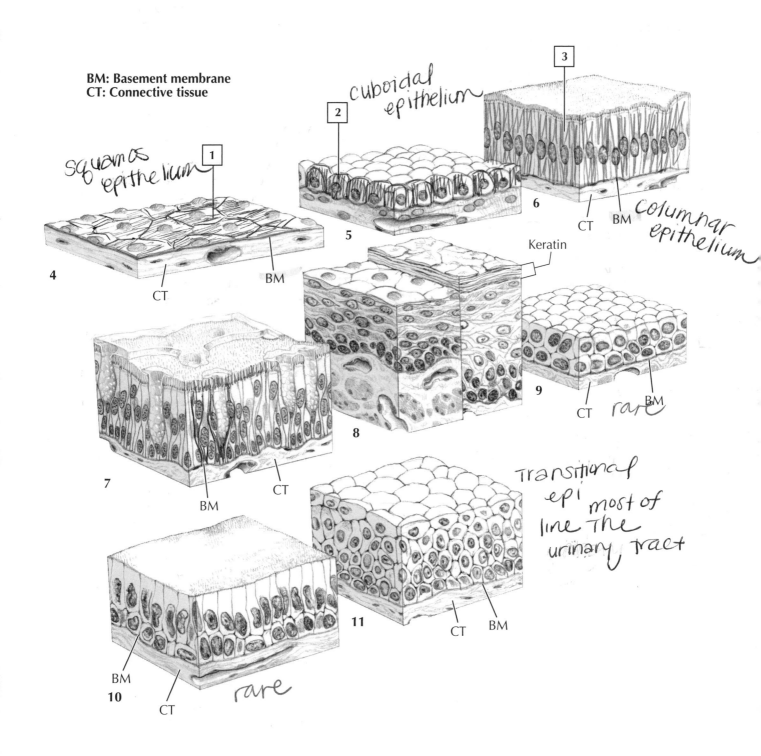

squamos epithelium

cuboidal epithelium

columnar epithelium

Keratin

1

2

3

4

CT

BM

5

6

CT   BM

7

BM   CT

8

9

CT   rare   BM

10

BM

CT

rare

11

CT   BM

Transitional epi most of line The urinary tract

Connective tissue comprises a diverse group of specialized cells and tissues. Connective tissues function in:

• Support
• Transport
• Storage
• Immune defense
• Thermoregulation

Two major groupings of connective tissues are recognized:

• **Connective tissue proper**: includes loose and dense connective tissue (arranged in either an irregular or a regular conformation)
• **Specialized connective tissue**: includes cartilage, bone, adipose tissue (fat), hemopoietic tissue, blood, and lymph

supporting CT

fluid CT

Connective tissue proper includes a variety of cell types and fibers enmeshed in a ground substance that comprises an **extracellular matrix**. **Loose connective tissue** is found largely under epithelia lining both the body's surface and its internal organ systems. Along with the skin, it is often the first line of defense against infection. **Dense connective tissue** has many fibers but few cells and includes tendons, ligaments, the submucosa, and reticular layers that offer support.

The fibrous elements in connective tissue include:

• **Collagen fibers**: numerous in connective tissues; offer flexibility and strength
• **Elastic fibers**: interwoven fibers that offer flexibility and retain their shape if stretched
• **Reticular fibers**: thinner collagen fibers that provide strength but are the least common of the fibrous elements

Clinical Note:

Tumors of the connective tissues are called sarcomas. Although there are over 25 different types of collagen, types I through IV are the most common. Type I accounts for 90% of the body's collagen and is common in the skin, muscle tendons, ligaments, and bone. Type II collagen is found in cartilage. Type III collagen is found in loose connective tissue and forms a loose reticular meshwork or supportive scaffold for the tissues and organs. Type IV collagen is found in the basement membrane supporting the epithelium.

COLOR each of most common cellular elements in connective tissue, using a different color for each type, as they appear in the different varieties of connective tissue:

1. **Plasma cells**: secrete immunoglobulins and are derived from B lymphocytes
2. **Macrophages**: phagocytic cells (engulf pathogens and cell debris) derived from monocytes in the blood
3. **Lymphocytes**: the principal cells of the immune system
4. **Mast cells**: respond early to immune challenges and secrete powerful vasoactive and chemotactic substances
5. **Adipocytes**: store and release triglycerides as needed by the body (fat cells), and produce hormones and growth factors
6. **Fibroblasts**: abundant cells that synthesize all the fibrous elements and elaborate the matrix
7. **Eosinophils**: respond to allergens and parasitic infections, and are phagocytes
8. **Myofibroblasts**: are capable of contraction and function similar to fibroblasts and smooth muscle cells
9. **Neutrophils**: respond to injury and immune challenges, and are capable of phagocytosis

Plate 1-6

Orientation and Introduction

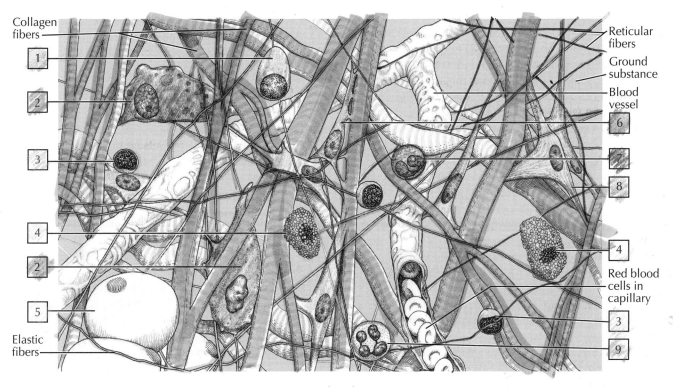

Collagen fibers

Reticular fibers

Ground substance

Blood vessel

Elastic fibers

Red blood cells in capillary

A. Connective tissue proper

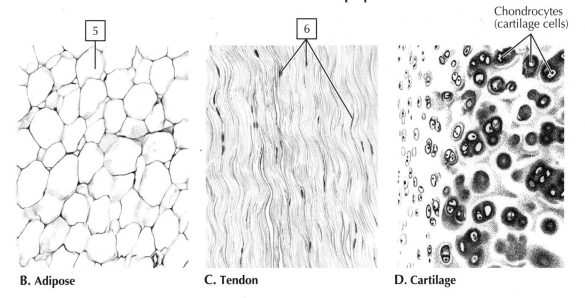

Chondrocytes (cartilage cells)

B. Adipose

C. Tendon

D. Cartilage

1 Skeleton

The human skeleton is divided into two descriptive regions: axial and appendicular.

COLOR each skeleton region a different color to differentiate them from one another:

1. **Axial skeleton: the bones of the skull, vertebral column (spine), ribs, and sternum (they form the "axis" or central line of the body)**

2. **Appendicular skeleton: the bones of the limbs, including the pectoral (shoulder) and pelvic girdles (they comprise the upper and lower limbs that attach to the axial skeleton)**

The axial skeleton includes 80 bones:
- The skull and associated bones (auditory ossicles and hyoid bone) account for 29 bones
- The thoracic cage (sternum and ribs) accounts for 25 bones
- The vertebral column accounts for 26 bones

The appendicular skeleton includes 134 bones:
- The pectoral girdle (paired clavicles and scapulae) accounts for 4 bones
- The upper limbs account for 64 bones
- The pelvic girdle (coxal or hip bone) accounts for 2 bones
- The lower limbs account for 64 bones

The skeletal system is composed of a living, dynamic, rigid connective tissue that forms the bones and cartilages of the human skeleton. Although we say the skeleton has 214 bones (including 8 sesamoid bones of the hands and feet), this number may actually vary somewhat. Cartilage is attached to some bones, especially where flexibility is important, and covers many of the articular (joint) surfaces of bones. About 99% of the body's calcium is stored in bones, and many bones possess a central cavity that contains bone marrow, a collection of hemopoietic (blood-forming) cells. Most individual bones can be classified into one of five shapes.

COLOR using a different color for each shape, the five different types of bones:

3. **Flat bone**
4. **Irregular bone**
5. **Short bone**
6. **Long bone**
7. **Sesamoid bone**

Functions of the skeletal system and bones include:
- Support
- Protecting vital tissues or organs
- Providing a mechanism, along with muscles, for movement
- Storing calcium
- Providing a supply of blood cells

Most articular surfaces of bone are covered by **hyaline cartilage**, the most common type of cartilage. A second type of cartilage is **fibrocartilage** and it is found where more support is needed (meniscus of the knee joint, intervertebral discs between the bodies of the vertebrae). The third type of cartilage is **elastic cartilage** and it is found where flexibility is needed (auricle of the ear, epiglottis).

Clinical Note:

Osteoporosis (porous bone) is the most common bone disease and results from an imbalance in bone resorption and formation, which places the bones at great risk for fracture. Approximately 10 million Americans (80% of them women) have osteoporosis.

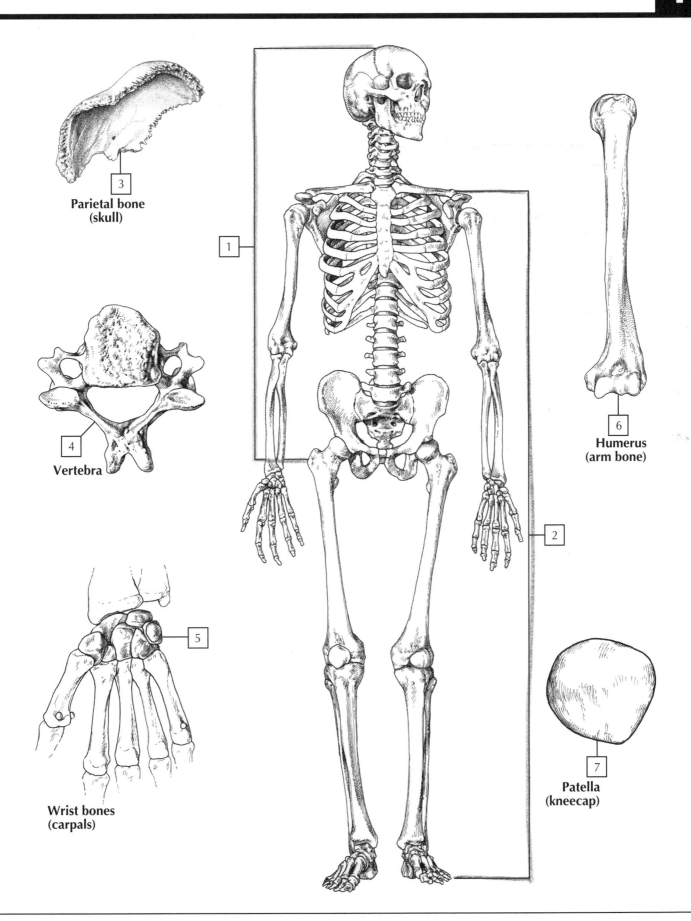

Parietal bone
(skull)

Vertebra

Wrist bones
(carpals)

Humerus
(arm bone)

Patella
(kneecap)

Joints are articulations between bones. Three types of joints are identified in humans:

- **Fibrous (synarthroses)**: bones joined by fibrous connective tissue (examples include sutures of some skull bones, fibrous connections between some long bones, and gomphoses [teeth in the jaw])
- **Cartilaginous (amphiarthroses)**: bones joined by either cartilage or cartilage and fibrous tissue; include primary (epiphysial plates of growing bones) and secondary types (intervertebral disc between adjacent vertebra of the spine)
- **Synovial (diarthroses)**: bones joined by a joint cavity filled with synovial fluid, surrounded by a capsule, with articular cartilage covering the opposed surfaces

Generally, the more movement that occurs at a joint, the more vulnerable that joint is to injury or dislocation. Joints that allow little or no movement offer greater support and strength.

Clinical Note:

Osteoarthritis is characterized by the progressive loss of articular cartilage and failure of repair. It can affect any synovial joint but most often involves the foot, hip, spine, and hand. Once the articular cartilage is degraded and lost, the exposed bony surfaces, called the subchondral (beneath the cartilage) bone, rub against one another, undergo some remodeling, and often cause significant pain.

COLOR the following features of each of the three major types of joints:

1. **Suture: a type of fibrous joint that allows little movement**

2. **Interosseous membrane: also a type of fibrous joint that permits some movement**

3. **Epiphysial plate: a cartilaginous joint that is immovable**

4. **Intervertebral disc: a cartilaginous joint that permits some movement**

5. **Synovial joint: the most common type of joint, which permits a range of movements (color the fibrous capsule, synovial membrane, articular cartilage, and synovial joint cavity each a different color)**

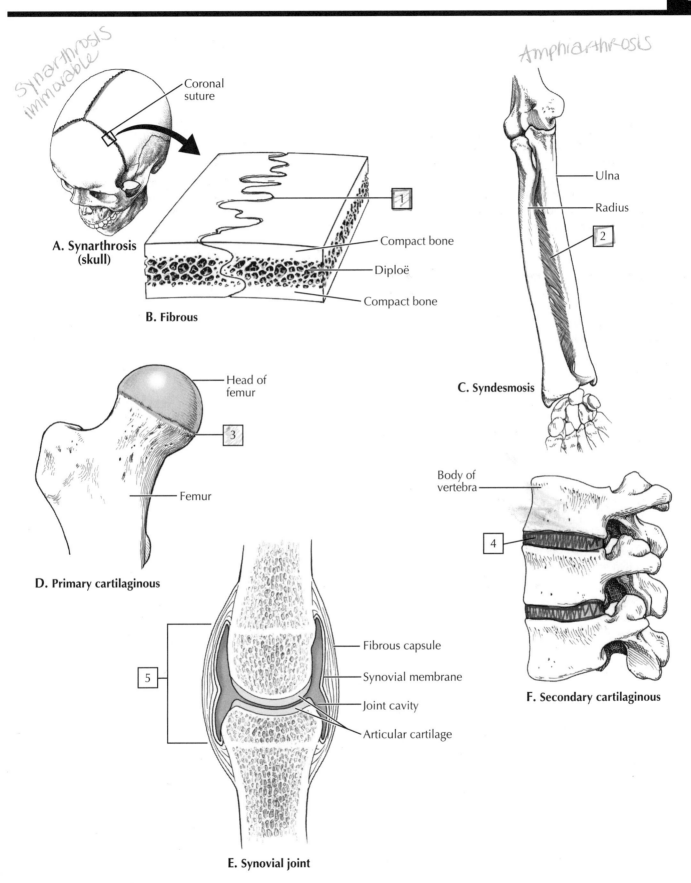

Synarthrosis immovable

Amphiarthrosis

Coronal suture

A. Synarthrosis (skull)

1

Compact bone

Diploë

Compact bone

B. Fibrous

Ulna

Radius

2

C. Syndesmosis

Head of femur

3

Femur

D. Primary cartilaginous

Body of vertebra

4

F. Secondary cartilaginous

5

Fibrous capsule

Synovial membrane

Joint cavity

Articular cartilage

E. Synovial joint

Generally, synovial joints offer considerable movement. They are classified according to their shape and the type of movement that they permit (uniaxial, biaxial, or multiaxial; movements in one, two, or multiple planes, respectively). The six types of synovial joints include:

- **Hinge (ginglymus)**: uniaxial joints that permit flexion and extension, similar to the elbow joint
- **Pivot (trachoid)**: uniaxial joints that permit rotation, similar to the joint between the atlas and axis (first two cervical vertebrae) of the neck that pivots from side to side as if shaking your head to signify "no"
- **Saddle**: biaxial joint for flexion, extension, abduction, adduction, and circumduction, similar to the joint at the base of the thumb (carpometacarpal joint)
- **Condyloid (ellipsoid)**: biaxial joint for flexion, extension, abduction, adduction, and circumduction, similar to the finger joints
- **Plane (gliding)**: joint for a simple gliding movement, similar to the joint at the shoulder between the clavicle and scapula (acromioclavicular joint)
- **Ball-and-socket (spheroid)**: multiaxial joint for flexion, extension, abduction, adduction, medial and lateral rotation, and circumduction, similar to the hip joint

COLOR the distal bone of each joint, as it usually undergoes the greatest amount of movement when that synovial joint moves:

- [ ] 1. **Ulna of the elbow's *hinge* joint**
- [ ] 2. **Axis of the atlanto-axial *pivot* joint**
- [ ] 3. **Metacarpal of the thumb's *saddle* joint**
- [ ] 4. **Tibia of the knee's *condyloid* joint**
- [ ] 5. **Femur of the hip's *ball-and-socket* joint: acetabulum of the pelvis forms the "socket" of this joint**
- [ ] 6. **Scapula of the acromioclavicular *plane* joint at the shoulder: plane joint between the acromion of the scapula and clavicle**

Within the synovial joint cavity a small amount of **synovial fluid**, a filtrate of blood flowing in the capillaries of the synovial membrane, lubricates the joint. This fluid has the consistency of albumen (egg white).

As muscles pass over a joint, their tendons may be cushioned by a fibrous sac called a **bursa**, which is lined by a synovial membrane (synovium) and contains a small amount of synovial fluid. These fluid-filled "bags" cushion the tendon as it slides over the bone and acts like a ball bearing to reduce some of the friction. Humans have over 150 bursae in different locations in the subcutaneous tissues associated with muscle tendons, bones, and joints at sites where cushioning helps to protect the tendon.

Clinical Note:

Movement at the joint can lead to inflammation of the tendons surrounding the joint and secondary inflammation of the bursa (**bursitis**) that cushions the joint and tendon. This inflammation is painful and can lead to a significant increase in the amount of synovial fluid in the bursa.

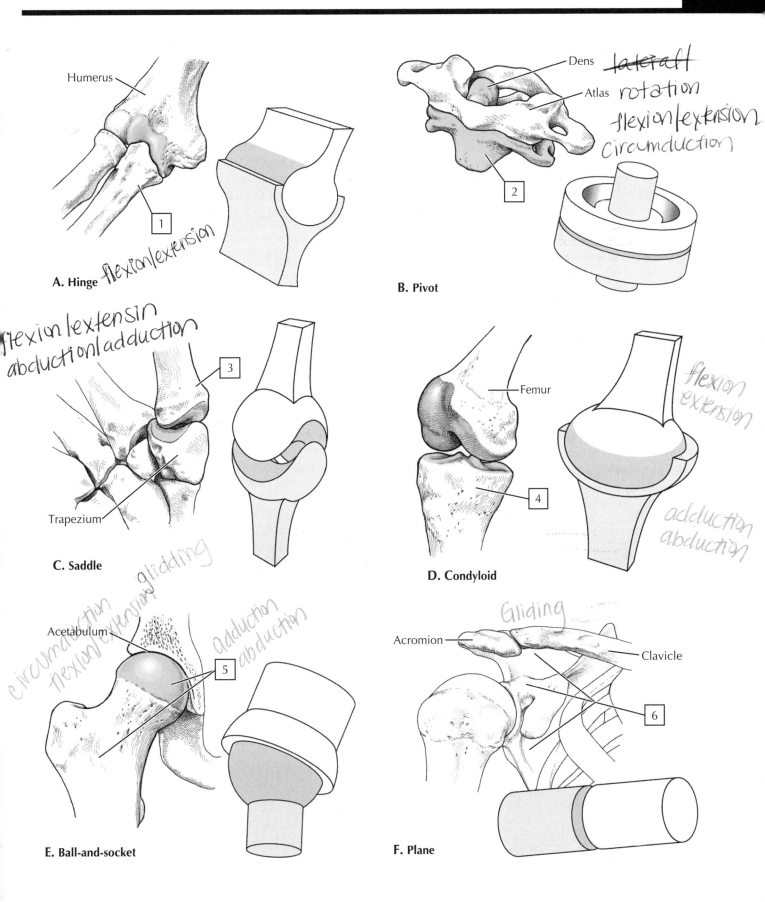

Humerus

1

A. Hinge flexion/extension

Dens — lateral
Atlas — rotation
flexion/extension
circumduction

2

B. Pivot

flexion/extensin
abduction/adduction

3

Trapezium

C. Saddle

Femur

flexion extension

4

adduction abduction

D. Condyloid

circumduction flexion/extension gliding

Acetabulum

adduction abduction

5

E. Ball-and-socket

Gliding

Acromion

Clavicle

6

F. Plane

Muscle cells (fibers) produce contractions (shorten in length) that result in movements, maintain posture, produce changes in shape, or move fluids through hollow tissues or organs. There are three different types of muscle:

- **Skeletal**: striated fibers that are attached to bone and are responsible for movement of the skeleton at its joints
- **Cardiac**: striated fibers that make up the walls of the heart
- **Smooth**: unstriated fibers that line various organs, attach to hair follicles, and line blood vessels

Muscle contractions occur in response to nerve stimulation at neuromuscular junctions, to paracrine stimulation (by localized release of various stimulating agents) in the local environment of the muscle, and to endocrine (via hormones) stimulation (see Plate 11-1).

Skeletal muscle is divided into bundles or fascicles. These fascicles are composed of fibers. The fibers are composed of myofibrils, and myofibrils contain myofilaments.

COLOR the elements of skeletal muscle, using a different color for each element:

☐ 1. **Muscle fascicles: which are surrounded by a connective tissue sheath known as the perimysium; epimysium is the connective tissue sheath that surrounds multiple fascicles to form a complete muscle "belly"**

☐ 2. **Muscle fibers: which are composed of a muscle cell that is a syncytium because it is multinucleated (the muscle fibers are surrounded by the endomysium)**

☐ 3. **Muscle myofibrils: which are longitudinally oriented and extend the full length of the muscle fiber cell**

☐ 4. **Muscle myofilaments: which are the individual myosin (thick filaments) and actin (thin filaments) filaments that slide over one another during muscle contraction**

Skeletal muscle moves bones at their joints and possesses an **origin** (the muscle's fixed or proximal attachment) and an **insertion** (the muscle's moveable or distal attachment). At the gross level, the shape of the muscle allows anatomists to classify them.

COLOR each of the five different conformations that characterize the gross appearance of skeletal muscle.

☐ 5. **Fusiform: thick in the center and tapered at the ends**

☐ 6. **Quadrate: four-sided muscle**

☐ 7. **Flat: parallel fibers**

☐ 8. **Circular: form sphincters that close off tubes**

☐ 9. **Pennate: feathered in appearance (unipennate, bipennate, or multipennate forms)**

Cardiac muscle has similarly arranged myofilaments as skeletal muscle but also possesses other structural features that distinguish it from skeletal muscle. Moreover, cardiac muscle has unique contraction properties, including an intrinsic rhythmic contraction and specialized conduction features that coordinate its contraction.

Smooth muscle usually occurs in bundles or sheets of elongated cells with a fusiform or tapered appearance. Smooth muscle is specialized for slow, prolonged contraction, and it also can contract in a wavelike fashion known as peristalsis.

In general, skeletal muscle does not undergo mitosis and responds to an increase demand by hypertrophy (increasing size but not numbers of cells). Cardiac muscle normally does not undergo mitosis and responds to an increased demand by hypertrophy. Smooth muscle can undergo mitosis and responds to an increased demand by hypertrophy and hyperplasia (increase in cell number). It also has the ability to regenerate.

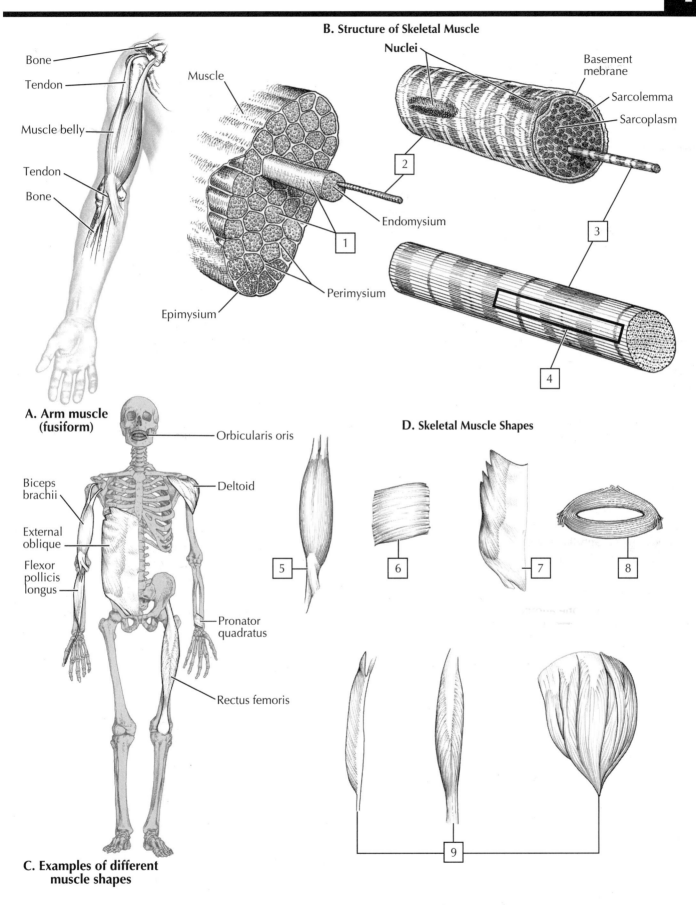

B. Structure of Skeletal Muscle

Bone

Tendon

Muscle belly

Tendon

Bone

A. Arm muscle (fusiform)

Muscle

Endomysium

Perimysium

Epimysium

1

Nuclei

Basement mebrane

Sarcolemma

Sarcoplasm

2

3

4

Orbicularis oris

Deltoid

Biceps brachii

External oblique

Flexor pollicis longus

Pronator quadratus

Rectus femoris

C. Examples of different muscle shapes

D. Skeletal Muscle Shapes

5

6

7

8

9

The nervous system integrates and regulates many body activities, sometimes at discrete locations (specific targets) and sometimes more globally. The nervous system usually acts quite rapidly and can also modulate effects of the endocrine and immune systems.

The nervous system comprises two structural divisions:
- **Central nervous system (CNS)** (brain and spinal cord)
- **Peripheral nervous system (PNS)** (somatic, autonomic, and enteric nerves in the periphery)

The **brain** includes the:
- **Cerebral cortex**: highest center for sensory and motor processing
- **Diencephalon**: includes the thalamus (relay and processing) and hypothalamus (emotions, autonomic control, and hormone production)
- **Cerebellum**: coordinates smooth motor activities and processes muscle position
- **Brainstem (midbrain, pons, and medulla)**: conveys motor and sensory information and mediates important autonomic functions

Peripheral nerves arise from the spinal cord and form networks of nerves; each network is called a **plexus**. The 31 pairs of spinal nerves contribute to four major nerve plexuses.

COLOR the four major nerve plexuses formed by the spinal nerves, using a different color for each plexus:

☐ 5. **Cervical plexus: largely innervates muscles of the neck**

☐ 6. **Brachial plexus: largely innervates muscles of the shoulder and upper limb**

☐ 7. **Lumbar plexus: largely innervates muscles of the anterior and medial thigh**

☐ 8. **Lumbosacral plexus: largely innervates muscles of the buttock, pelvis, perineum, and lower limb**

COLOR the subdivisions of the cerebral cortex, using a different color for each lobe:

☐ 1. **Cortex, frontal lobe: processes motor, visual, speech, and personality modalities**

☐ 2. **Cortex, parietal lobe: processes sensory information**

☐ 3. **Cortex, temporal lobe: processes language, auditory, and memory modalities**

☐ 4. **Cortex, occipital lobe: processes vision**

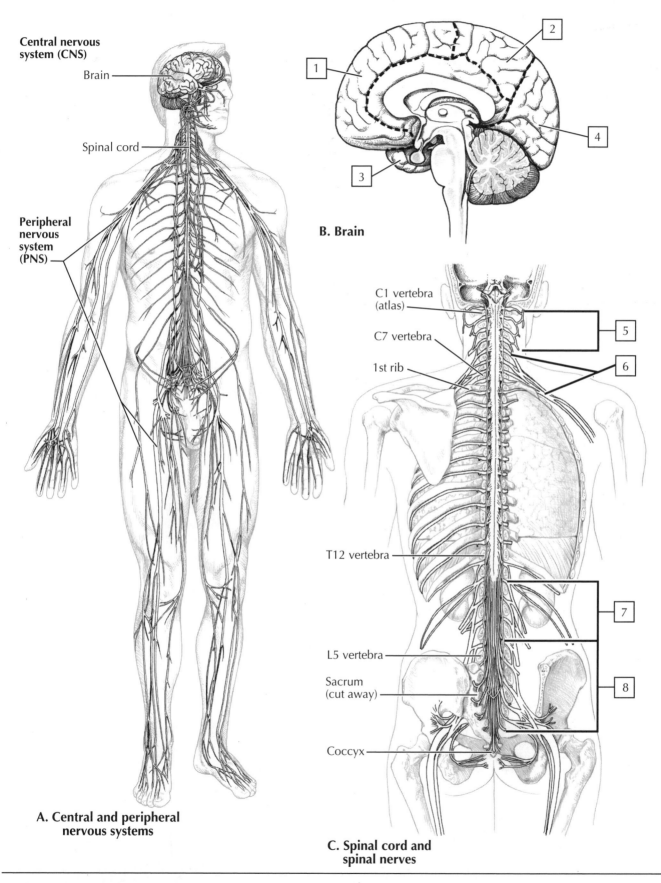

Central nervous system (CNS)

Brain

Spinal cord

Peripheral nervous system (PNS)

1

2

3

4

B. Brain

C1 vertebra (atlas)

C7 vertebra

1st rib

5

6

T12 vertebra

7

L5 vertebra

Sacrum (cut away)

8

Coccyx

A. Central and peripheral nervous systems

C. Spinal cord and spinal nerves

1 Skin (Integument)

The skin is the largest organ in the body, accounting for about 15% to 20% of the total body mass. The skin consists of two layers: epidermis and dermis.

COLOR the brackets that delineate the two layers of the skin, using two different colors:

- ☐ 1. **Epidermis: an outer protective layer consisting of a keratinized stratified squamous epithelium derived from embryonic ectoderm**
- ☐ 2. **Dermis: a dense connective tissue layer that gives skin most of its thickness and support and is derived from embryonic mesoderm**

The outer epidermal layer itself consists of four layers.

COLOR the four layers of the epidermis, listed below from outermost to innermost, using different colors than previously used:

- ☐ 3. **Stratum corneum: an anuclear cell layer that is thick and contains flattened cells filled almost entirely with keratin filaments**
- ☐ 4. **Stratum granulosum: a layer one to three cells thick whose cells contain keratohyalin granules containing a protein that will aggregate the keratin filaments of the next layer**
- ☐ 5. **Stratum spinosum: several cell layers thick and composed of cells with cytoplasmic processes, which they lose as they ascend toward the surface of the skin**
- ☐ 6. **Stratum basale: a single germinal cell layer that is mitotically active and provides cells for the layers superficial to it**

The epidermis is renewed by cells from the basal layer that rise up through the skin to the surface.

The dermis is divided into a papillary and reticular layer and contains epidermal skin appendages. Dermal papillae extend up into the underside of the epidermis and increase the surface area for the attachment of the epidermis to the underlying dermal layer. The reticular dermis lies deeper and is thicker and less cellular than the papillary layer. Deep within the dermis and subcutaneous tissue lie atriovenous shunts that participate in thermoregulation along with the sweat glands.

COLOR the epidermal skin appendages found in the dermal layer:

- ☐ 7. **Sebaceous glands**
- ☐ 8. **Hair follicles**
- ☐ 9. **Sweat glands (several types)**

Additionally, the dermis contains capillaries, specialized receptors and nerves, pigment cells, immune cells, and smooth muscle (arrector pili muscles attached to the hair follicles).

Also, if you wish, color the small arteries and veins red and blue, respectively, and a nerve fiber yellow. **Note that from this point forward, arteries will always be colored red, veins blue, and nerves yellow.**

Beneath the dermis lies a loose connective tissue layer, the hypodermis or subcutaneous tissue (superficial fascia), of variable thickness that often contains a significant amount of adipose (fat) cells.

Skin functions include:
- Protection, via both mechanical abrasion and immune responses
- Temperature regulation, via vasodilatation or vasoconstriction, and by sweat gland activity (water evaporation as a cooling mechanism)
- Sensation, via touch (mechanoreceptors such as pacinian and Meissner's corpuscles), pain (nociceptors), and temperature receptors (thermoreceptors)
- Endocrine, via secretion of hormones, cytokines, and growth factors
- Exocrine, via secretion of sweat from sweat glands and oily sebum from sebaceous glands

Clinical Note:
Psoriasis is a chronic inflammatory skin disorder that affects approximately 1% to 3% of the population and is characterized by defined red plaques, capped with a surface scale of desquamated epidermis.

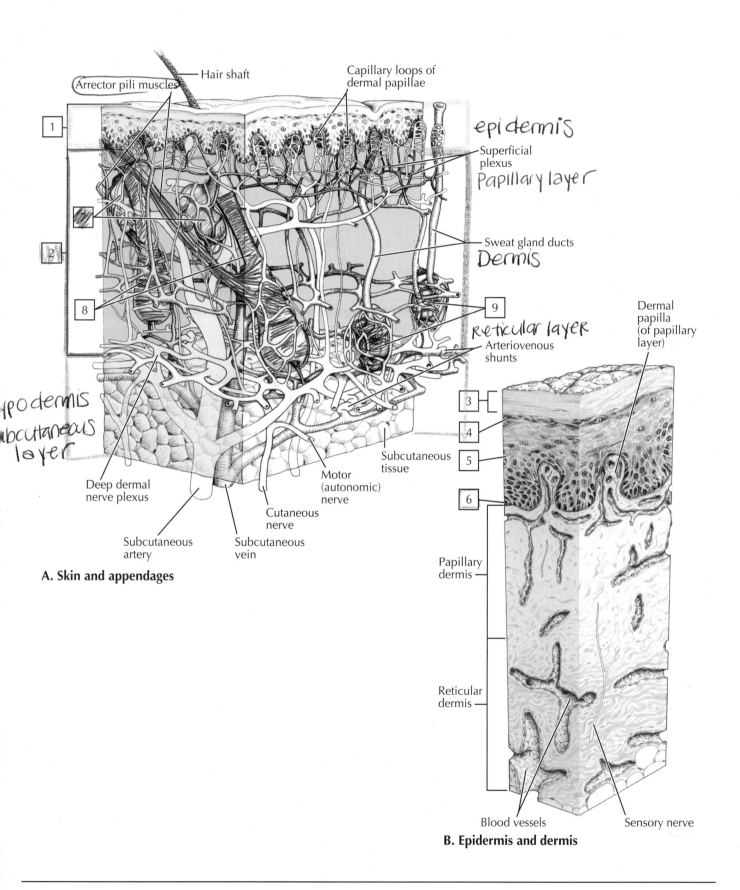

Hair shaft

Arrector pili muscles

Capillary loops of dermal papillae

epidermis

Superficial plexus

Papillary layer

Sweat gland ducts

Dermis

1

2

8

9

Reticular layer

Arteriovenous shunts

Dermal papilla (of papillary layer)

3

4

5

6

Subcutaneous tissue

Papillary dermis

Reticular dermis

ypodermis
ubcutaneous
layer

Deep dermal nerve plexus

Subcutaneous artery

Subcutaneous vein

Cutaneous nerve

Motor (autonomic) nerve

A. Skin and appendages

Blood vessels

Sensory nerve

B. Epidermis and dermis

1 Body Cavities

Organ systems and other visceral structures are often segregated into body cavities. These cavities can protect the viscera and also may allow for some expansion and contraction in size. Two major collections of body cavities are recognized:

- **Dorsal cavities**: include the brain, surrounded by the meninges and bony cranium, and the spinal cord, surrounded by the same meninges as the brain and also surrounded by the vertebral column
- **Ventral cavities**: include the **thoracic** and **abdominopelvic** cavities, separated from each other by the abdominal diaphragm (skeletal muscle important in respiration)

The CNS (brain and spinal cord) is surrounded by three membranes (see Plate 4-18):

- **Pia mater**: a delicate, transparent inner layer that intimately covers the brain and spinal cord
- **Arachnoid mater**: a fine, weblike membrane beneath the outer dura mater
- **Dura mater**: a thick, tough outermost layer that is vascularized and richly innervated by sensory nerve fibers

COLOR the brain and spinal cord, using a different color for each and for their coverings:

☐ 1. **Brain and its dural lining (1A)**

☐ 2. **Spinal cord and its dural lining (2A)**

The thoracic cavity contains **two pleural cavities** (right and left; see Plate 7-5) and a single midline space called the **mediastinum** (middle space). The heart and structures lying posterior to it, including the descending thoracic aorta and esophagus, lie within the thoracic cavity. The heart itself resides in its sac, called the **pericardial sac** (see Plate 5-3), which also has a parietal and visceral layer.

COLOR the two pleural cavities and the serous membrane lining these cavities:

☐ 3. **Parietal pleura: lines the thoracic walls and abuts the mediastinum medially**

☐ 4. **Visceral pleura: encases the lungs themselves and reflects off of the lung surface to be continuous with the parietal pleura**

☐ 5. **Heart and its surrounding pericardium (5A)**

The abdominopelvic cavity also is lined by a serous membrane, called the **peritoneum**, which likewise has a parietal and visceral layer.

COLOR the abdominopelvic cavity and its peritoneal membranes (see Plate 8-5):

☐ 6. **Parietal peritoneum: lining the body walls**

☐ 7. **Visceral peritoneum: reflects off of the body walls and covers the abdominal visceral (organs) structures**

Clinical Note:
Each of these spaces—the pleural, pericardial, and peritoneal—are considered "potential" spaces, because between the parietal and visceral layers we usually find only a small amount of serous lubricating fluid that keeps the surfaces of the organs moist and slick. This lubrication reduces friction from movements, such as during respiration, the heartbeat, or peristalsis. However, during inflammation or because of trauma, fluids can collect in these spaces (pus or blood) and restrict movement of the viscera. In that case, these potential spaces become real spaces and may necessitate the removal of the offending fluid, to prevent compromise of organ function or exacerbation of an ongoing infection.

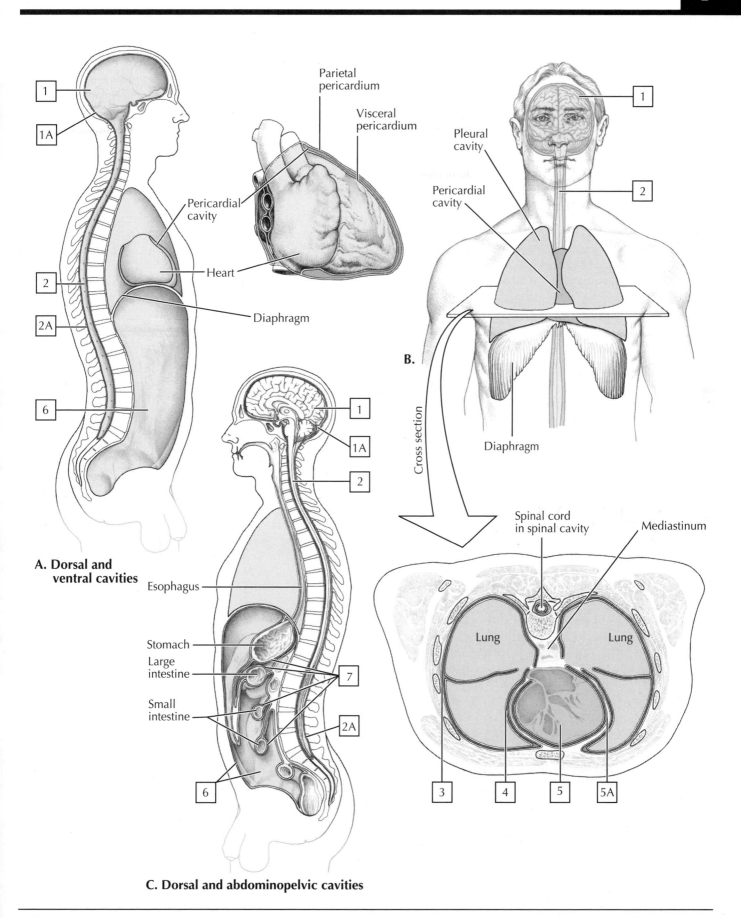

Parietal pericardium

Visceral pericardium

Pericardial cavity

Heart

Diaphragm

A. Dorsal and ventral cavities

Esophagus

Stomach

Large intestine

Small intestine

Pleural cavity

Pericardial cavity

B.

Diaphragm

Cross section

Spinal cord in spinal cavity

Mediastinum

Lung

Lung

C. Dorsal and abdominopelvic cavities

REVIEW QUESTIONS

1. Write the correct term of relationship for each of the following:
   A. Nearer to the head: _____
   B. Closer to the surface: _____
   C. Divides body into equal right and left halves: _____

2. Which term below best describes the position of the hand when the palm is facing toward the ground?
   A. Abduction
   B. Extension
   C. Plantar flexion
   D. Pronation

3.
   A. Which intracellular organelle produces ATP? _____
   B. Which intracellular organelle has pores in its membrane? _____
   C. Which intracellular organelle is a condensation of RNA? _____

4. List the three types of epithelium based on cell shape. _____

5. List the three types of joints found in humans. _____

6. List the three types of muscle found in humans. _____

7. What two structures comprise the central nervous system in humans? _____

8. The spinal cord is covered by: (A) Pia mater, (B) Arachnoid mater, and (C) Dura mater. Using a red pencil, circle the covering that lies closest to the spinal cord. With a blue pencil, circle the layer that is richly innervated and vascularized. With a green pencil, circle the layer that lies between the other two layers.

ANSWER KEY

1A. Superior (cranial)

1B. Superficial

1C. Median plane

2D. Pronation

3A. Mitochondria

3B. Nucleus

3C. Nucleolus

4. Squamous, cuboidal, columnar

5. Fibrous, cartilaginous, synovial

6. Skeletal, cardiac, smooth

7. Brain and spinal cord

8. Red: Pia mater

   Blue: Dura mater

   Green: Arachnoid mater

2

Chapter 2 **Skeletal System**

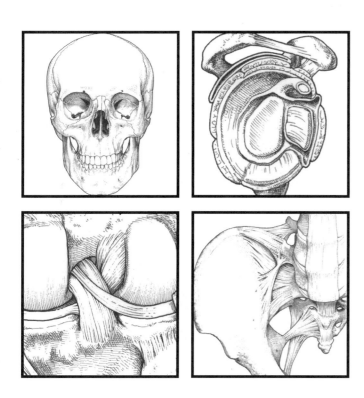

2 Bone Structure and Classification

Bone is a specialized form of connective tissue, consisting of cells and matrix. The matrix is mineralized with calcium phosphate (hydroxyapatite crystals), giving it a hard texture and serving as a significant reservoir for calcium. Bone is classified as:
- **Compact:** dense bone that forms the outer layer of a bone
- **Spongy:** cancellous bone that contains a meshwork of thin trabeculae or spicules of bone tissue, and is found in the epiphyses of and metaphyses of long bones

A typical long bone has the following structural elements:
- **Diaphysis:** the shaft of the bone
- **Epiphysis:** two expanded ends of the bone that are covered by articular cartilage
- **Metaphysis:** lies between the diaphysis and epiphysis, and is a conical region adjacent to the area where active bone growth will occur
- **Marrow cavity:** the central portion of the shaft of many bones, it contains stem cells that produce blood cells

COLOR each of the following features of a long bone, using a different color for each feature:
- [ ] 1. **Epiphysis (highlight the bracket)**
- [ ] 2. **Metaphysis (highlight the bracket)**
- [ ] 3. **Diaphysis (highlight the bracket)**
- [ ] 4. **Articular cartilage (hyaline cartilage)**
- [ ] 5. **Spongy bone**
- [ ] 6. **Periosteum: a thin fibrous connective tissue sheath or capsule that surrounds the shaft of a bone but is not found on the articular surfaces, which are covered by articular cartilage**
- [ ] 7. **Marrow cavity**
- [ ] 8. **Compact bone**

Bone formation occurs largely by the deposition of matrix (osteoid) that later becomes calcified, and by resorption of bone.

Thus it is a dynamic process just like any other living tissue in the body. Three major types of cells participate in this process:
- **Osteoblasts:** cells that form new bone by laying down osteoid
- **Osteocytes:** mature bone cells, formerly osteoblasts, that become surrounded by bone matrix and are responsible for maintaining the bone matrix
- **Osteoclasts:** large cells that enzymatically dissolve bone matrix and are commonly found at sites of active bone remodeling

COLOR the following features of compact bone:
- [ ] 9. **Osteon**
- [ ] 10. **Vein (color blue)**
- [ ] 11. **Artery (color red)**
- [ ] 12. **Lamellae of bone matrix: with osteocytes embedded within the lamellae**
- [ ] 13. **Osteocytes**

An **osteon** (haversian system) is the cyclindrical unit of bone and consists of a central canal (haversian canal), which contains the neurovascular bundle supplying the osteon. This canal is surrounded by concentric lamellae of bone matrix and radially oriented small canaliculi that contain the processes of osteocytes, which are the bone cells. Compact bone is organized into these haversian systems, but spongy bone is trabecular and its arrangement is not nearly as concentric or uniformly organized (see left side of image B).

Clinical Note:
Rickets is a disease process in which calcium deficiency during active growth leads to matrix formation that is not normally mineralized with calcium. It can occur from a lack of dietary calcium, vitamin D deficiency, or both, because vitamin D is necessary for the normal absorption of calcium by the small intestine.

Plate 2-1

Skeletal System

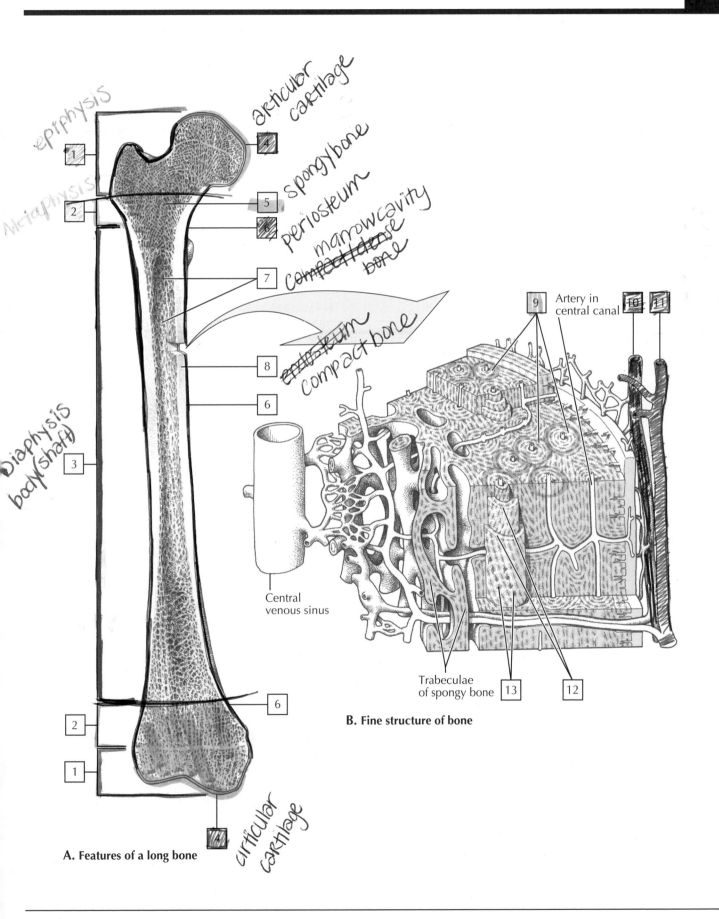

epiphysis

articular cartilage

Metaphysis

spongy bone

periosteum

marrow cavity

compact dense bone

Diaphysis body (shaft)

periosteum

compact bone

Artery in central canal

Central venous sinus

Trabeculae of spongy bone

articular cartilage

A. Features of a long bone

B. Fine structure of bone

2 External Features of the Skull

The skull is divided into the **neurocranium** or calvaria (contains the brain and its meningeal coverings) and the **viscerocranium** (facial skeleton). The skull is composed of 22 bones (excluding the middle ear ossicles), with 8 forming the cranium and 14 forming the face. The orbits (eye sockets) lie between the calvaria (skull cap) and the facial skeleton and are formed by contributions from 7 different bones.

COLOR the bones of the calvaria, using either solid colors, or diagonal lines or stippling of different colors for the larger bones:

- ☐ **1. Frontal**
- ☐ **2. Parietal (paired bones)**
- ☐ **3. Sphenoid**
- ☐ **4. Temporal (paired bones)**
- ☐ **5. Occipital**
- ☐ **6. Ethmoid**

The bones of the calvaria are attached to each other by sutures, a type of fibrous joint that is immobile. The sutures include:

- Coronal suture
- Lambdoid suture
- Sagittal suture
- Squamous suture
- Sphenoparietal suture
- Sphenosquamous suture
- Parietomastoid suture
- Occipitomastoid suture

COLOR the bones of the facial skeleton (all paired bones except the vomer and mandible), using different colors or patterns from those used to highlight the bones of the calvaria:

- ☐ **7. Nasal**
- ☐ **8. Lacrimal**
- ☐ **9. Zygomatic**
- ☐ **10. Maxilla**
- ☐ **11. Inferior nasal concha**
- ☐ **12. Vomer**
- ☐ **13. Mandible**
- ☐ **14. Palatine**

Clinical Note:

The lateral aspect of the skull, where the frontal, parietal, sphenoid, and temporal bones converge, is called the **pterion**. The skull is thin here and trauma to the side of the head in this region can lead to intracranial bleeding (epidural hematoma) from a lacerated middle meningeal artery, which lies between the inner aspect of these bones and the dura covering the brain.

 See Netter: *Atlas of Human Anatomy,* 6th Edition, Plates 4, 6, 9, and 10.

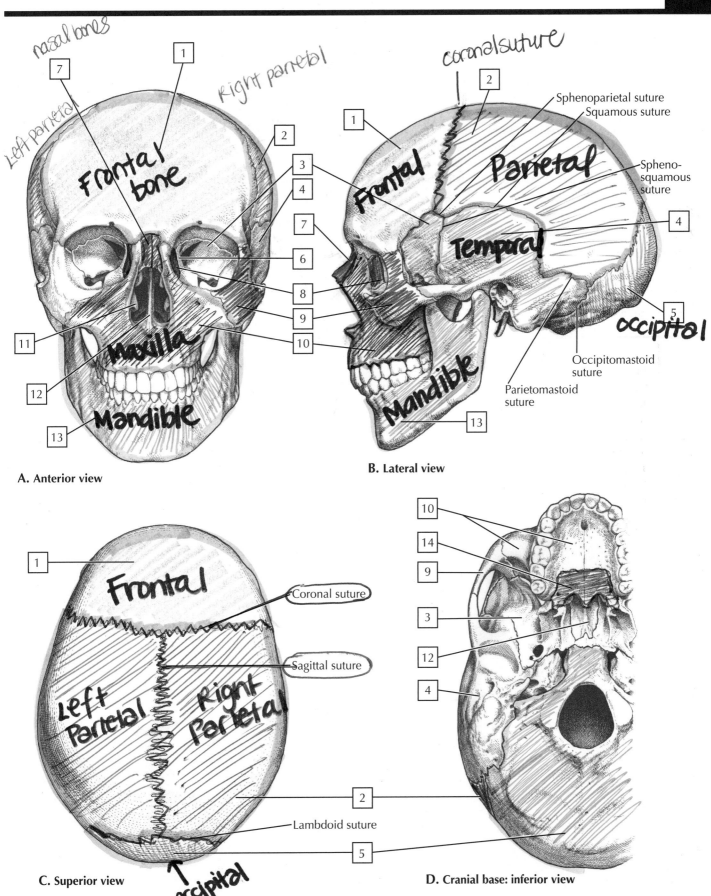

nasal bones

Left parietal Right parietal

coronal suture

7

1

2

Frontal bone

Sphenoparietal suture
Squamous suture

2

1

3

4

Frontal

Parietal

Sphenosquamous suture

7

4

6

Temporal

8

9

5

11

occipital

10

Maxilla

Occipitomastoid suture

12

Parietomastoid suture

Mandible

Mandible

13

13

A. Anterior view

B. Lateral view

1

Frontal

Coronal suture

Sagittal suture

Left Parietal

Right Parietal

10

14

9

3

12

4

2

Lambdoid suture

5

occipital

2

5

C. Superior view

D. Cranial base: inferior view

The nasal septum is formed by:
• The perpendicular plate of the ethmoid
• Vomer
• Palatine bones
• Septal cartilages

The lateral nasal wall is formed by seven bones.

COLOR the bones that make up the lateral nasal wall, using a different color for each bone:

1. Nasal bone
2. Ethmoid (superior and middle conchae)
3. Lacrimal bone
4. Inferior concha (a separate bone)
5. Maxilla
6. Palatine bone
7. Sphenoid bone

The inferior aspect of the skull (cranial base or floor) is divided into three cranial fossae:
• Anterior: contains the orbital roof and frontal lobes of the brain
• Middle: contains the temporal lobes of the brain
• Posterior: contains the cerebellum, pons, and medulla of the brain

Numerous holes appear in the cranial floor, and they are called **foramina**. Important structures, especially cranial nerves arising from the brain, pass through the foramen to access the exterior. These important structures are labeled on the illustration of the cranial base.

COLOR the leader line and foramen (hole) for each identified foramen and the structures that pass through that foramen.

A. Skull: sagittal aspect

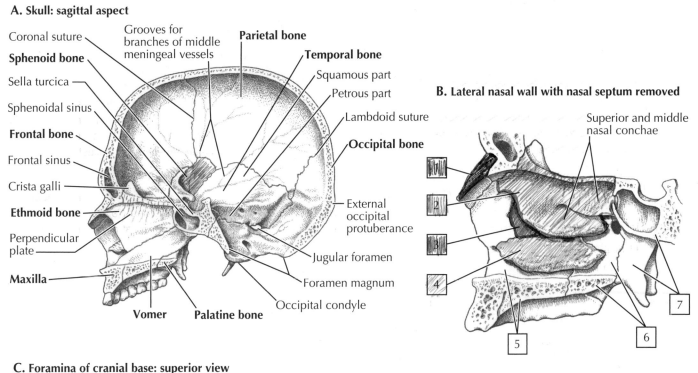

Coronal suture
Sphenoid bone
Sella turcica
Sphenoidal sinus
Frontal bone
Frontal sinus
Crista galli
Ethmoid bone
Perpendicular plate
Maxilla

Grooves for branches of middle meningeal vessels
Parietal bone
Temporal bone
Squamous part
Petrous part
Lambdoid suture
Occipital bone

External occipital protuberance
Jugular foramen
Foramen magnum

Vomer
Palatine bone
Occipital condyle

B. Lateral nasal wall with nasal septum removed

Superior and middle nasal conchae

C. Foramina of cranial base: superior view

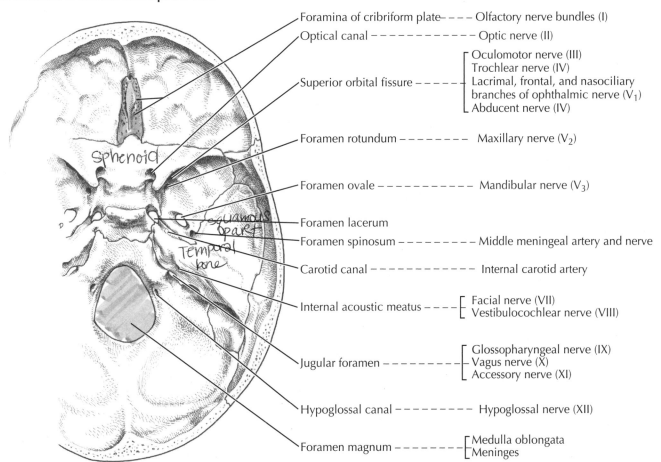

Foramina of cribriform plate – – – Olfactory nerve bundles (I)

Optical canal – – – – – – – – – – – Optic nerve (II)

Superior orbital fissure – – – – –
⌈ Oculomotor nerve (III)
| Trochlear nerve (IV)
| Lacrimal, frontal, and nasociliary
| branches of ophthalmic nerve (V₁)
⌊ Abducent nerve (IV)

Foramen rotundum – – – – – – – – Maxillary nerve (V₂)

Foramen ovale – – – – – – – – – – Mandibular nerve (V₃)

Foramen lacerum

Foramen spinosum – – – – – – – – Middle meningeal artery and nerve

Carotid canal – – – – – – – – – – – Internal carotid artery

Internal acoustic meatus – – – –
⌈ Facial nerve (VII)
⌊ Vestibulocochlear nerve (VIII)

Jugular foramen – – – – – – – – –
⌈ Glossopharyngeal nerve (IX)
| Vagus nerve (X)
⌊ Accessory nerve (XI)

Hypoglossal canal – – – – – – – – Hypoglossal nerve (XII)

Foramen magnum – – – – – – – –
⌈ Medulla oblongata
⌊ Meninges

Features of the mandible (lower jaw) are summarized in the table below. The mandible articulates with the temporal bone and, in chewing or speaking, it is only the mandible or lower jaw that moves; the upper jaw or maxilla remains stationary. The lower teeth are contained in the alveolar portion of the mandible.

FEATURE	CHARACTERISTICS
Mandibular head	Articulates with mandibular fossa of temporal bone
Mandibular foramen	Inferior alveolar nerve, artery, and vein enter mandible at this opening
Teeth	16 teeth: 4 incisors, 2 canines, 4 premolars (bicuspid), 6 molars (third molars called wisdom teeth)

COLOR the mandibular teeth, using a different color for each type (note that there are 16 teeth in the mandible and 16 teeth in the maxilla):

- [ ] 1. Molars (the third molars are called wisdom teeth) (6 teeth)
- [ ] 2. Premolars (bicuspids) (4 teeth)
- [ ] 3. Canines (2 teeth)
- [ ] 4. Incisors (4 teeth)

The **temporomandibular joint (TMJ)** is actually two synovial joints in one, separated by an articular disc. The articular surfaces of most synovial joints are covered by hyaline cartilage, but the TMJ surfaces are covered by fibrocartilage. The TMJ is a modified hinge type of synovial joint, and its features are summarized in the table below.

LIGAMENT	ATTACHMENT	COMMENT
Capsule	Temporal fossa and tubercle to mandibular head	Permits side-to-side motion, protrusion, and retrusion
Lateral (TMJ)	Temporal to mandible	Thickened fibrous band of capsule
Articular disc	Between temporal bone and mandible	Divides joint into two synovial compartments

COLOR the following features of the TMJ:

- [ ] 5. Joint capsule
- [ ] 6. Lateral (temporomandibular) ligament
- [ ] 7. Articular disc (fibrocartilage)

Clinical Note:
Because of its vulnerable location, the mandible is the second most commonly fractured facial bone (the nasal bone is the first). Dislocation of the TMJ can occur when the mandibular condyle moves anterior to the articular eminence (just anterior to the "open position" seen in part E). Sometimes, just a wide yawn is enough to cause dislocation, which can be quite painful.

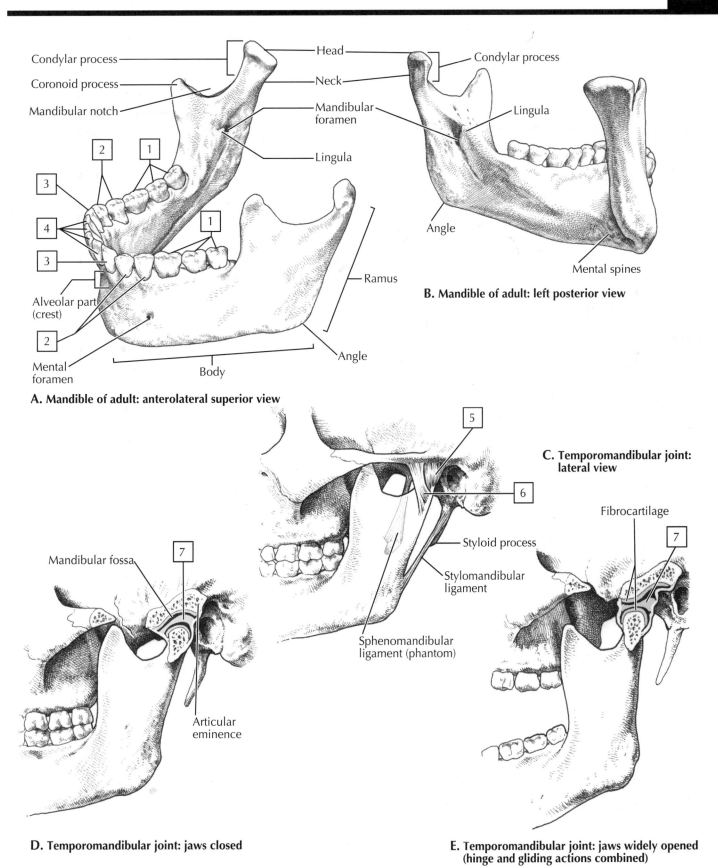

Condylar process
Coronoid process
Mandibular notch

Head
Neck

2 1
3
4
1
3
2

Alveolar part
(crest)

Mental
foramen

Body

Ramus

Angle

A. Mandible of adult: anterolateral superior view

Condylar process
Mandibular
foramen
Lingula

Lingula

Angle

Mental spines

B. Mandible of adult: left posterior view

5

**C. Temporomandibular joint:
lateral view**

6

Styloid process

Stylomandibular
ligament

Sphenomandibular
ligament (phantom)

Fibrocartilage

7

Mandibular fossa

7

Articular
eminence

D. Temporomandibular joint: jaws closed

**E. Temporomandibular joint: jaws widely opened
(hinge and gliding actions combined)**

The vertebral column (spine) forms the central axis of the human body, highlighting the segmental nature of all vertebrates, and is composed of 33 vertebrae distributed as follows:

- **Cervical vertebrae:** 7 total, with the first two called the atlas (C1) and axis (C2)
- **Thoracic vertebrae:** 12 total, each articulating with a pair of ribs
- **Lumbar vertebrae:** 5 total, large vertebrae to support the body's weight
- **Sacrum:** 5 fused vertebrae
- **Coccyx:** 4 total vertebrae, Co1 often not fused but Co2-Co4 are fused, a remnant of our embryonic tail

Viewed from the lateral aspect, one can identify the:

- **Cervical curvature (cervical lordosis):** acquired secondarily when the infant can support the weight of its own head
- **Thoracic curvature (thoracic kyphosis):** a primary curvature present in the fetus
- **Lumbar curvature (lumbar lordosis):** acquired secondarily when the infant assumes an upright posture
- **Sacral curvature:** a primary curvature present in the fetus

A "typical" vertebra has several consistent features:

- **Body:** weight-bearing portion that tends to increase in size as one descends the spine
- **Arch:** projection formed by paired pedicles and laminae
- Transverse processes: lateral extensions from the union of the pedicle and lamina
- **Articular processes (facets):** two superior and two inferior facets for articulation
- **Spinous process:** projection that extends posteriorly from the union of two laminae
- **Vertebral notches:** superior and inferior features that in articulated vertebrae form intervertebral foramina
- **Intervertebral foramina:** traversed by spinal nerve roots and associated vessels
- **Vertebral foramen (canal):** formed from the vertebral arch and body, the foramen contains the spinal cord and its meningeal coverings
- **Transverse foramina:** apertures that exist in transverse processes of cervical vertebrae and transmit vertebral vessels

COLOR the following features of a typical vertebra, using a different color for each feature:

- [ ] **1. Body**
- [ ] **2. Transverse process**
- [ ] **3. Articular facets**
- [ ] **4. Spinous process**
- [ ] **5. Arch**

Additionally, adjacent articulated vertebrae are secured by ligaments, and their individual vertebral bodies are separated by fibrocartilaginous intervertebral discs (IVD). The IVD acts as a shock absorber and compresses and expands slightly in response to weight bearing. The central portion of the IVD is a gelatinous **nucleus pulposus** that is surrounded by concentric layers of fibrocartilage called the **anulus fibrosus**. As the result of excessive pressure or dehydration associated with aging, the anulus can begin to weaken and the nucleus pulposus can herniate ("slipped disc") through the cartilaginous lamellae and impinge on a nerve root as it exits the spinal cord (see Plate 2-7).

COLOR the key ligaments observed in a lateral "cutaway" view of several adjacent vertebrae:

- [ ] **6. Intervertebral discs: fibrocartilaginous discs between adjacent bodies**
- [ ] **7. Anterior longitudinal ligament: connects adjacent bodies and the IVD along their anterior aspect**
- [ ] **8. Posterior longitudinal ligament: connects adjacent bodies and IVD along their posterior aspect**
- [ ] **9. Supraspinous ligament: between adjacent spinous processes**
- [ ] **10. Interspinous ligament: between adjacent spinous processes**
- [ ] **11. Ligamenta flava: connect adjacent laminae; contain elastic fibers**

Clinical Note:
Accentuated curvatures of the spine may occur congenitally or be acquired. **Scoliosis** is an accentuated lateral and rotational curve of the thoracic or lumbar spine, more common in adolescent girls. Hunchback is an accentuated **kyphosis** of the thoracic spine, usually from poor posture or osteoporosis. Swayback is an **accentuated lordosis** of the lumbar spine, usually from weakened trunk muscles or obesity, but also commonly seen in late pregnancy.

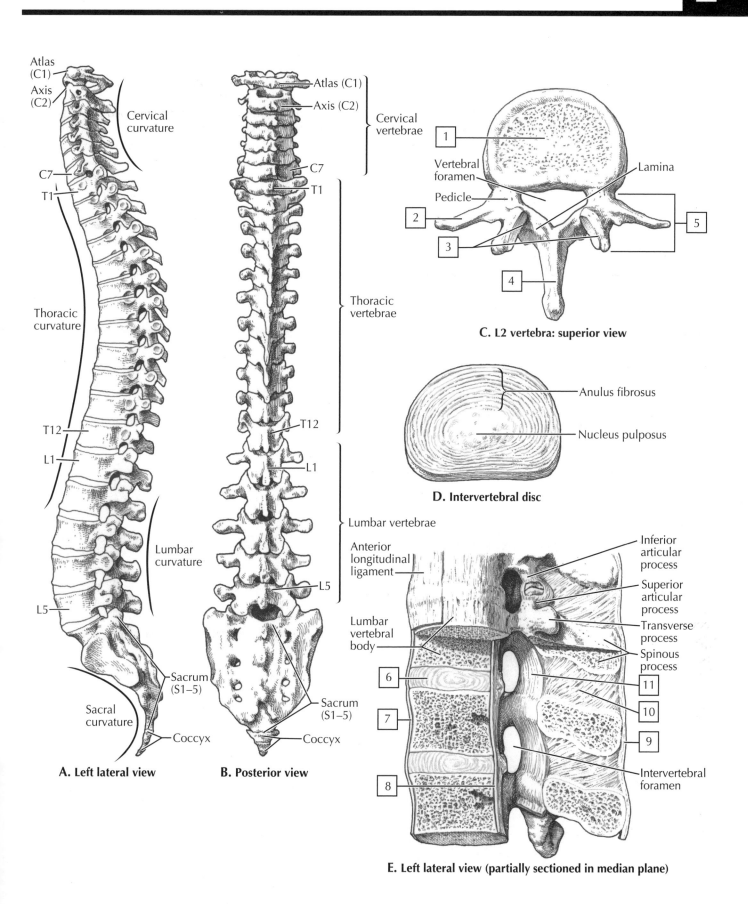

Atlas (C1)
Axis (C2)
Cervical curvature
C7
T1
Thoracic curvature
T12
L1
L5
Sacral curvature
Sacrum (S1–5)
Coccyx

A. Left lateral view

Atlas (C1)
Axis (C2)
Cervical vertebrae
C7
T1
Thoracic vertebrae
T12
L1
Lumbar vertebrae
L5
Sacrum (S1–5)
Coccyx

B. Posterior view

Cervical vertebrae
Vertebral foramen
Pedicle
Lamina

1
2
3
4
5

C. L2 vertebra: superior view

Anulus fibrosus
Nucleus pulposus

D. Intervertebral disc

Anterior longitudinal ligament
Lumbar vertebral body

Inferior articular process
Superior articular process
Transverse process
Spinous process

6
7
8

11
10
9

Intervertebral foramen

E. Left lateral view (partially sectioned in median plane)

The **cervical spine** is composed of seven cervical vertebrae. The first two cervical vertebrae are unique and are termed the **atlas** (C1) and **axis** (C2). The atlas (C1) holds the head on the neck and gets its name from the god Atlas, who held the world on his shoulders. The axis (C2) is the point of articulation where the head turns on the neck, providing an axis of rotation. The cervical region is a fairly mobile portion of the spine, allowing for flexion and extension as well as rotation and lateral bending. Features of the seven cervical vertebrae are summarized in the table below.

The **thoracic spine** is composed of 12 thoracic vertebrae. The 12 pairs of ribs articulate with the thoracic vertebrae, and this region of the spine is more rigid and inflexible than the neck. Key features of the thoracic vertebrae include:

- Heart-shaped body, with facets for rib articulation
- Small circular vertebral foramen (the spinal cord passes through the vertebral foramen)
- Long transverse processes, which have costal facets for rib articulation (T1-T10 only)
- Long spinous processes, which slope posteriorly and overlap the next vertebra below

ATLAS (C1)	OTHER CERVICAL VERTEBRAE (C3 TO C7)
Ringlike bone; superior facet articulates with occipital bone	Large triangular vertebral foramen
Two lateral masses with facets	Foramen transversarium, through which the vertebral artery passes
No body or spinous process	C3 to C5: short bifid spinous process
C1 rotates on articular facets of C2	C6 to C7: long spinous process
Vertebral artery runs in groove on posterior arch	C7 called vertebra prominens
	Narrow intervertebral foramina
	Nerve roots at risk of compression
AXIS (C2)	
Dens projects superiorly	
Strongest cervical vertebra	

COLOR the following features of the cervical vertebrae (parts *A-C*), using a different color for each feature:

- [ ] 1. Posterior arch of the atlas
- [ ] 2. Vertebral canal: the spinal cord passes through the vertebral canal
- [ ] 3. Dens of the axis
- [ ] 4. Foramen transversarium
- [ ] 5. Intervertebral discs (note that no IVD exists between the atlas and axis)
- [ ] 6. Body (note that the atlas does not possess a body)
- [ ] 7. Transverse process
- [ ] 8. Bifid spine
- [ ] 9. Lamina

COLOR the following features of the thoracic vertebrae (parts *D* and *E*):

- [ ] 10. Body
- [ ] 11. Superior costal (rib) facet
- [ ] 12. Vertebral canal
- [ ] 13. Spinous process
- [ ] 14. Transverse costal facet
- [ ] 15. Inferior costal facet

Cervical vertebrae

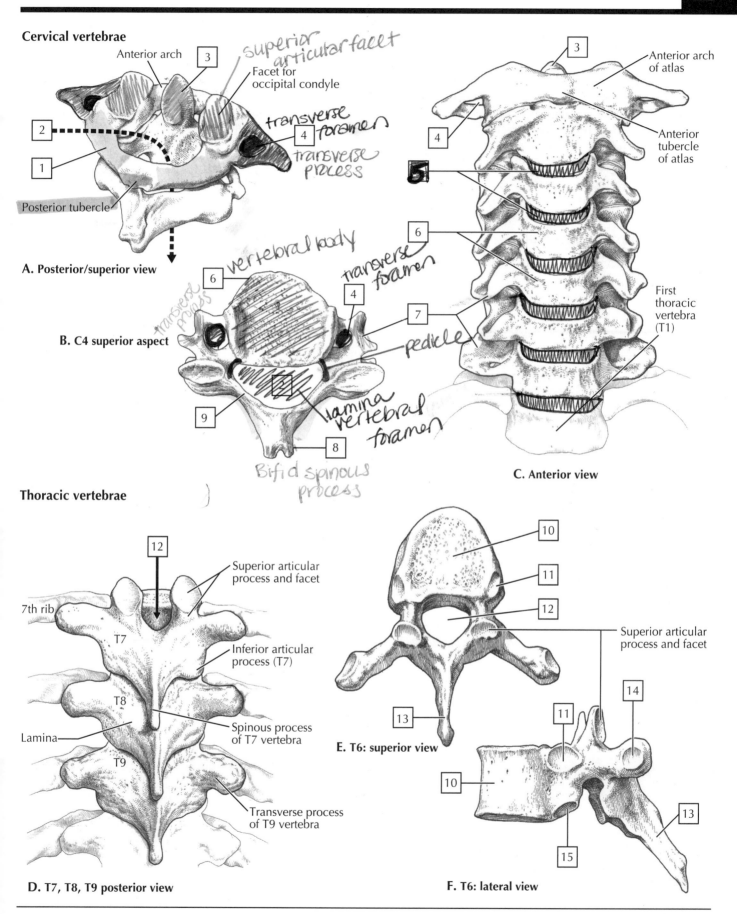

Anterior arch

3

superior articular facet

Facet for occipital condyle

2

transverse foramen

4

transverse process

1

Posterior tubercle

A. Posterior/superior view

6 *vertebral body*

transverse process

4 *transverse foramen*

7

pedicle

9

lamina
vertebral
foramen

8

Bifid spinous process

B. C4 superior aspect

3

Anterior arch of atlas

4

Anterior tubercle of atlas

5

6

6

7

First thoracic vertebra (T1)

C. Anterior view

Thoracic vertebrae

12

Superior articular process and facet

7th rib

T7

Inferior articular process (T7)

T8

Spinous process of T7 vertebra

Lamina

T9

Transverse process of T9 vertebra

D. T7, T8, T9 posterior view

10

11

12

Superior articular process and facet

13

E. T6: superior view

11

14

10

13

15

F. T6: lateral view

The **lumbar spine** is composed of five lumbar vertebrae. They are comparatively large for bearing the weight of the trunk and also fairly mobile, but not nearly as mobile as the cervical spine. The **sacrum** is composed of five fused vertebrae that form a single wedge-shaped bone. The sacrum provides support for the pelvis. The **coccyx** is a remnant of our embryonic tail and usually consists of four vertebrae, with the last three being fused into a single bone. The coccyx lacks vertebral arches and has no vertebral canal. The general features of all of these vertebrae are summarized in the table below.

THORACIC VERTEBRAE	LUMBAR VERTEBRAE
Heart-shaped body, with facets for rib articulation	Kidney-shaped body, massive for support
Small circular vertebral foramen	Midsized triangular vertebral foramen
Long transverse processes, which have facets for rib articulation in T1-T10	Facets face medial or lateral direction, which permits good flexion and extension
Long spinous processes, which slope posteriorly and overlap next vertebra	Spinous process is short
	L5 is largest vertebra

SACRUM	COCCYX
Large, wedge-shaped bone, which transmits body weight to pelvis	Co1 often not fused
Five fused vertebrae, with fusion complete by puberty	Co2 to Co4 fused
Four pairs of sacral foramina on dorsal and ventral (pelvic) side	No pedicles, laminae, spines
Sacral hiatus, the opening of sacral vertebral foramen	Remnant of our embryonic tail

COLOR the following features of the lumbar (part **A**), sacral (parts **B, C,** and **E**), and coccygeal (parts **B, C,** and **E**) vertebrae, using a different color for each feature:

- [ ] 1. **Intervertebral foramen: traversed by a spinal nerve as it leaves the spinal cord and passes out to the periphery**
- [ ] 2. **Intervertebral disc**
- [ ] 3. **Body**
- [ ] 4. **Superior articular process**
- [ ] 5. **Spinous process**
- [ ] 6. **Lumbosacral articular surface: articulates with the body of the L5 vertebra**
- [ ] 7. **Anterior sacral foramina: for the passage of spinal nerves**
- [ ] 8. **Coccygeal vertebrae**
- [ ] 9. **Median sacral crest: equivalent of vertebral spinous processes elsewhere along the vertebral column**

COLOR the following features of image (part **D**) of the articulated lower spine (lumbar, sacrum, and coccygeal vertebrae):

- [ ] 10. **Anterior longitudinal ligament**
- [ ] 11. **Intervertebral discs**
- [ ] 12. **Spinal nerves (color yellow)**
- [ ] 13. **Interspinous ligament**
- [ ] 14. **Supraspinous ligament**

Clinical Note:

Stress- or age-related changes can lead to dehydration of the intervertebral discs (IVD). In this process, the central nucleus pulposus herniates through the anulus fibrosus, and if the herniation is posterolateral, which is most common, it can compress the spinal nerve or its root as it exits the intervertebral foramen.

COLOR

- [ ] 15. **The herniating nucleus pulposus as it compresses a spinal nerve**

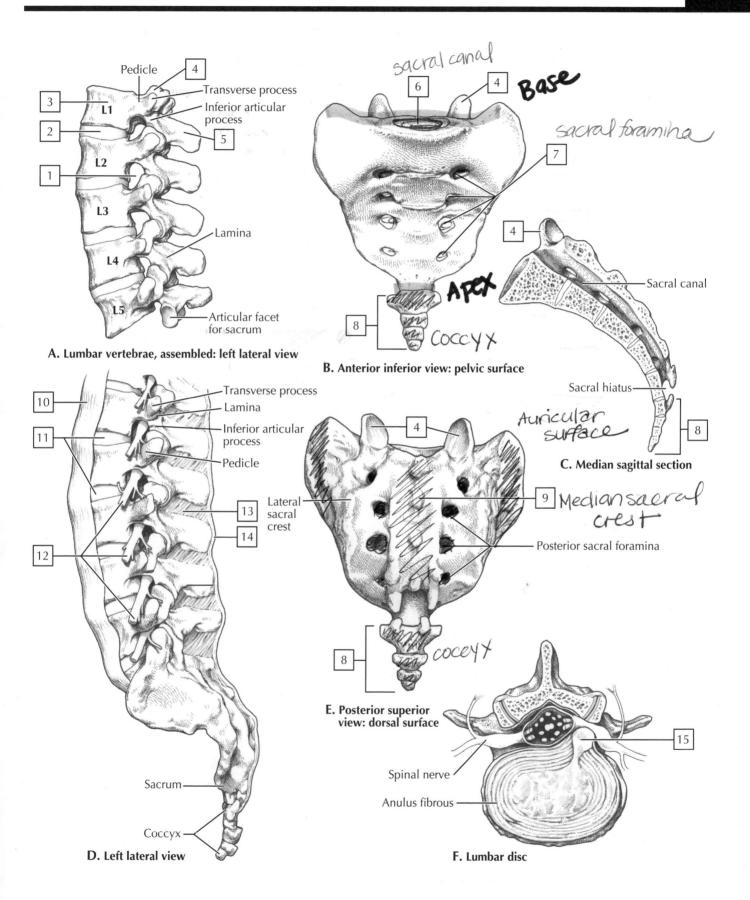

Pedicle

4

3 **L1**

Transverse process

Inferior articular
process

2

5

1 **L2**

L3

Lamina

L4

L5

Articular facet
for sacrum

A. Lumbar vertebrae, assembled: left lateral view

sacral canal

6 4 *Base*

sacral foramina

7

4

Sacral canal

8 *APEX*

COCCYX

B. Anterior inferior view: pelvic surface

Sacral hiatus

*Auricular
surface*

8

C. Median sagittal section

10

Transverse process
Lamina
Inferior articular
process
Pedicle

11

4

13

14

Lateral
sacral
crest

9 *Median sacral
crest*

Posterior sacral foramina

12

8 *coccyx*

**E. Posterior superior
view: dorsal surface**

15

Spinal nerve

Sacrum

Anulus fibrous

Coccyx

D. Left lateral view

F. Lumbar disc

The thoracic cage is part of the axial skeleton and includes the midline sternum and 12 pairs of ribs, each with a(n):

- **Head:** it articulates with the inferior costal facet of the vertebral body above and with the superior costal facet of the body of its own vertebra (for example, rib 3 with T3 vertebra)
- **Neck**
- **Tubercle:** it articulates with the transverse process of its own vertebra
- **Angle**

Ribs 1 to 7 articulate with the sternum directly and are called "true ribs."

Ribs 8 to 10 articulate with costal cartilages of the ribs above and are called "false ribs."

Ribs 11 to 12 articulate with vertebrae only and are called "floating ribs."

LIGAMENT	ATTACHMENT	COMMENT
Sternoclavicular (Saddle-type Synovial) Joint with an Articular Disc		
Capsule	Clavicle and manubrium	Allows elevation, depression, protraction, retraction, circumduction
Sternoclavicular	Clavicle and manubrium	Consists of anterior and posterior ligaments
Interclavicular	Between both clavicles	Connects two sternoclavicular joints
Costoclavicular	Clavicle to first rib	Anchors clavicle to first rib
Sternocostal (Primary Cartilaginous [Synchondroses]) Joints		
First sternocostal	First rib to manubrium	Allows no movement at this joint
Radiate sternocostal	Ribs 2-7 with sternum	Permits some gliding or sliding movement at these synovial plane joints
Costochondral (Primary Cartilaginous) Joints		
Cartilage	Costal cartilage to rib	Allows no movement at these joints
Interchondral (Synovial Plane) Joints		
Interchondral	Between costal cartilages	Allows some gliding movement

Functionally, the thoracic cage participates in breathing, via its muscle attachments, protection of the vital thoracic organs, including the heart and lungs, and as a conduit for the passage of important structures to and from the head and also the abdomen. The opening at the top of the thoracic cage is the **superior thoracic aperture,** and that at the bottom is called the **inferior thoracic aperture.** The inferior aperture is largely covered by the abdominal diaphragm, an important skeletal muscle used in breathing.

The upper limb attaches to the thoracic cage at the pectoral girdle, which includes the:

- **Clavicle:** acts as a strut to keep the limb at the side of the body wall
- **Scapula:** a flat triangular bone that has 16 different muscles attached to it that largely act on the shoulder joint

COLOR the following features of the thoracic cage, using a different color for each feature:

- [ ] 1. **Costal cartilages**
- [ ] 2. **Clavicle**
- [ ] 3. **Sternum and its three parts:**
  - 3A. *Manubrium*
  - 3B. *Body*
  - 3C. *Xiphoid process*
- [ ] 4. **Superior costal facet: articulation for head of rib of same number as the vertebra**
- [ ] 5. **Inferior costal facet: articulation for head of rib one number greater than the vertebra number**
- [ ] 6. **Parts of a typical rib (6A, head; 6B, neck; 6C, tubercle; and 6D, angle and remainder of the rib)**

Clinical Note:

Thoracic trauma often includes **rib fractures** (the 1st, 11th, and 12th ribs are usually spared), crush injuries (commonly with rib fractures), and penetrating chest wounds (stab and gunshot). The pain associated with rib fractures is often intense because of the expansion and contraction of the rib cage during respiration.

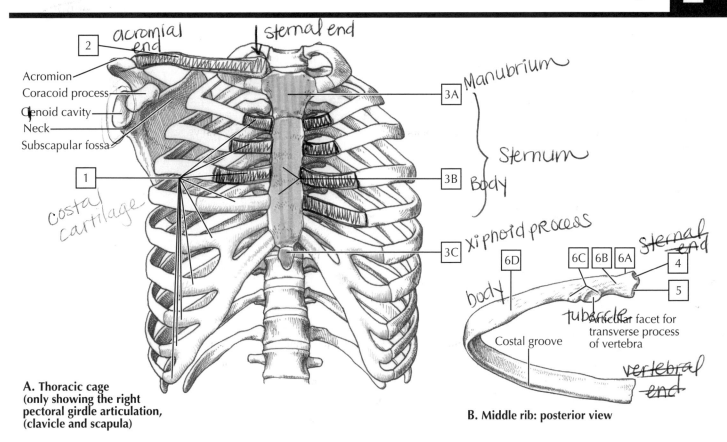

acromial end

sternal end

2

Acromion
Coracoid process
Glenoid cavity
Neck
Subscapular fossa

Manubrium

3A

Sternum

Body

3B

Xiphoid process

3C

costal cartilage

1

**A. Thoracic cage
(only showing the right
pectoral girdle articulation,
(clavicle and scapula)**

body

6D

6C 6B 6A

sternal end

4

5

tubercle

Articular facet for
transverse process
of vertebra

Costal groove

vertebral end

B. Middle rib: posterior view

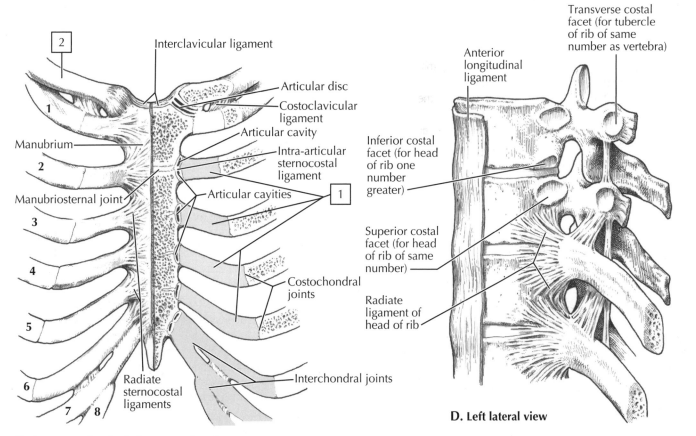

2

Interclavicular ligament

1

Manubrium

2

Manubriosternal joint

3

4

5

6

7   8

Articular disc

Costoclavicular
ligament

Articular cavity

Intra-articular
sternocostal
ligament

Articular cavities

1

Costochondral
joints

Radiate
sternocostal
ligaments

Interchondral joints

C. Sternocostal articulations: anterior view

Transverse costal
facet (for tubercle
of rib of same
number as vertebra)

Anterior
longitudinal
ligament

Inferior costal
facet (for head
of rib one
number
greater)

Superior costal
facet (for head
of rib of same
number)

Radiate
ligament of
head of rib

D. Left lateral view

The **craniovertebral joints** are synovial joints that offer a relatively wide range of motion compared with most joints of the spine and include the:

- Atlanto-occipital joint, between the **atlas** (C1) and the occipital bone of the skull; allows for flexion and extension, as in nodding the head to signify "yes"
- Atlanto-axial joint, between the atlas and the **axis** (C2); allows for rotational movement, as in shaking the head to signify "no"

LIGAMENT	ATTACHMENT	COMMENT
Atlanto-occipital (Biaxial Condyloid Synovial) Joint		
Articular capsule	Surround facets and occipital condyles	Allows flexion and extension
Anterior and posterior membranes	Anterior and posterior arches of C1 to foramen magnum	Limits movement of joint
Atlanto-axial (Uniaxial Synovial) Joint		
Tectorial membrane	Axis body to margin of foramen magnum	Is continuation of posterior longitudinal ligament
Apical	Dens to occipital bone	Is very small
Alar	Dens to occipital condyles	Limits rotation
Cruciate	Dens to lateral masses	Resembles a cross; allows rotation

COLOR the following ligaments of the craniovertebral joints (parts **A-D**), using a different color for each ligament:

1. Capsule of the atlanto-occipital joint
2. Capsule of the atlanto-axial joint
3. Posterior longitudinal ligament
4. Alar ligaments
5. Cruciate ligament: superior and inferior bands and transverse ligament of the atlas

Joints of the **vertebral arches** are plane synovial joints between the superior and inferior articular facets that allow some gliding or sliding movement.

Joints of the **vertebral bodies** are secondary cartilaginous joints between adjacent vertebral bodies. These stable, weight-bearing joints also serve as shock absorbers.

The **intervertebral discs** consist of an outer fibrocartilaginous **anulus fibrosus** and inner gelatinous **nucleus pulposus.** The lumbar discs are the thickest and the upper thoracic spine discs the thinnest. Anterior and posterior longitudinal ligaments help to stabilize these joints.

LIGAMENT	ATTACHMENT	COMMENT
Zygapophysial (Plane Synovial) Joints		
Articular capsule	Surrounds facets	Allows gliding motion C5-C6 is most mobile L4-L5 permits most flexion
Intervertebral (Secondary Cartilaginous [Symphyses]) Joints		
Anterior longitudinal (AL)	Anterior bodies and intervertebral discs	Is strong and prevents hyperextension
Posterior longitudinal (PL)	Posterior bodies and intervertebral discs	Is weaker than AL and prevents hyperflexion
Ligamenta flava	Connect adjacent laminae of vertebrae	Limit flexion and are more elastic
Interspinous	Connect spines	Are weak
Supraspinous	Connect spinous tips	Are stronger and limit flexion
Ligamentum nuchae	C7 to occipital bone	Is cervical extension of supraspinous ligament and is strong
Intertransverse	Connect transverse processes	Are weak ligaments
Intervertebral discs	Between adjacent bodies	Are secured by AL and PL ligaments

COLOR the following ligaments of the vertebral arches and bodies (parts *E* and *F*), using a different color for each ligament:

6. Intervertebral disc
7. Anterior longitudinal ligament
8. Posterior longitudinal ligament
9. Ligamentum flavum (appears yellow because it contains elastic fibers)
10. Interspinous ligament
11. Supraspinous ligament
12. Radiate ligament of the head of a rib

Clinical Note:

Whiplash is a nonmedical term for a cervical hyperextension injury (muscular, ligament, and/or bone damage), which is usually associated with a rear-end vehicular accident. The relaxed neck is thrown backward, or hyperextended, as the vehicle accelerates rapidly forward. Rapid recoil of the neck into extreme flexion occurs next. Properly adjusted headrests can significantly reduce the occurrence of hyperextension injury.

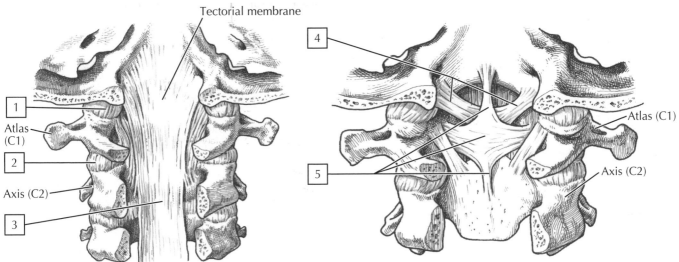

Tectorial membrane

1

Atlas (C1)

2

Axis (C2)

3

4

Atlas (C1)

5

Axis (C2)

A. Upper part of vertebral canal with spinous processes and parts of vertebral arches removed to expose ligaments on posterior vertebral bodies: posterior view

B. Principal part of tectorial membrane removed to expose deeper ligament: posterior view

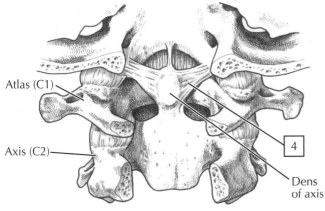

Atlas (C1)

Axis (C2)

4

Dens of axis

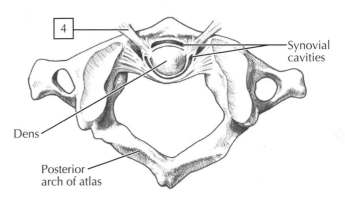

4

Synovial cavities

Dens

Posterior arch of atlas

C. Cruciate ligament removed to show deepest ligaments: posterior view

D. Median atlanto-axial joint: superior view

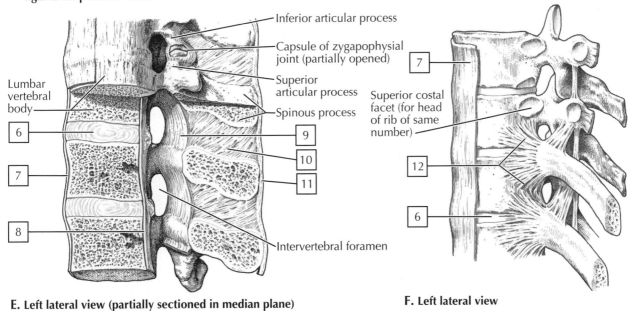

Inferior articular process

Capsule of zygapophysial joint (partially opened)

Superior articular process

Spinous process

Lumbar vertebral body

6

7

8

9

10

11

Intervertebral foramen

7

Superior costal facet (for head of rib of same number)

12

6

E. Left lateral view (partially sectioned in median plane)

F. Left lateral view

The **pectoral girdle** is the attachment point of the upper limb to the thoracic wall. The only direct articulation is between the clavicle and the sternum, with the other end of the clavicle articulating with the **scapula** at the acromion. The bone of the arm, called the **humerus**, articulates with the scapula at the glenoid cavity, forming the shoulder or glenohumeral joint. The distal end of the humerus contributes to the elbow joint. Numerous muscles act on the shoulder joint, giving this joint tremendous mobility. The triangular-shaped scapula, for instance, is the site of attachment for 16 different muscles! The features of the clavicle, scapula, and humerus are summarized in the table below.

COLOR each of the following bones of the pectoral girdle (part *A*), using a different color for each bone:

☑ 1. Clavicle
☐ 2. Scapula
☑ 3. Humerus

CLAVICLE	SCAPULA	HUMERUS
Cylindrical bone with slight S-shaped curve	Flat triangular bone	Long bone
Middle third: narrowest portion	Shallow glenoid cavity	Proximal head: articulates with glenoid cavity of scapula
First bone to ossify but last to fuse	Attachment locations for 17 muscles	Distal medial and lateral condyles: articulate at elbow with ulna and radius
Formed by intramembranous ossification	Fractures are relatively uncommon	Surgical neck is a common fracture site, which endangers axillary nerve
Most commonly fractured bone		
Acts as strut to keep limb away from trunk		

COLOR each of the following features of the pectoral girdle bones (parts *B* and *C*), using a different color for each feature:

☑ 4. **Coracoid process of the scapula**
☑ 5. **Spine of the scapula**
☐ 6. **Trochlea of the distal humerus: for articulation with the ulna at the elbow**
☐ 7. **Acromial facet of the clavicle: articulates with the scapula at the acromion**
☐ 8. **Sternal facet of the clavicle: articulates with the manubrium of the sternum**

Clinical Note:

The **clavicle** is the most commonly fractured bone in the body, especially in children. The fractures usually occur from a fall on an outstretched hand or from direct trauma to the shoulder. Fractures of the clavicle usually occur in the middle third of the bone.

Plate 2-10   See Netter: *Atlas of Human Anatomy*, 6th Edition, Plates 404 to 406.

Skeletal System

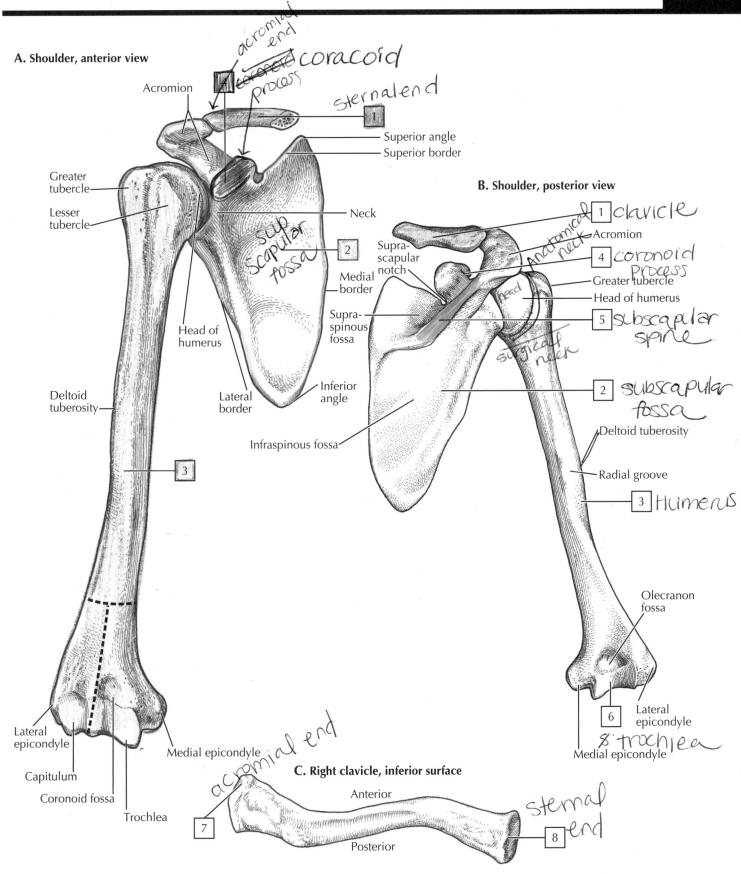

A. Shoulder, anterior view

acromial end
coronoid process coracoid process
sternal end

Acromion

1

Superior angle
Superior border

Greater tubercle

Lesser tubercle

Neck

sub scapular fossa

2

B. Shoulder, posterior view

1 clavicle
Acromion
anatomical neck
4 coronoid process
Greater tubercle
Head of humerus
5 subscapular spine

Head of humerus

Medial border

Supra-scapular notch

Supra-spinous fossa

head

surgical neck

2 subscapular fossa

Deltoid tuberosity

Deltoid tuberosity

Radial groove

3 Humerus

Infraspinous fossa

Inferior angle

Lateral border

3

Olecranon fossa

Lateral epicondyle

Medial epicondyle

Lateral epicondyle

Capitulum

Coronoid fossa

Trochlea

Medial epicondyle

6

8 trochlea

acromial end

C. Right clavicle, inferior surface

Anterior

sternal end

7

Posterior

8

The **shoulder,** or **glenohumeral joint,** is a multiaxial synovial ball-and-socket joint that allows tremendous mobility of the upper limb. Because of the shallow nature of this ball-and-socket joint and its relatively loose capsule, the shoulder joint is one of the most commonly dislocated joints in the body. The **acromio-clavicular joint** is a plane synovial joint that permits some gliding movement when the arm is raised and the scapula rotates. The shoulder joint is reinforced by four **rotator cuff muscles,** whose tendons help stabilize the joint (also see Plate 3-17 on rotator cuff muscles):

- Supraspinatus
- Infraspinatus
- Teres minor
- Subscapularis

Bursae help to reduce friction by separating the muscle tendons from the fibrous capsule of the glenohumeral joint. Additionally, although the glenoid cavity of the scapula is shallow, a rim of fibrocartilage, called the glenoid labrum ("lip"), lines the peripheral margin of the cavity like a collar and deepens the "socket." Note also that the tendon of the long head of the biceps muscle passes deep to the joint capsule to insert on the supraglenoid tubercle of the scapula. Features of the shoulder joint ligaments and bursae are summarized in the table below.

LIGAMENT OR BURSA	ATTACHMENT	COMMENT
Acromioclavicular (Synovial Plane) Joint		
Capsule and articular disc	Surrounds joint	Allows gliding movement as arm is raised and scapula rotates
Acromioclavicular	Acromion to clavicle	
Coracoclavicular (conoid and trapezoid ligaments)	Clavicle to coracoid process	Reinforces the joint
Glenohumeral (Multiaxial Synovial Ball-and-Socket) Joint		
Capsule	Surrounds joint	Permits flexion, extension, abduction, adduction, circumduction; most frequently dislocated joint
Coracohumeral	Coracoid process to greater tubercle of humerus	
Glenohumeral	Supraglenoid tubercle to lesser tubercle of humerus	Composed of superior, middle, and inferior thickenings
Transverse humeral	Spans greater and lesser tubercles of humerus	Holds long head of biceps tendon in intertubercular groove
Glenoid labrum	Margin of glenoid cavity of scapula	Is fibrocartilaginous ligament that deepens glenoid cavity
Bursae		
Subacromial		Between coraco-acromial arch and suprascapular muscle
Subdeltoid		Between deltoid muscle and capsule
Subscapular		Between subscapularis tendon and scapular neck

COLOR the following ligaments, tendons, and the bursae labelled in C and D (color these blue) associated with the shoulder joint, using a different color for each:

- [ ] 1. **Supraspinatus tendon**
- [ ] 2. **Subscapularis tendon**
- [ ] 3. **Biceps brachii tendon (long head)**
- [ ] 4. **Capsular ligaments of the shoulder**
- [ ] 5. **Infraspinatus tendon**
- [ ] 6. **Teres minor tendon**

Clinical Note:

Movement at the shoulder joint, or almost any joint, can lead to inflammation of the tendons surrounding that joint and secondary inflammation of the bursa that cushions the joint from the overlying muscle or tendon. At the shoulder, the supraspinatus muscle tendon is especially vulnerable because it can become pinched by the greater tubercle of the humerus, the acromion, and the coraco-acromial ligament.

About 95% of shoulder joint dislocations occur in an anterior direction. Often this can happen with a throwing motion, which places stress on the capsule and anterior elements of the rotator cuff (especially the subscapularis tendon).

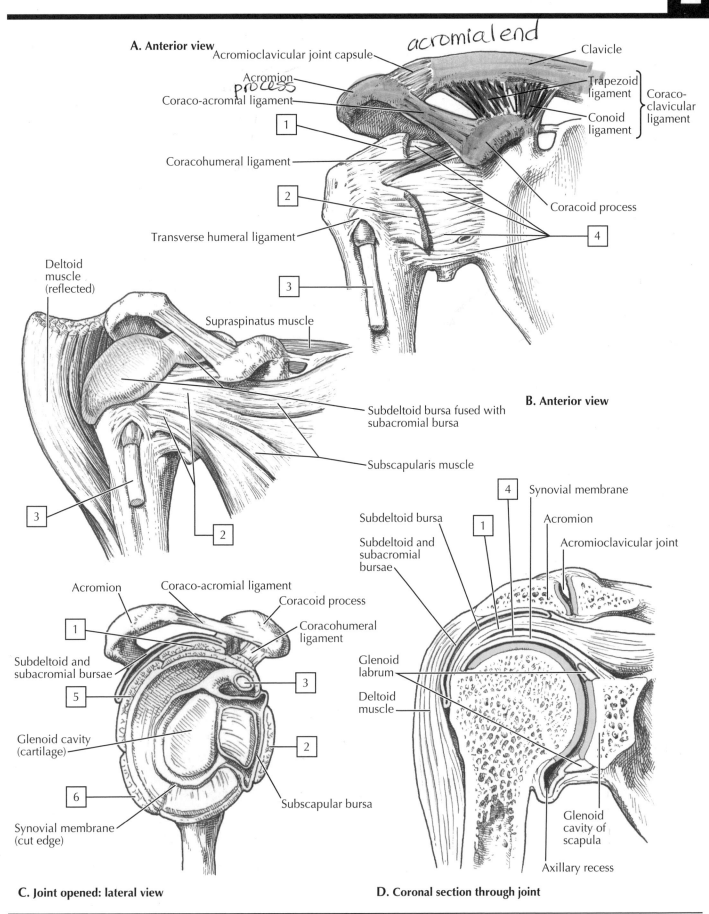

A. Anterior view

acromial end

Acromioclavicular joint capsule

Clavicle

Acromion
process

Trapezoid ligament

Coraco-acromial ligament

Conoid ligament

Coraco-clavicular ligament

1

Coracohumeral ligament

Coracoid process

2

4

Transverse humeral ligament

3

Deltoid muscle (reflected)

Supraspinatus muscle

B. Anterior view

Subdeltoid bursa fused with subacromial bursa

3

Subscapularis muscle

2

Subdeltoid bursa

4

Synovial membrane

Acromion

Subdeltoid and subacromial bursae

1

Acromioclavicular joint

Glenoid labrum

Acromion

Coraco-acromial ligament

Coracoid process

1

Coracohumeral ligament

Subdeltoid and subacromial bursae

5

3

Deltoid muscle

Glenoid cavity (cartilage)

2

6

Subscapular bursa

Synovial membrane (cut edge)

Glenoid cavity of scapula

Axillary recess

C. Joint opened: lateral view

D. Coronal section through joint

The forearm extends from the elbow proximally to the wrist distally and is composed of two bones, the **radius** laterally and the **ulna** medially. The radius is the shorter of the two bones. The region just anterior to the elbow is known as the **cubital fossa** (a cubit is an ancient term for linear measurement and was the length from the elbow to the tip of the middle finger) and is a common site for venipuncture (access to a vein to withdraw blood or administer fluids).

An interosseous membrane connects the radius and ulna and is a type of fibrous joint. The movements of supination (palm facing forward in anatomical position) and pronation (palm facing backward) are unique movements of the wrist and hand but occur exclusively in the forearm with the radius crossing over the ulna (pronation) or back alongside the ulna (supination) (see parts **A-C**).

COLOR each bone and note each bone's labeled features:

- [ ] **1. Radius**
- [ ] **2. Ulna**

The elbow joint is composed of the following joints, and its ligaments and features are summarized in the table below:
- Humero-ulnar: for flexion and extension, the ulnar trochlear notch articulates with the trochlea of the humerus
- Humero-radial: for flexion and extension, the head of the radius articulates with the capitulum of the humerus
- Proximal radio-ulnar: for supination and pronation, the radial head articulates with the radial notch of the ulna

LIGAMENT	ATTACHMENT	COMMENT
Humero-ulnar (Uniaxial Synovial Hinge [Ginglymus]) Joint		
Capsule	Surrounds joint	Provides flexion and extension
Ulnar (medial) collateral	Medial epicondyle of humerus to coronoid process and olecranon of ulna	Is triangular ligament with anterior, posterior, and oblique bands
Humeroradial Joint		
Capsule	Surrounds joint	Capitulum of humerus to head of radius
Radial (lateral) collateral	Lateral epicondyle of humerus to radial notch of ulna and anular ligament	Is weaker than ulnar collateral ligament but provides posterolateral stability
Proximal Radio-ulnar (Uniaxial Synovial Pivot) Joint		
Anular ligament	Surrounds radial head and radial notch of ulna	Keeps radial head in radial notch; allows pronation and supination

COLOR the following key ligaments of the elbow joint (parts **D-F**), using a different color for each ligament:

- [ ] **3. Radial collateral ligament: on the lateral side of the elbow**
- [ ] **4. Anular ligament: surrounds the radial head in the proximal radio-ulnar articulation**
- [ ] **5. Ulnar collateral ligament: on the medial side of the elbow**

Clinical Note:
Elbow dislocations are third in frequency after shoulder and finger dislocations. Dislocation often occurs from a fall on an outstretched hand, and a dislocation in the posterior direction is the most common type.

Plate 2-12 See Netter: *Atlas of Human Anatomy*, 6th Edition, Plates 422, 424, and 425.

Skeletal System

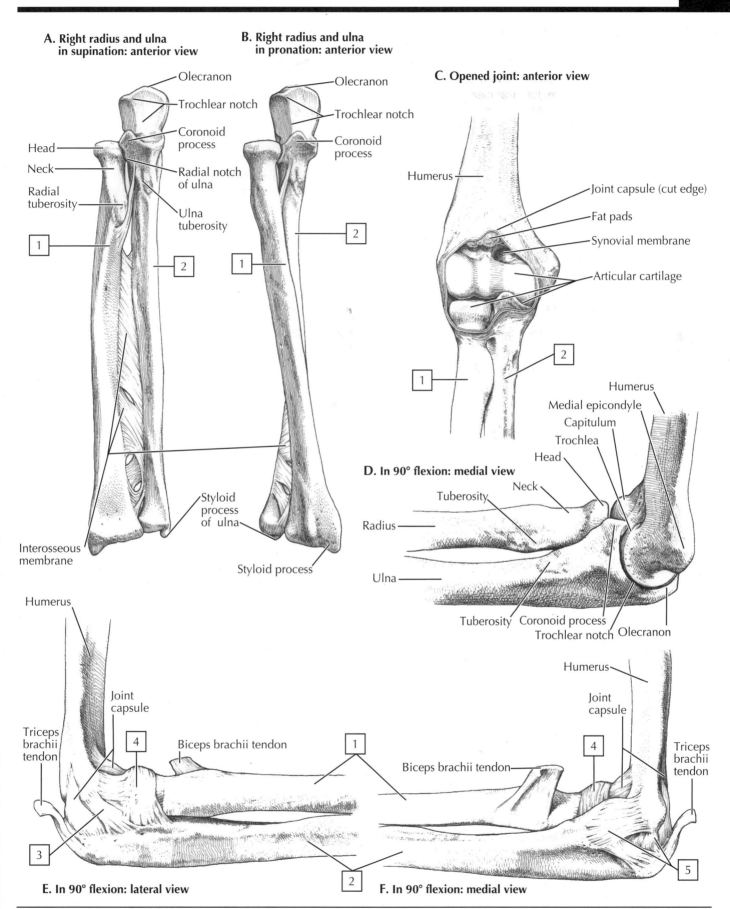

A. Right radius and ulna in supination: anterior view

Olecranon
Trochlear notch
Coronoid process
Head
Neck
Radial notch of ulna
Radial tuberosity
Ulna tuberosity
1
2
Interosseous membrane

B. Right radius and ulna in pronation: anterior view

Olecranon
Trochlear notch
Coronoid process
2
1
Styloid process of ulna
Styloid process

C. Opened joint: anterior view

Humerus
Joint capsule (cut edge)
Fat pads
Synovial membrane
Articular cartilage
1
2

D. In 90° flexion: medial view

Humerus
Medial epicondyle
Capitulum
Trochlea
Head
Neck
Tuberosity
Radius
Ulna
Tuberosity
Coronoid process
Trochlear notch
Olecranon

E. In 90° flexion: lateral view

Humerus
Joint capsule
4
Biceps brachii tendon
Triceps brachii tendon
1
2
3

F. In 90° flexion: medial view

Humerus
Joint capsule
4
Biceps brachii tendon
Triceps brachii tendon
1
2
5

The wrist and hand are composed of the following 29 bones:
- 8 carpal (wrist) bones, arranged in proximal and distal rows of 4 bones each
- 5 metacarpals, which span the palm of the hand
- 14 phalanges, 2 for the thumb (1st digit) and 3 each for the remaining 4 digits
- 2 sesamoid bones, situated at the distal end of the thumb metacarpal

These bones and their features are summarized in the table below.

FEATURE	CHARACTERISTICS
Proximal Row of Carpals	
Scaphoid (boat shaped)	Lies beneath anatomical snuffbox
Lunate (moon or crescent shaped)	Is most commonly fractured carpal
Triquetrum (triangular)	All three bones (scaphoid, lunate, triquetrum) articulate with distal radius
Pisiform (pea shaped)	
Distal Row of Carpals	
Trapezium (four sided)	Distal row articulates with proximal row of carpals and with metacarpals 1-5
Trapezoid	
Capitate (round bone)	
Hamate (hooked bone)	
Metacarpals	
Numbered 1-5	Possess a base, shaft, and head
(thumb to little finger)	Are triangular in cross section
	Fifth metacarpal most commonly fractured
Two sesamoid bones	Are associated with head of first metacarpal
Phalanges	
Three for each digit except thumb	Possess a base, shaft, and head
	Termed proximal, middle, and distal
	Distal phalanx of middle finger commonly fractured

The carpal bones are not aligned in a flat plane but form an arch, the **carpal arch**, with its concave aspect facing anteriorly. Tendons from forearm muscles, vessels, and nerves pass through or across this arch to gain access to the hand. A tight band of connective tissue, the flexor retinaculum, spans the carpal arch forming a "carpal tunnel" for the structures passing through this archway.

COLOR the following bones of the wrist and hand, using different colors for each carpal bone, a uniform color for the metacarpals, another uniform color for all the phalanges of the digits, and a new color for the sesamoid bones:

1. **Scaphoid:** some clinicians refer to this bone as the navicular ("little ship")
2. **Trapezium**
3. **Trapezoid**
4. **Lunate**
5. **Triquetrum**
6. **Pisiform**
7. **Hamate**
8. **Capitate**
9. **Metacarpals**
10. **Phalanges of each digit**
11. **Sesamoid bones (two at the distal end of the thumb metacarpal)**

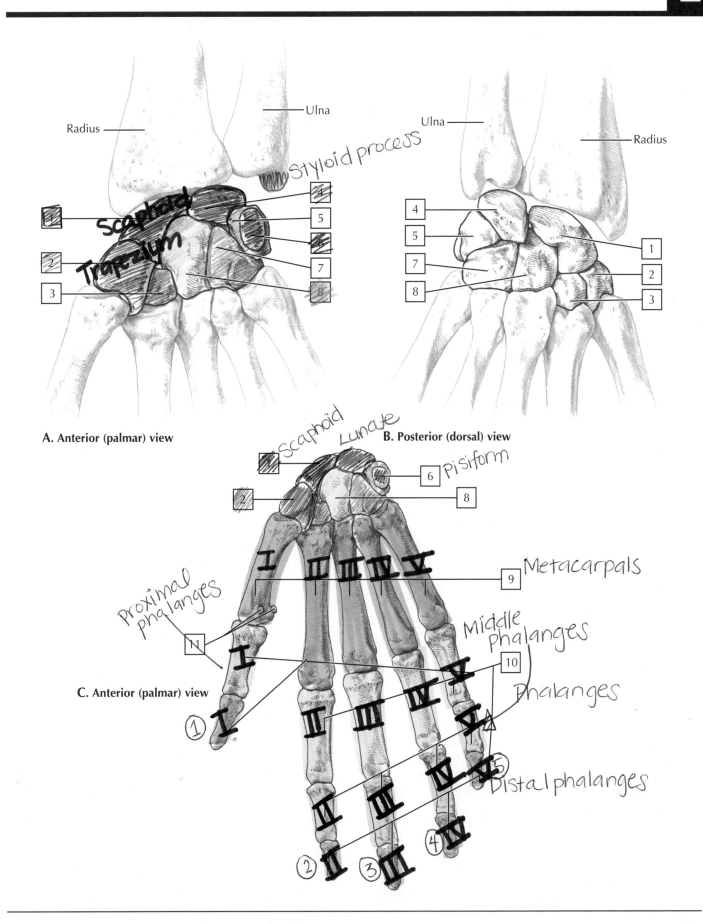

Radius

Ulna

Styloid process

Scaphoid

Trapezium

A. Anterior (palmar) view

Ulna

Radius

B. Posterior (dorsal) view

Scaphoid

Lunate

Pisiform

Metacarpals

Proximal phalanges

Middle phalanges

Phalanges

Distal phalanges

C. Anterior (palmar) view

The classification and ligaments of the wrist and finger joints are summarized in the following table. The wrist joint is a radiocarpal (biaxial synovial ellipsoid) joint between the distal radius of the forearm and the scaphoid, lunate and triquetrum carpals, and the articular disc at the distal ulna. On the facing page, note the finger movements associated with these joints.

COLOR the following major ligaments, using a different color for each ligament:

- [ ] 1. Palmar radiocarpal ligaments
- [ ] 2. Dorsal radiocarpal ligament
- [ ] 3. Articular disc of the wrist joint
- [ ] 4. Capsule of a metacarpophalangeal joint
- [ ] 5. Capsule of a proximal interphalangeal joint
- [ ] 6. Capsule of a distal interphalangeal joint
- [ ] 7. Collateral ligament of a metacarpophalangeal joint
- [ ] 8. Palmar ligament (plate)

LIGAMENT	ATTACHMENT	COMMENT
Radiocarpal (Biaxial Synovial Ellipsoid) Joint		
Capsule and disc	Surrounds joint; radius to scaphoid, lunate, and triquetrum	Provides little support; allows flexion, extension, abduction, adduction, circumduction
Palmar (volar) radiocarpal ligaments	Radius to scaphoid, lunate, and triquetrum	Are strong and stabilizing
Dorsal radiocarpal	Radius to scaphoid, lunate, and triquetrum	Is weaker ligament
Radial collateral	Radius to scaphoid and triquetrum	Stabilizes proximal row of carpals
Distal Radiocarpal (Uniaxial Synovial Pivot) Joint		
Capsule	Surrounds joint; ulnar head to ulnar notch of radius	Is thin superiorly; allows pronation, supination
Palmar and dorsal radio-ulnar	Extends transversely between the two bones	Articular disc binds bones together
Intercarpal (Synovial Plane) Joints		
Proximal row of carpals	Adjacent carpals	Permits gliding and sliding movements
Distal row of carpals	Adjacent carpals	Are united by anterior, posterior, and interosseous ligaments
Midcarpal (Synovial Plane) Joints		
Palmar (volar) intercarpal	Proximal and distal rows of carpals	Is location for one third of wrist extension and two thirds of flexion; permits gliding and sliding movements
Carpal collaterals	Scaphoid, lunate, and triquetrum to capitate and hamate	Stabilize distal row (ellipsoid synovial joint)
Carpometacarpal (CMC) (Plane Synovial) Joints (Except Thumb)		
Capsule	Carpals to metacarpals of digits 2-5	Surrounds joints; allows some gliding movement
Palmar and dorsal CMC	Carpals to metacarpals of digits 2-5	Dorsal ligament strongest
Interosseous CMC	Carpals to metacarpals of digits 2-5	
Thumb (Biaxial Saddle) Joint		
Same ligaments as CMC	Trapezium to first metacarpal	Allows flexion, extension, abduction, adduction, circumduction
		Is common site for arthritis
Metacarpophalangeal (Biaxial Condyloid Synovial) Joint		
Capsule	Metacarpal to proximal phalanx	Surrounds joint; allows flexion, extension, abduction, adduction, circumduction
Radial and ulnar collaterals	Metacarpal to proximal phalanx	Are tight in flexion and loose in extension
Palmar (volar) plate	Metacarpal to proximal phalanx	If broken digit, cast in flexion or ligament will shorten during healing
Interphalangeal (Uniaxial Synovial Hinge) Joints		
Capsule	Adjacent phalanges	Surrounds joints; allows flexion and extension
Two collaterals	Adjacent phalanges	Are oriented obliquely
Palmar (volar) plate	Adjacent phalanges	Prevents hyperextension

Plate 2-14   See Netter: *Atlas of Human Anatomy*, 6th Edition, Plates 441, 442, and 445.

Skeletal System

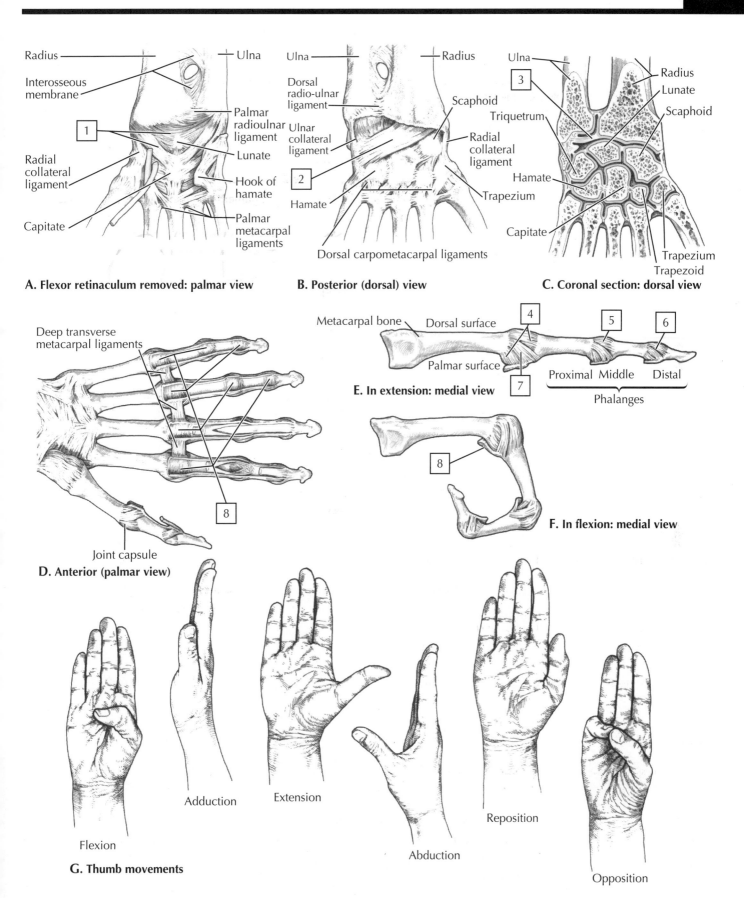

A. Flexor retinaculum removed: palmar view

Radius
Interosseous membrane
1
Radial collateral ligament
Capitate
Ulna
Palmar radioulnar ligament
Lunate
Hook of hamate
Palmar metacarpal ligaments

B. Posterior (dorsal) view

Ulna
Dorsal radio-ulnar ligament
Ulnar collateral ligament
2
Hamate
Radius
Scaphoid
Radial collateral ligament
Trapezium
Dorsal carpometacarpal ligaments

C. Coronal section: dorsal view

Ulna
3
Triquetrum
Hamate
Capitate
Radius
Lunate
Scaphoid
Trapezium
Trapezoid

D. Anterior (palmar view)

Deep transverse metacarpal ligaments
8
Joint capsule

E. In extension: medial view

Metacarpal bone
Dorsal surface
4
5
6
Palmar surface
7
Proximal Middle Distal
Phalanges

F. In flexion: medial view

8

G. Thumb movements

Flexion
Adduction
Extension
Abduction
Reposition
Opposition

The **pelvic girdle** is the attachment point of the lower limb to the trunk of the body. The bony pelvis includes the:
- **Pelvic bone:** a fusion of three separate bones called the **ilium, ischium,** and **pubis,** which all join each other in the acetabulum (a cup-shaped feature for articulation with the head of the femur, our thigh bone); the two pelvic bones (right and left) articulate with the sacrum posteriorly and at the pubic symphysis anteriorly
- **Sacrum:** a fusion of five sacral vertebrae of the spine
- **Coccyx:** the terminal end of the spine and a remnant of our embryonic tail

COLOR the pelvic girdle, using a different color for each of the following bones (parts *A* and *B*):

- [ ] 1. **Ischium**
- [ ] 2. **Ilium**
- [ ] 3. **Pubis**

The three pelvic bones fuse into a single bone during late adolescence. Also, gender differences exist in the structure of the pelvis and represent adaptations for childbirth. For example, the female pelvis has wider iliac crests and a broader pubic arch than the male pelvis has. Finally, the pelvis articulates with the sacrum at the sacro-iliac (plane synovial) joint, which is reinforced by strong ligaments that provide stability and support. The joints and ligaments of the pelvic girdle are summarized in the table below.

COLOR the following key ligaments of the pelvic articulations (parts *C* and *D*), using a different color for each ligament:

- [ ] 4. **Posterior sacro-iliac ligaments**
- [ ] 5. **Sacrospinous ligament: divides the sciatic notch into the greater and lesser sciatic foramina**
- [ ] 6. **Sacrotuberous ligament**
- [ ] 7. **Anterior sacro-iliac ligaments**
- [ ] 8. **Pubic symphysis: fibrocartilage that permits some expansion during childbirth**

FEATURE	CHARACTERISTICS
Coxal (hip) bone	
	Fusion of three bones on each side to form the pelvis, which articulates with the sacrum to form the pelvic girdle
Ilium	Body fused to ischium and pubis, all meeting in the acetabulum (socket for articulation with femoral head)
	Ala (wing): weak spot of ilium
Ischium	Body fused with other two bones; ramus fused with pubis
Pubis	Body fused with other two bones; ramus fused with ischium
Femur (proximal)	
Long bone	Longest bone in the body and very strong
Head	Point of articulation with acetabulum of coxal bone
Neck	Common fracture site
Greater trochanter	Point of the hip; attachment site for several gluteal muscles
Lesser trochanter	Attachment site of iliopsoas tendon (strong hip flexor)

LIGAMENT	ATTACHMENT	COMMENT
Lumbosacral Joint*		
Intervertebral (IV) disc	Between L5 and sacrum	Allows little movement
Iliolumbar	Transverse process of L5 to crest of ilium	Can be involved in avulsion fracture
Sacro-iliac (Plane Synovial) Joint		
Sacro-iliac	Sacrum to ilium	Allows little movement; consists of posterior (strong), anterior (provides rotational stability), and interosseous (strongest) ligaments
Sacrococcygeal (Symphysis) Joint		
Sacrococcygeal	Between coccyx and sacrum	Allows some movement; consists of anterior, posterior, and lateral ligaments; contains an IV disc between S5 and C1
Pubic Symphysis		
Pubic	Between pubic bones	Allows some movement, fibrocartilage disc
Accessory Ligaments		
Sacrotuberous	Iliac spines and sacrum to ischial tuberosity	Provides vertical stability
Sacrospinous	Ischial spine to sacrum and coccyx	Divides sciatic notch into greater and lesser sciatic foramina

*Other ligaments include those binding any two vertebrae and facet joints.

Plate 2-15   See Netter: *Atlas of Human Anatomy*, 6th Edition, Plates 333 and 473.

Skeletal System

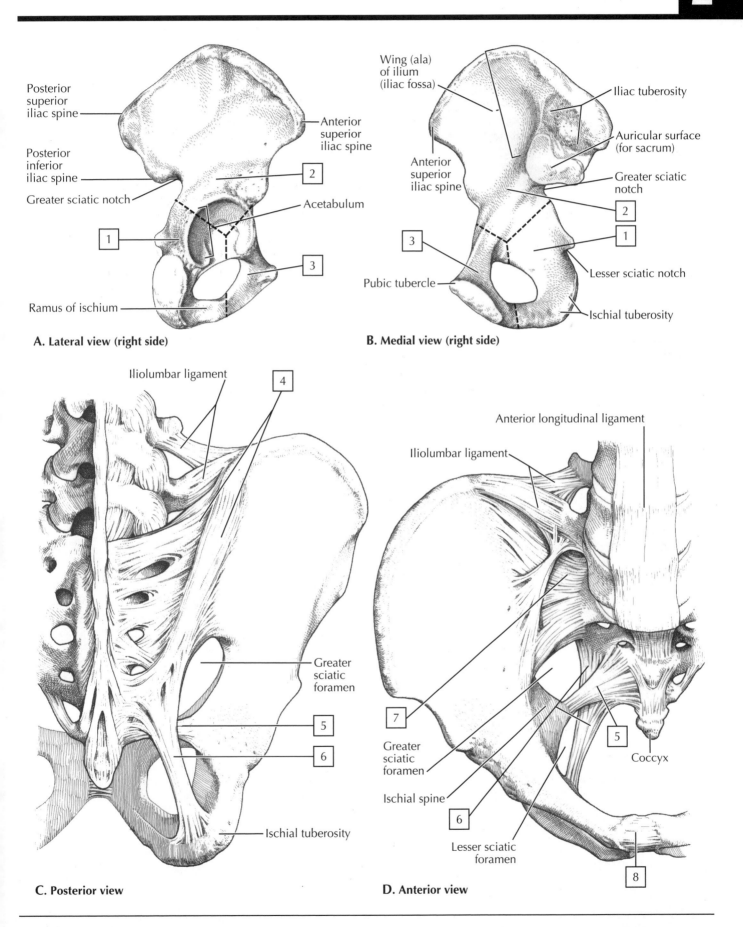

Posterior superior iliac spine

Posterior inferior iliac spine

Greater sciatic notch

Ramus of ischium

Anterior superior iliac spine

2

Acetabulum

1

3

A. Lateral view (right side)

Wing (ala) of ilium (iliac fossa)

Iliac tuberosity

Anterior superior iliac spine

Auricular surface (for sacrum)

Greater sciatic notch

2

3

1

Pubic tubercle

Lesser sciatic notch

Ischial tuberosity

B. Medial view (right side)

Iliolumbar ligament

4

Greater sciatic foramen

5

6

Ischial tuberosity

C. Posterior view

Anterior longitudinal ligament

Iliolumbar ligament

7

Greater sciatic foramen

Ischial spine

5

Coccyx

6

8

Lesser sciatic foramen

D. Anterior view

The hip joint is a multiaxial synovial ball-and-socket joint between the head of the femur and the acetabulum of the pelvic bone. Unlike the ball-and-socket shoulder joint, the hip joint is designed for stability and support at the expense of some mobility. Similar to the shoulder joint, the acetabulum is rimmed by a fibrocartilaginous "lip" called the **acetabular labrum** that deepens the socket. The features of the hip joint are summarized in the table below. The primary hip joint ligaments include three major ligaments that surround the hip joint and one internal ligament to the head of femur.

COLOR the following ligaments of the hip joint, using a different color for each ligament or feature:

☐ 1. **Iliofemoral ligament (Y ligament of Bigelow):** positioned anteriorly

☐ 2. **Pubofemoral ligament: positioned anteriorly and inferiorly**

☐ 3. **Ischiofemoral ligament: positioned posteriorly**

☐ 4. **Acetabular labrum: fibrocartilage around the rim of the socket**

☐ 5. **Articular cartilage on the head of the femur**

☐ 6. **Ligament of the head of the femur: attaches to the acetabular notch and transverse acetabular ligament**

LIGAMENT	ATTACHMENT	COMMENT
Hip (Multiaxial Synovial Ball-and-Socket) Joint		
Capsular	Acetabular margin to femoral neck	Encloses femoral head and part of neck; acts in flexion, extension, abduction, adduction, circumduction
Iliofemoral	Iliac spine and acetabulum to intertrochanteric line	Is strongest ligament; forms inverted Y (of Bigelow); limits hyperextension and lateral rotation
Ischiofemoral	Acetabulum to femoral neck posteriorly	Limits extension and medial rotation; is weaker ligament
Pubofemoral	Pubic ramus to lower femoral neck	Limits extension and abduction
Labrum	Acetabulum	Fibrocartilage, deepens socket
Transverse acetabular	Acetabular notch interiorly	Cups acetabulum to form a socket for femoral head
Ligament of head of femur	Acetabular notch and transverse ligament to femoral head	Artery to femoral head runs in ligament

Clinical Note:

Hip fractures are common injuries. In the young, the fracture often results from trauma, whereas in the elderly the cause is often related to osteoporosis and associated with a fall. The neck of the femur is a common site for such fractures.

Plate 2-16 See Netter: *Atlas of Human Anatomy*, 6th Edition, Plates 474 and 491.

Skeletal System

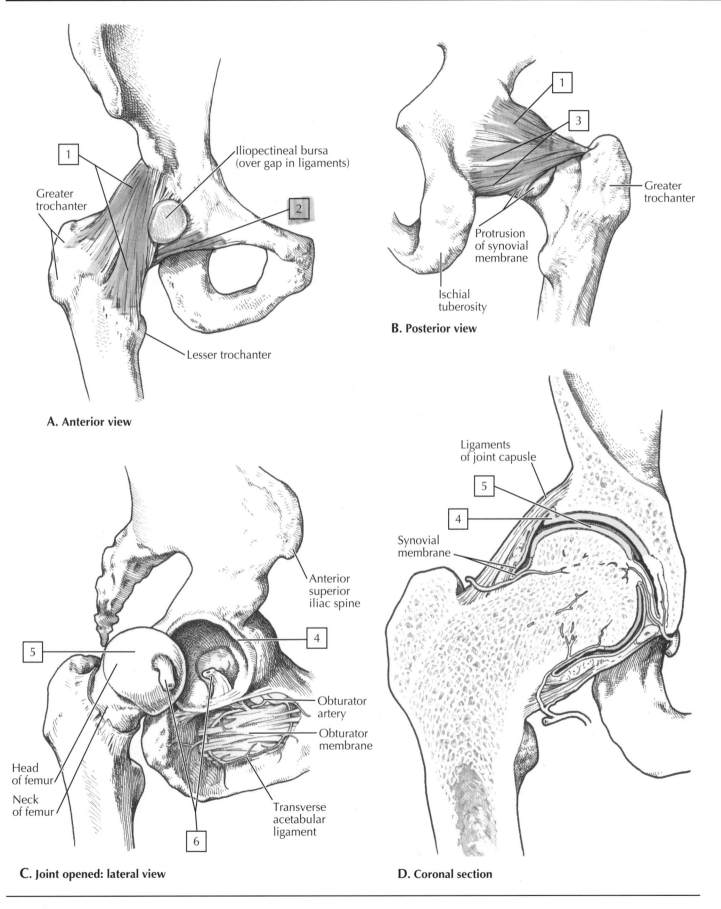

Iliopectineal bursa
(over gap in ligaments)

1

2

Greater
trochanter

Lesser trochanter

A. Anterior view

1

3

Greater
trochanter

Protrusion
of synovial
membrane

Ischial
tuberosity

B. Posterior view

Anterior
superior
iliac spine

4

Obturator
artery

Obturator
membrane

5

Head
of femur

Neck
of femur

6

Transverse
acetabular
ligament

C. Joint opened: lateral view

Ligaments
of joint capusle

5

4

Synovial
membrane

D. Coronal section

The **femur** is the bone of the thigh (anatomically, the thigh is the region between the hip and knee and the leg is the region between the knee and ankle). The femur is the longest bone in the body and transmits the weight of the body from the knee to the pelvis. The major features of the femur are summarized in the table below.

The bones of the leg are the **tibia** and **fibula**. The tibia is the larger of the two leg bones and is medially placed in the leg, and its shaft can be palpated just beneath the skin from the base of the knee to the ankle joint. The articulation of the distal femur and proximal tibia forms the knee joint, and a large sesamoid bone called the **patella** lies anterior to this joint and is embedded in the tendon of the quadriceps femoris muscle. The fibula is not a weight-bearing bone, is found laterally in the leg, and is primarily a bone for muscle attachment. Features of the tibia and fibula are summarized in the table below.

COLOR the following bones of the thigh and leg, using a different color for each bone:

☐ **1. Femur**
☐ **2. Patella**
☐ **3. Tibia**
☐ **4. Fibula**

Clinical Note:

Most **fractures** of the femur occur across the neck of femur within the articular capsule. Tibial fractures occur most frequently where the tibial shaft is narrowest, which is about one third of the way down the shaft. Fibular fractures are most common just proximal to the lateral malleolus, just above the ankle joint on the lateral side.

FEATURE	CHARACTERISTICS
Femur	
Long bone	Longest bone in the body; very strong
Head	Point of articulation with acetabulum of coxal bone
Neck	Common fracture site
Greater trochanter	Point of hip; attachment site for several gluteal muscles
Lesser trochanter	Attachment site of iliopsoas tendon (strong hip flexor)
Distal condyles	Medial and lateral (smaller) sites that articulate with tibial condyles
Patella	
	Sesamoid bone (largest) embedded in quadriceps femoris tendon
Tibia	
Long bone	Large, weight-bearing bone
Proximal facets	Large plateau for articulation with femoral condyles
Tibial tuberosity	Insertion site for patellar ligament
Inferior articular surface	Surface for cupping talus at the ankle joint
Medial malleolus	Prominence on medial aspect of ankle
Fibula	
Long bone	Slender bone, primarily for muscle attachment
Neck	Possible damage to common fibular nerve if fracture occurs here

Plate 2-17   See Netter: *Atlas of Human Anatomy*, 6th Edition, Plates 476 and 500.

Skeletal System

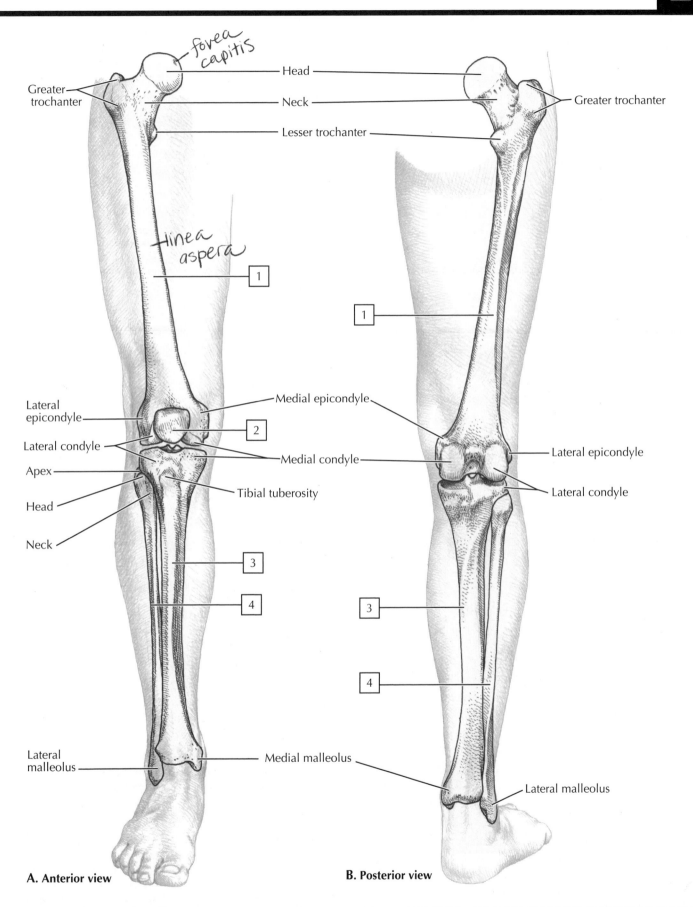

fovea capitis

Greater trochanter

Head

Neck

Lesser trochanter

Greater trochanter

linea aspera

1

1

Lateral epicondyle

Medial epicondyle

2

Lateral condyle

Medial condyle

Lateral epicondyle

Apex

Lateral condyle

Head

Tibial tuberosity

Neck

3

3

4

4

Lateral malleolus

Medial malleolus

Lateral malleolus

A. Anterior view

B. Posterior view

The knee is a biaxial condylar synovial joint and is the most sophisticated joint in the body. It participates in flexion, extension, and some gliding and medial rotation when it is flexed. When in full extension, the femur rotates medially on the tibia, and the ligaments tighten to "lock" the knee. Features of this joint are summarized in the table below. Only the major ligaments are shown in these illustrations.

COLOR the following extracapsular and intracapsular ligaments of the knee joint, using a different color for each ligament:

☐ 1. **Medial meniscus: fibrocartilage disc on the tibia that deepens the articular surface and acts as a shock absorber or cushion**

☐ 2. **Tibial (medial) collateral ligament**

☐ 3. **Posterior cruciate ligament**

☐ 4. **Anterior cruciate ligament**

☐ 5. **Lateral meniscus: similar disc of fibrocartilage on the lateral side of the tibia**

☐ 6. **Fibular (lateral) collateral ligament**

LIGAMENT	ATTACHMENT	COMMENT
Knee (Biaxial Condylar Synovial) Joint		
Capsule	Surrounds femoral and tibial condyles, and patella	Is fibrous, weak (offers little support); flexion, extension, some gliding, and medial rotation
Extracapsular Ligaments		
Tibial collateral	Medial femoral epicondyle to medial tibial condyle	Limits extension and abduction of leg; attached to medial meniscus
Fibular collateral	Lateral femoral epicondyle to fibular head	Limits extension and adduction of leg; overlies popliteus tendon
Patellar	Patella to tibial tuberosity	Acts in extension of quadriceps tendon
Arcuate popliteal	Fibular head to capsule	Passes over popliteus muscle
Oblique popliteal	Semimembranosus tendon to posterior knee	Limits hyperextension and lateral rotation
Intracapsular Ligaments		
Medial meniscus	Interarticular area of tibia, lies over medial facet, attached to tibial collateral	Is semicircular (C-shaped); acts as cushion; often torn
Lateral meniscus	Interarticular area of tibia, lies over lateral facet	Is more circular and smaller than medial meniscus; acts as cushion
Anterior cruciate	Anterior intercondylar tibia to lateral femoral condyle	Prevents posterior slipping of femur on tibia; torn in hyperextension
Posterior cruciate	Posterior intercondylar tibia to medial femoral condyle	Prevents anterior slipping of femur on tibia; shorter and stronger than anterior cruciate
Transverse	Anterior aspect of menisci	Binds and stabilizes menisci
Posterior meniscofemoral (ligament of Wrisberg)	Posterior lateral meniscus to medial femoral condyle	Is strong
Patellofemoral (Biaxial Synovial Saddle) Joint		
Quadriceps tendon	Muscles to superior patella	Is part of extension mechanism
Patellar	Patella to tibial tuberosity	Acts in extension of quadriceps tendon; patella stabilized by medial and lateral ligament (retinaculum) attachment to tibia and femur

Clinical Note:

Rupture of the weaker anterior cruciate ligament (ACL) is a common athletic injury, usually related to twisting of the knee while the foot is firmly on the ground. Because the ACL prevents hyperextension of the knee, movement of the tibia forward on the femur while keeping the foot stable (anterior drawer sign) is used to assess ACL integrity. Often, **ACL injuries** may also be accompanied by a tear of the tibial collateral ligament or the medial meniscus. The medial meniscus attaches to the tibial collateral ligament. The combination of these three ligament tears—ACL, tibial collateral ligament, and medial meniscus—is known as the "unhappy triad."

Plate 2-18 See Netter: *Atlas of Human Anatomy*, 6th Edition, Plates 495, 496, and 498.

Skeletal System

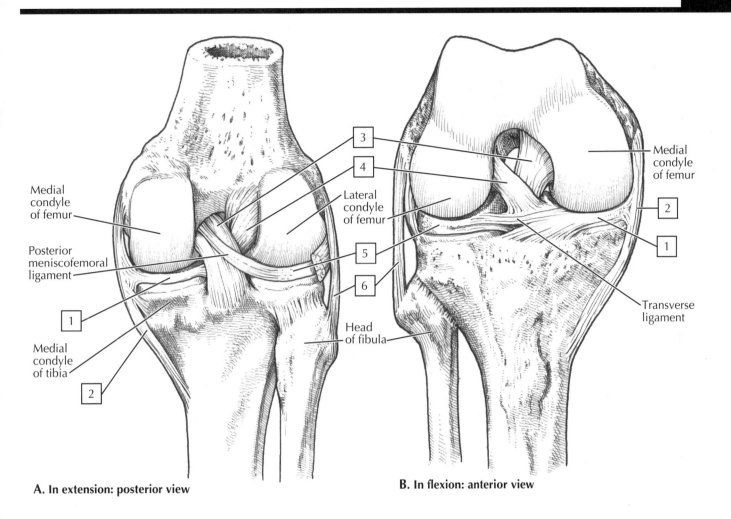

A. In extension: posterior view

Medial condyle of femur

Posterior meniscofemoral ligament

Medial condyle of tibia

3

4

5

6

Lateral condyle of femur

Head of fibula

Medial condyle of femur

Transverse ligament

B. In flexion: anterior view

1

2

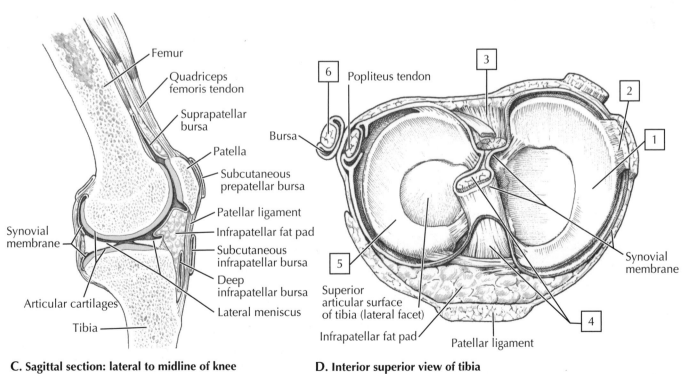

Femur

Quadriceps femoris tendon

Suprapatellar bursa

Patella

Subcutaneous prepatellar bursa

Patellar ligament

Infrapatellar fat pad

Subcutaneous infrapatellar bursa

Deep infrapatellar bursa

Lateral meniscus

Synovial membrane

Articular cartilages

Tibia

C. Sagittal section: lateral to midline of knee

Bursa

Popliteus tendon

6

3

2

1

Synovial membrane

5

Superior articular surface of tibia (lateral facet)

Infrapatellar fat pad

Patellar ligament

4

D. Interior superior view of tibia

The ankle and foot are composed of the following 28 bones:
- 7 tarsal (ankle) bones, arranged in a proximal group of 2 tarsals (talus and calcaneus), a distal row of 4 tarsals (cuboid and 3 cuneiforms), and a single intermediate tarsal (navicular) between these groups
- 5 metatarsals, which span the middle portion of the sole of the foot
- 14 phalanges, 2 for the big toe (hallucis) and 3 each for the other 4 toes
- 2 sesamoid bones, situated on the plantar surface of the distal first metatarsal

The bones of the foot are not aligned in a single flat plane with each bone in contact with the ground. Rather, the foot has two arches, each supported by ligaments and muscles:
- Longitudinal arch, formed by the posterior portion of the calcaneus (heel) and the heads of the five metatarsals; this arch is highest on the medial side of the foot
- Transverse arch, formed by the cuboid, cuneiforms, and the bases of the metatarsals; this arch runs from side to side

COLOR the following bones of the ankle and foot, using a different color for each tarsal, a uniform color for the metatarsals, another uniform color for the phalanges, and a new color for the sesamoid bones.

☐ 1. Calcaneus
☐ 2. Talus
☐ 3. Navicular
☐ 4. Cuneiforms (color all three the same color)
☐ 5. Cuboid
☐ 6. Metatarsals
☐ 7. Phalanges
☐ 8. Sesamoid bones

FEATURE	CHARACTERISTICS
Talus (ankle bone)	Transfers weight from tibia to foot; no muscle attachment
Trochlea	Articulates with tibia and fibula
Head	Articulates with navicular bone
Calcaneus (heel bone)	Articulates with talus superiorly and cuboid anteriorly
Sustentaculum tali	Medial shelf that supports talar head
Navicular	"Boat shaped," between talar head and three cuneiforms
Tuberosity	If large, can cause medial pain in tight-fitting shoe
Cuboid	Most lateral tarsal bone
Groove	For fibularis (peroneus) longus tendon
Cuneiform	Three wedge-shaped bones
Metatarsals	
Numbered 1 to 5, from great toe (big toe) to little toe	Possess base, shaft, and head
	Fibularis brevis tendon inserts on 5th metatarsal
Two sesamoid bones	Associated with flexor hallucis brevis tendons
Phalanges	
Three for each digit except great toe	Possess base, shaft, and head
	Termed proximal, middle, and distal
	Stubbed 5th toe common injury

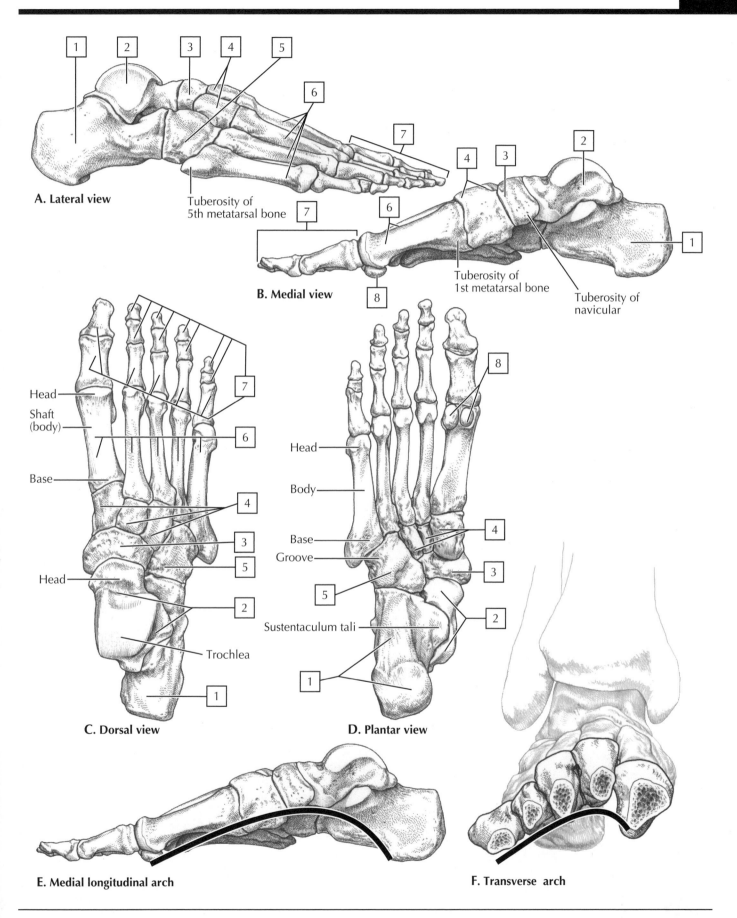

A. Lateral view

Tuberosity of
5th metatarsal bone

B. Medial view

Tuberosity of
1st metatarsal bone

Tuberosity of
navicular

Head

Shaft
(body)

Base

Head

Trochlea

C. Dorsal view

Head

Body

Base

Groove

Sustentaculum tali

D. Plantar view

E. Medial longitudinal arch

F. Transverse arch

The classification and ligaments of the ankle and foot joints are summarized in the table below. The ankle joint is primarily a ta-locrural (talus with the distal tibia of the leg) joint (weight-bearing) and laterally, a talofibular (talus with the distal fibula of the leg) joint.

COLOR the following major ligaments, using a different color for each ligament:

☐ 1. **Anterior talofibular**

☐ 2. **Posterior talofibular**

☐ 3. **Calcaneofibular: these first three ligaments together form the "lateral collateral" ligament of the ankle**

☐ 4. **Long plantar**

☐ 5. **Medial (deltoid) ligament: composed of four separate ligaments extending from the tibia to the talus or calcaneus**

☐ 6. **Plantar calcaneonavicular: called the "spring" ligament, it helps support the medial arch of the foot**

☐ 7. **Capsule of a proximal interphalangeal joint**

☐ 8. **Capsule of a metatarsophalangeal joint**

Clinical Note:
Calcaneal fractures are the most common tarsal fracture, usually caused by forceful landing on the heel, as in jumping from a great height. The talus is driven down into the calcaneus, which cannot withstand the force because the calcaneus is spongy bone. Most **ankle sprains** are inversion injuries where one lands on the lateral aspect of the foot, the sole is turned medially, and the components of the lateral collateral ligament are stretched or torn.

LIGAMENT	ATTACHMENT	COMMENT
Distal Tibiofibular (Fibrous [Syndesmosis]) Joint		
Anterior tibiofibular	Anterior distal tibia and fibula	Runs obliquely
Posterior tibiofibular	Posterior distal tibia and fibula	Is weaker than anterior ligament
Inferior transverse	Medial malleolus to fibula	Is deep continuation of posterior ligament
Talocrural (Uniaxial Synovial Hinge [Ginglymus]) Joint		
Capsule	Tibia to talus	Functions in plantarflexion and dorsiflexion
Medial (deltoid)	Medial malleolus to talus, calcaneus, and navicular	Limits eversion of foot; maintains medial long arch; has four parts
Lateral (collateral)	Lateral malleolus to talus and calcaneus	Is weak and often sprained; resists inversion of foot; has three parts
INTERTARSAL JOINTS		
Talocalcaneal (Subtalar Plane Synovial) Joints		
Capsule	Margins of articulation	Functions in inversion and eversion
Talocalcaneal	Talus to calcaneus	Has medial, lateral, and posterior parts
Interosseous	Talus to calcaneus	Is strong; binds bones together
Talocalcaneonavicular (Partial Ball-and-Socket Synovial) Joint		
Capsule	Encloses part of joint	Functions in gliding and rotational movements
Plantar calcaneonavicular	Sustentaculum tali to navicular bone	Is strong plantar support for head of talus (called spring ligament)
Dorsal talonavicular	Talus to navicular	Is dorsal support to talus
Calcaneocuboid (Plane Synovial) Joint		
Capsule	Encloses joint	Functions in inversion and eversion
Calcaneocuboid	Calcaneus to cuboid	Are dorsal, plantar (short plantar, strong), and long plantar ligaments
Tarsometatarsal (Plane Synovial) Joints		
Capsule	Encloses joint	Functions in gliding or sliding movements
Tarsometatarsal	Tarsals to metatarsals	Are dorsal, plantar, interosseous ligaments
Intermetatarsal (Plane Synovial) Joints		
Capsule	Base of metatarsals	Provides little movement, supports transverse arch
Intermetatarsal	Adjacent metatarsals	Are dorsal, plantar, interosseous ligaments
Deep transverse	Adjacent metatarsals	Connect adjacent heads
Metatarsophalangeal (Multiaxial Condyloid Synovial) Joints		
Capsule	Encloses joint	Functions in flexion, extension, some abduction and adduction, and circumduction
Collateral	Metatarsal heads to base of proximal phalanges	Are strong ligaments
Plantar (plates)	Plantar side of capsule	Are part of weight-bearing surface
Interphalangeal (Uniaxial Hinge Synovial) Joints		
Capsule	Encloses each joint	Functions in flexion and extension
Collateral	Head of one to base of other	Support the capsule
Plantar (plates)	Plantar side of capsule	Support the capsule

Plate 2-20   See Netter: *Atlas of Human Anatomy,* 6th Edition, Plates 514 and 515.

Skeletal System

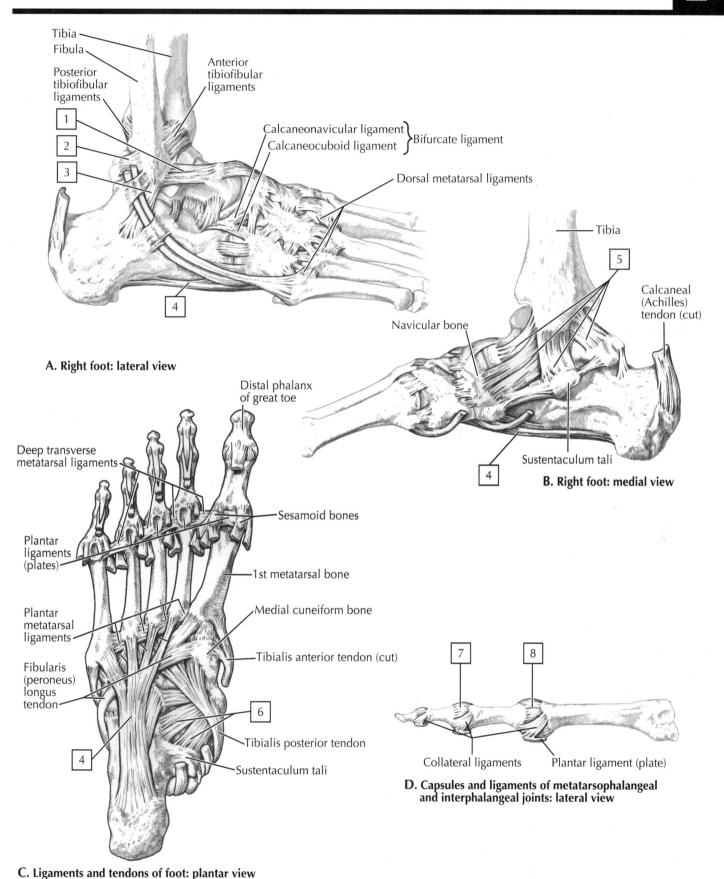

Tibia
Fibula
Posterior tibiofibular ligaments
Anterior tibiofibular ligaments

1
2
3

Calcaneonavicular ligament
Calcaneocuboid ligament } Bifurcate ligament

Dorsal metatarsal ligaments

4

A. Right foot: lateral view

Tibia

5

Calcaneal (Achilles) tendon (cut)

Navicular bone

4

Sustentaculum tali

B. Right foot: medial view

Distal phalanx of great toe

Deep transverse metatarsal ligaments

Sesamoid bones

Plantar ligaments (plates)

1st metatarsal bone

Medial cuneiform bone

Plantar metatarsal ligaments

Tibialis anterior tendon (cut)

Fibularis (peroneus) longus tendon

6

4

Tibialis posterior tendon

Sustentaculum tali

C. Ligaments and tendons of foot: plantar view

7   8

Collateral ligaments   Plantar ligament (plate)

D. Capsules and ligaments of metatarsophalangeal and interphalangeal joints: lateral view

1. Color the bones of the human skull indicated by the letters on the image:
   Frontal bone (color green)
   Sphenoidal bone (color yellow)
   Zygomatic bone (color brown)
   Mandible (color blue)
   Occipital bone (color red)
   Temporal bone (color orange)

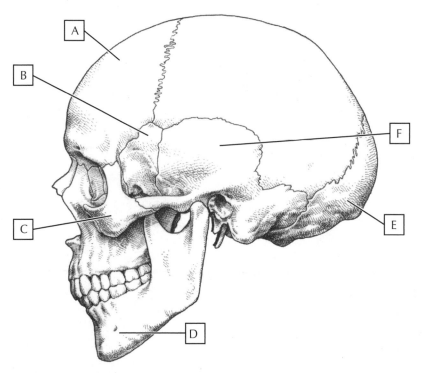

2. What is the name of the four teeth at the front of each jaw? _____

3. The arch of a thoracic vertebra is formed by which two paired elements? _____

4. What artery passes through the foramen transversarium of the cervical vertebra? _____

5. Which three bones form the pectoral girdle and arm of the upper limb? _____

6. Which carpal bone articulates with the metacarpal of the thumb? _____

7. What are the three bones that fuse to form the bony pelvis? _____

8. Most fractures of the femur involve which portion of the bone? _____

9. Which ligament of the knee, if torn, will result in excessive extension at the joint? _____

10. Which pair(s) of ribs is/are considered "floating ribs?" _____

1.

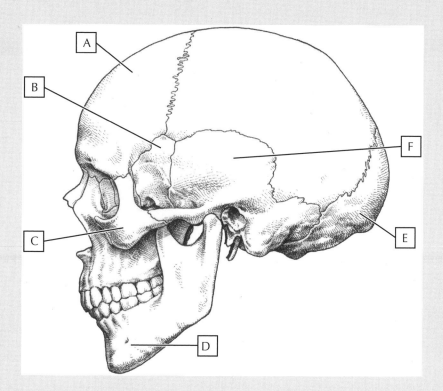

(A) Frontal bone
(B) Sphenoidal bone
(C) Zygomatic bone
(D) Mandible
(E) Occipital bone
(F) Temporal bone

2. Incisors

3. Pedicles and laminae

4. Vertebral artery

5. Clavicle, scapula, and humerus

6. Trapezium

7. Ilium, ischium, and pubis

8. Femoral neck

9. Anterior cruciate ligament (ACL)

10. 11th and 12th pairs of ribs are floating ribs

Chapter 3 **Muscular System**

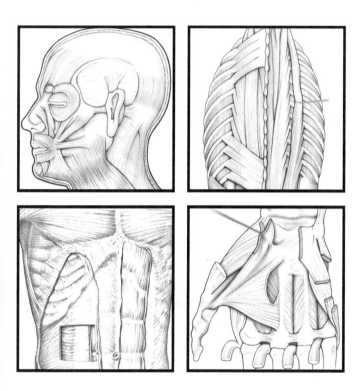

The muscles of facial expression are in several ways unique among the skeletal muscles of the body. They all originate embryologically from the second pharyngeal arch and are all innervated by terminal branches of the facial nerve (CN VII). Additionally, most arise from the bones of the face or fascia, and insert into the dermis of the skin overlying the scalp, face, and anterolateral neck. Some of the more important muscles of facial expression are summarized in the table below and may be colored on the images on the facing page.

All these muscles are supplied by the facial nerve (CN VII).

MUSCLE	ORIGIN	INSERTION	MAIN ACTIONS
Frontalis	Skin of forehead	Epicranial aponeurosis	Elevates eyebrows and forehead, and wrinkles forehead
Orbicularis oculi	Medial orbital margin, medial palpebral ligament, and lacrimal bone	Skin around margin of orbit; tarsal plate	Closes eyelids; orbital part forcefully and palpebral part for blinking
Nasalis	Superior part of canine ridge of maxilla	Nasal cartilages	Draws ala of nose toward septum to compress opening
Orbicularis oris	Median plane of maxilla superiorly and mandible inferiorly; other fibers from deep surface of skin	Mucous membrane of lips	Closes and protrudes lips (e.g., purses them during whistling)
Levator labii superioris	Frontal process of maxilla and infra-orbital region	Skin of upper lip and alar cartilage	Elevates lip, dilates nostril, raises angle of mouth
Platysma	Superficial fascia of deltoid and pectoral regions	Mandible, skin of cheek, angle of mouth, and orbicularis oris	Depresses mandible and tenses skin of lower face and neck
Mentalis	Incisive fossa of mandible	Skin of chin	Elevates and protrudes lower lip and wrinkles chin
Buccinator	Mandible, pterygomandibular raphe, and alveolar processes of maxilla and mandible	Angle of mouth	Presses cheek against molar teeth, thereby aiding chewing

COLOR some of the more important muscles of facial expression listed below, using a different color for each muscle:

☐ 1. Epicranius (frontalis and occipitalis): these two muscles are connected to one another by the galea aponeurotica (a broad, flat tendon)

☐ 2. Orbicularis oculi: a sphincter muscle that closes the eyelids (has a palpebral part in the eyelids and an orbital part attached to the bony orbital rim)

☐ 3. Levator labii superioris: elevates the lip and flares the nostrils

☐ 4. Nasalis: has a transverse and an alar part

☐ 5. Orbicularis oris: a sphincter muscle that purses our lips (the "kissing" muscle)

☐ 6. Depressor anguli oris: depresses our lip (the "sad" muscle, as it turns the corners of our lips downward)

☐ 7. Platysma: a broad, thin muscle that covers the anterolateral neck and tenses the skin of the lower face and neck

☐ 8. Buccinator: allows us to draw in our cheeks, thereby keeping food between our molars during chewing (sometimes we "bite" this muscle or "bite our cheek" when it contracts too vigorously)

☐ 9. Risorius: our "smiling" muscle (helped by the zygomaticus muscles)

Clinical Note:
Unilateral paralysis of the facial nerve (often from inflammation), called **Bell's palsy**, can lead to an asymmetry of the facial features, because the facial muscles are flaccid on the affected side of the face. People with Bell's palsy may not be able to frown or wrinkle the forehead, close their eyelids tightly, smile, purse their lips, or tense the skin of the neck.

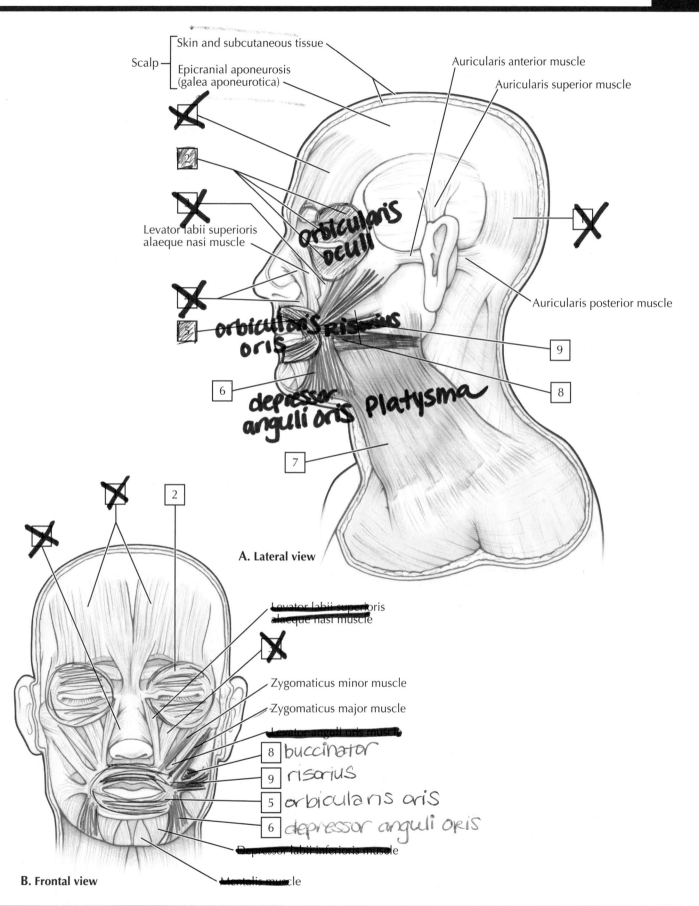

Scalp
- Skin and subcutaneous tissue
- Epicranial aponeurosis (galea aponeurotica)

Auricularis anterior muscle

Auricularis superior muscle

Levator labii superioris alaeque nasi muscle

orbicularis oculi (handwritten)

Auricularis posterior muscle

orbicularis oris (handwritten)

risorius (handwritten)

9

8

6

depressor anguli oris (handwritten)

Platysma (handwritten)

7

A. Lateral view

2

Levator labii superioris alaeque nasi muscle

Zygomaticus minor muscle

Zygomaticus major muscle

Levator anguli oris muscle

8 *buccinator* (handwritten)

9 *risorius* (handwritten)

5 *orbicularis oris* (handwritten)

6 *depressor anguli oris* (handwritten)

Depressor labii inferioris muscle

B. Frontal view

Mentalis muscle

The muscles of mastication include four pairs of muscles (left and right side) that attach to the mandible, are embryological derivatives of the first pharyngeal arch, are all innervated by the mandibular division of the trigeminal nerve (CN V$_3$), and are important in biting and chewing food.

COLOR each of the following muscles of mastication, using a different color for each:

☐ 1. **Temporalis:** a broad muscle arising from the temporal fossa and overlying fascia that elevates (closes) the mandible; you see this muscle contract on the side of your head when you are chewing.

☐ 2. **Masseter:** a powerful muscle that elevates the mandible and is evident in people who chew a lot of gum, because you can see the muscle contract; chronic gum chewers tend to have chubby cheeks because their masseter muscles are enlarged from chronic use.

☐ 3. **Lateral pterygoid:** located medial to the ramus of the mandible, it is important in the side-to-side movements required during masticating (grinding) the food

☐ 4. **Medial pterygoid:** located medial to the ramus of the mandible, it too participates in masticating the food, and because its muscle fibers run in the same direction as the masseter muscle, it also assists this muscle in closing the jaw

These muscles are summarized in the table below: all are innervated by the mandibular nerve (CN V$_3$).

MUSCLE	ORIGIN	INSERTION	MAIN ACTIONS
Temporalis	Floor of temporal fossa and deep temporal fascia	Coronoid process and ramus of mandible	Elevates mandible; posterior fibers retrude mandible
Masseter	Zygomatic arch	Ramus of mandible and coronoid process	Elevates and protrudes mandible; deep fibers retrude it
Lateral pterygoid	*Superior head*: infratemporal surface of greater wing of sphenoid *Inferior head*: lateral pterygoid plate	Neck of mandible, articular disc, and capsule of TMJ	Acting together, protrude mandible and depress chin; acting alone and alternately, produces side-to-side movements
Medial pterygoid	*Deep head*: medial surface of lateral pterygoid plate and palatine bone *Superficial head*: tuberosity of maxilla	Ramus of mandible, inferior to mandibular foramen	Elevates mandible; acting together, protrude mandible; acting alone, protrudes side of jaw; acting alternately, produces grinding motion

Clinical Note:
  Tetanus is a disease caused by a neurotropic toxin of *Clostridium tetani* that can affect the central nervous system and cause a painful tonic contraction of muscles, especially the masseter, leading to a condition called "lockjaw." There is a vaccination to prevent this disease, so it is important to always keep your immunizations up to date.

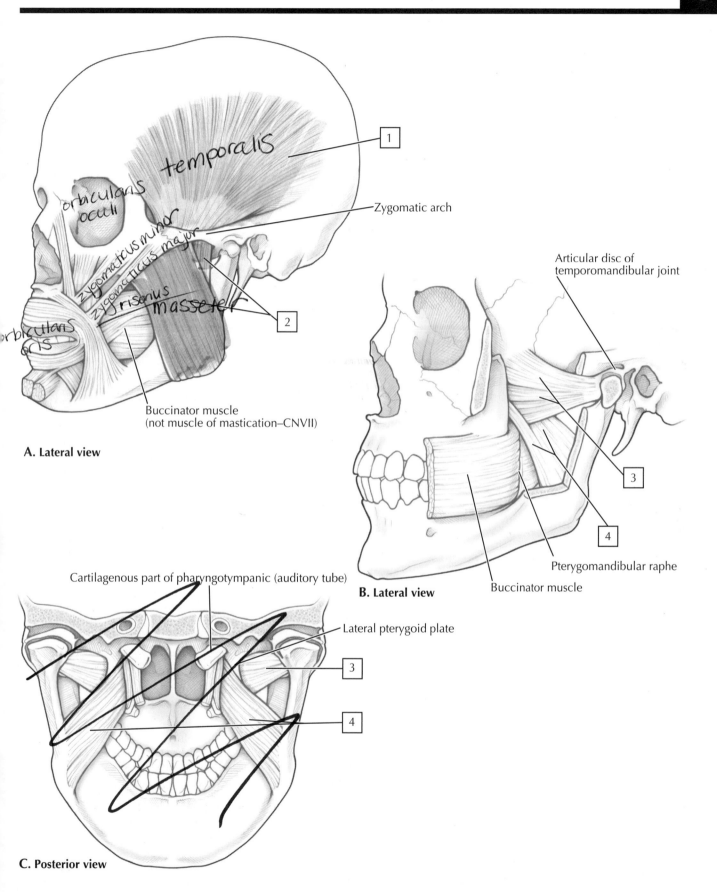

temporalis

orbicularis oculi

1

Zygomatic arch

zygomaticus minor

zygomaticus major

zygomaticus risonus

masseter

2

orbicularis oris

Buccinator muscle
(not muscle of mastication–CNVII)

A. Lateral view

Articular disc of
temporomandibular joint

3

4

Pterygomandibular raphe

Buccinator muscle

B. Lateral view

Cartilagenous part of pharyngotympanic (auditory tube)

Lateral pterygoid plate

3

4

C. Posterior view

The eyeball has two sets of muscles associated with its movements:
- **Extrinsic:** extra-ocular muscles, six skeletal muscles that move the globe or eyeball proper within the orbit
- **Intrinsic:** smooth muscles that affect the size of the pupil (dilate or constrict the pupil) or that affect the shape of the lens for accommodation (near vision) or distance vision (these smooth muscles will be discussed in Chapter 4, Plate 4-23).

COLOR the following extrinsic muscles, using a different color for each muscle:

☐ **1. Superior oblique**
☐ **2. Superior rectus**
☐ **3. Lateral rectus**
☐ **4. Inferior rectus**
☐ **5. Inferior oblique**
☐ **6. Medial rectus**

In addition to the six extra-ocular muscles, there is another skeletal muscle that works in concert with these muscles to elevate the upper eyelid, called the levator palpebrae superioris (its antagonist would be the orbicularis oculi, which closes the eyelids).

COLOR the following muscle:

☐ **7. Levator palpebrae superioris**

Together, the extra-ocular muscles and the levator palpebrae superioris are innervated by three different cranial nerves, the oculomotor (CN III), trochlear (CN IV), and abducent (CN VI) nerves. These muscles are summarized in the table below. The actions of the extra-ocular muscles are complex and involve multiple subtle movements (including rotational movements), so the movements described in the table are those described anatomically. The movements tested clinically by a physician, where the isolated primary movement of each muscle is observed (elevation, depression, abduction, or adduction), are shown in part *D* (also see Clinical Note).

MUSCLE	ORIGIN	INSERTION	INNERVATION	MAIN ACTIONS
Levator palpebrae superioris	Lesser wing of sphenoid bone, anterosuperior optic canal	Tarsal plate and skin of upper eyelid	Oculomotor nerve	Elevates upper eyelid
Superior rectus	Common tendinous ring	Sclera just posterior to cornea	Oculomotor nerve	Elevates, adducts, and rotates eyeball medially
Inferior rectus	Common tendinous ring	Anterior sclera	Oculomotor nerve	Depresses, adducts, and rotates eyeball medially
Medial rectus	Common tendinous ring	Anterior sclera	Oculomotor nerve	Adducts eyeball
Lateral rectus	Common tendinous ring	Anterior sclera	Abducent nerve	Abducts eyeball
Superior oblique	Body of sphenoid bone	Passes through a trochlea and inserts into sclera	Trochlear nerve	Medially rotates, depresses, and abducts eyeball
Inferior oblique	Floor of orbit	Sclera deep to lateral rectus muscle	Oculomotor nerve	Laterally rotates, elevates, and abducts eyeball

Clinical Note:

Because the extra-ocular muscles act as synergists and antagonists and may be responsible for multiple movements, the physician tests the isolated action of each muscle by tracking eye movement while moving her finger in an H pattern. The image at the bottom of the facing page illustrates which muscle is being tested as this happens. For example, when the finger is held up and to the right of the patient's eyes, the patient must primarily use the superior rectus (SR) muscle of his right eye and the inferior oblique (IO) muscle of his left eye to focus on the finger. "Pure" abduction is performed by the lateral rectus (LR) and "pure" adduction by the medial rectus (MR) muscles. In all other cases, three muscles together can abduct (SR, LR, and IR) or adduct (IO, MR, and SO) the eyeball, and two muscles together can elevate (SR and IO) or depress (IR and SO) the globe. If weakness of a muscle is observed, then the physician must determine if it is a muscle problem and/or a nerve problem (damage to the nerve innervating the muscle).

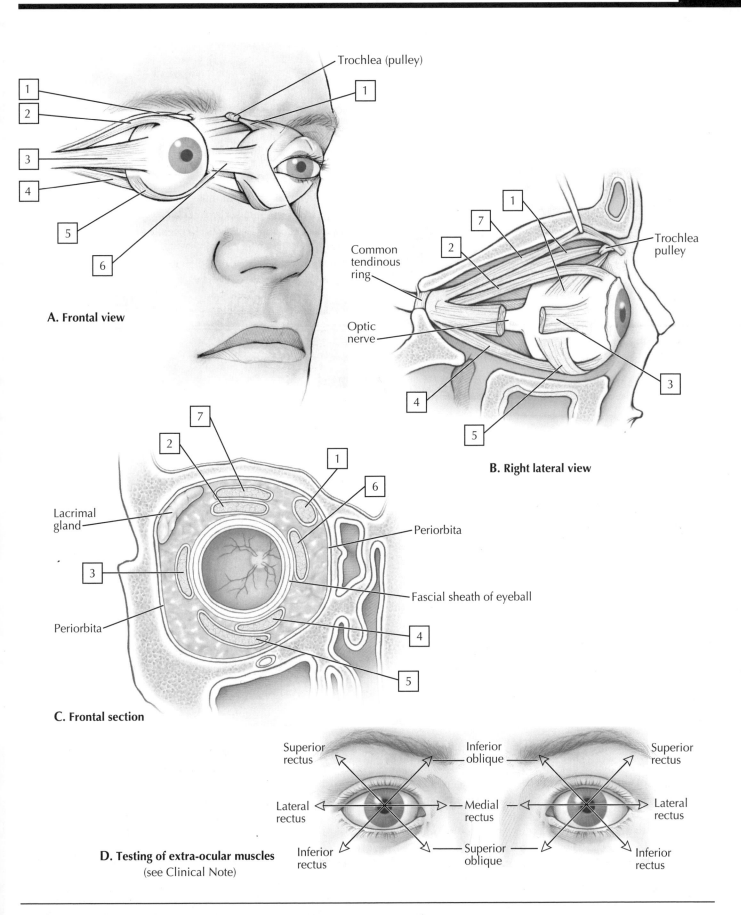

Trochlea (pulley)

1

1

2

3

4

5

6

A. Frontal view

Common
tendinous
ring

Optic
nerve

1

7

2

3

4

5

Trochlea
pulley

B. Right lateral view

7

2

1

6

Lacrimal
gland

3

Periorbita

Periorbita

Fascial sheath of eyeball

4

5

C. Frontal section

Superior
rectus

Inferior
oblique

Superior
rectus

Lateral
rectus

Medial
rectus

Lateral
rectus

Inferior
rectus

Superior
oblique

Inferior
rectus

D. Testing of extra-ocular muscles
(see Clinical Note)

The muscles of the **tongue** are all skeletal muscles and include:
- **Intrinsic muscles:** composed of longitudinal, transverse, and vertical bundles of skeletal muscle that allow one to curl, elongate, and flatten the tongue
- **Extrinsic muscles:** four muscles that move the tongue (protrude, elevate, depress, or retract) that all have the suffix "glossus" in their name, referring to the tongue

All of the tongue muscles are innervated by the **hypoglossal nerve** (CN XII) except the palatoglossus, which is innervated by the vagus nerve (CN X). The principal muscle of the tongue is the genioglossus, which blends with the intrinsic longitudinal muscle fibers to anchor the tongue to the floor of the mouth. Ounce for ounce, the genioglossus (and its intrinsic muscle component) is the strongest muscle in the body!

COLOR the following muscles of the tongue, using a different color for each muscle:

- [ ] **1. Genioglossus**
- [ ] **2. Hyoglossus**
- [ ] **3. Palatoglossus**
- [ ] **4. Styloglossus**

The muscles of the **palate** include four muscles, which all act on the soft palate (the anterior two thirds of the palate is "hard" [bone covered with mucosa], whereas the posterior palate is "soft" [fibromuscular]).

COLOR the following muscles of the palate, using a different color for each muscle:

- [ ] **5. Tensor veli palatini**
- [ ] **6. Levator veli palatini**
- [ ] **7. Palatopharyngeus**
- [ ] **8. Musculus uvulae (uvular muscle)**

The palatoglossus muscle, although grouped with the extrinsic tongue muscles, also acts on the soft palate, so it can be considered a palate muscle as well. The tongue and palate muscles are summarized in the table below.

MUSCLE	ORIGIN	INSERTION	INNERVATION	MAIN ACTIONS
Genioglossus	Mental spine of mandible	Dorsum of tongue and hyoid bone	Hypoglossal nerve	Depresses and protrudes tongue
Hyoglossus	Body and greater horn of hyoid bone	Lateral and inferior aspect of tongue	Hypoglossal nerve	Depresses and retracts tongue
Styloglossus	Styloid process and stylohyoid ligament	Lateral and inferior aspect of tongue	Hypoglossal nerve	Retracts tongue and draws it up for swallowing
Palatoglossus	Palatine aponeurosis of soft palate	Lateral aspect of tongue	Vagus nerve and pharyngeal plexus	Elevates posterior tongue
Levator veli palatini	Temporal (petrous portion) bone	Palatine aponeurosis	Vagus nerve via pharyngeal plexus	Elevates soft palate during swallowing
Tensor veli palatini	Scaphoid fossa of medial pterygoid plate, spine of sphenoid, and auditory tube	Palatine aponeurosis	Mandibular nerve (V_3)	Tenses soft palate and opens auditory tube during swallowing and yawning
Palatopharyngeus	Hard palate and superior palatine aponeurosis	Lateral pharyngeal wall	Vagus nerve via pharyngeal plexus	Tenses soft palate; pulls walls of pharynx superiorly, anteriorly, and medially during swallowing
Musculus uvulae	Nasal spine and palatine aponeurosis	Mucosa of uvula	Vagus nerve via pharyngeal plexus	Shortens, elevates, and retracts uvula

The oral surface of the tongue is covered with a stratified squamous epithelium that contains many papillae, including the:
- **Filiform papillae:** most numerous mucosal projections that increase the surface area of the tongue but do not contain taste buds
- **Fungiform papillae:** larger than filiform papillae, are rounded and cone-shaped, and contain taste buds
- **Foliate papillae:** rudimentary in humans, found largely along the lateral sides of the tongue near the terminal sulcus, but do contain taste buds
- **Circumvallate papillae:** large capped papillae found in a single row just anterior to the terminal sulcus, and contain taste buds

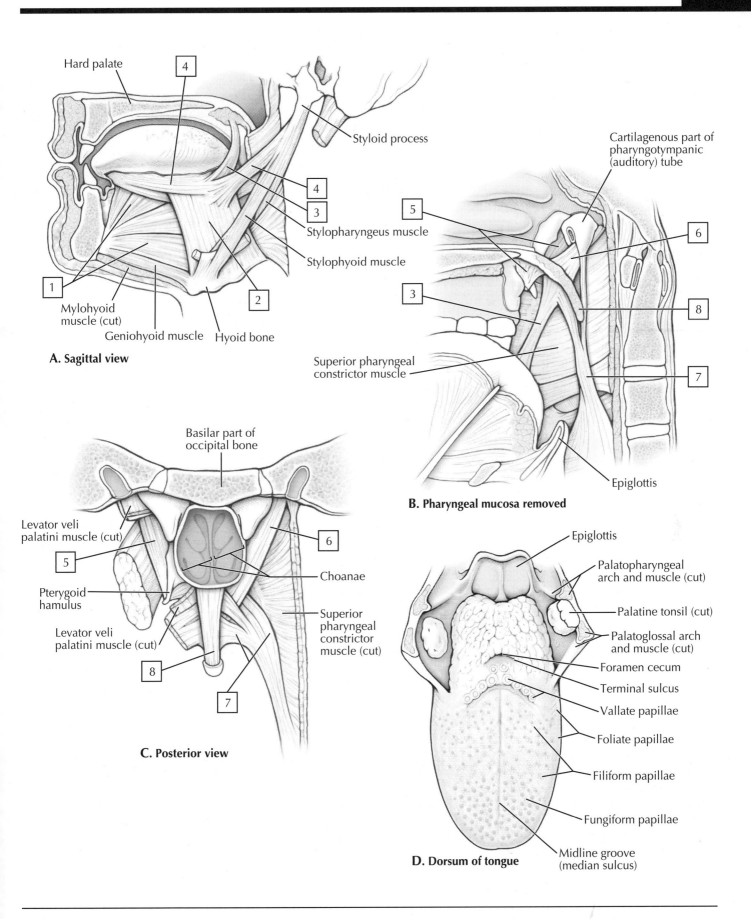

A. Sagittal view

Hard palate

Styloid process

4

4

3

Stylopharyngeus muscle

Stylophyoid muscle

1

2

Mylohyoid muscle (cut)

Geniohyoid muscle

Hyoid bone

B. Pharyngeal mucosa removed

Cartilagenous part of pharyngotympanic (auditory) tube

5

6

3

8

7

Superior pharyngeal constrictor muscle

Epiglottis

C. Posterior view

Basilar part of occipital bone

Levator veli palatini muscle (cut)

5

Choanae

Pterygoid hamulus

Levator veli palatini muscle (cut)

8

Superior pharyngeal constrictor muscle (cut)

7

6

D. Dorsum of tongue

Epiglottis

Palatopharyngeal arch and muscle (cut)

Palatine tonsil (cut)

Palatoglossal arch and muscle (cut)

Foramen cecum

Terminal sulcus

Vallate papillae

Foliate papillae

Filiform papillae

Fungiform papillae

Midline groove (median sulcus)

The pharynx (throat) is a muscular tube found just posterior to the nasal and oral cavities that extends inferiorly to become continuous with the esophagus at about the level of the intervertebral disc between the C6 and C7 vertebral bodies. Muscles of the pharynx include the:

- **Superior pharyngeal constrictor:** located behind the nasal and oral cavities
- **Middle pharyngeal constrictor:** located behind the mandible and hyoid bone
- **Inferior pharyngeal constrictor:** located behind the thyroid and cricoid cartilages
- **Stylopharyngeus:** extends from the styloid process into the lateral wall of the pharynx
- **Salpingopharyngeus:** a small interior muscle of the pharynx

COLOR the following pharyngeal muscles, using a different color for each muscle:
- ☐ 1. Stylopharyngeus
- ☐ 2. Superior pharyngeal constrictor
- ☐ 3. Inferior pharyngeal constrictor
- ☐ 4. Middle pharyngeal constrictor

MUSCLE	ORIGIN	INSERTION	INNERVATION	MAIN ACTIONS
Superior pharyngeal constrictor	Hamulus, pterygomandibular raphe, mylohyoid line of mandible	Median raphe of pharynx	Vagus via pharyngeal plexus	Constricts wall of pharynx during swallowing
Middle pharyngeal constrictor	Stylohyoid ligament and horns of hyoid bone	Median raphe of pharynx	Vagus via pharyngeal plexus	Constricts wall of pharynx during swallowing
Inferior pharyngeal constrictor	Oblique line of thyroid cartilage, and cricoid cartilage	Median raphe of pharynx	Vagus via pharyngeal plexus	Constricts wall of pharynx during swallowing
Salpingopharyngeus	Auditory (pharyngotympanic) tube	Side of pharynx wall	Vagus via pharyngeal plexus	Elevates pharynx and larynx during swallowing and speaking
Stylopharyngeus	Medial aspect of styloid process	Posterior and superior border of thyroid cartilage	Glossopharyngeal nerve	Elevates pharynx and larynx during swallowing and speaking

Viewing the interior mucosal-lined wall of the pharynx reveals the three regions of the pharynx:

- **Nasopharynx:** posterior to the choanae, or openings of the nasal cavities, and soft palate
- **Oropharynx:** the region between the soft palate and the posterior third of the tongue
- **Laryngopharynx** (hypopharynx): from the epiglottis to the beginning of the esophagus

The pharyngeal muscles contract sequentially, beginning superiorly and moving inferiorly to "squeeze" a bolus of chewed food down the pharynx and into the upper esophagus. This process of swallowing is called **deglutition** and involves the interplay and coordinated movements of the tongue, soft palate, pharynx, and larynx to work properly. Deglutition includes the following steps:

- The bolus of food is pushed up against the hard palate by the tongue
- The soft palate is elevated to close off the nasopharynx
- The bolus is pushed back into the oropharynx by the action of the tongue

- As the bolus reaches the epiglottis, the larynx is elevated and the tip of the epiglottis is tipped downward over the laryngeal opening (aditus)
- Contractions of the pharyngeal constrictors squeeze the bolus into two streams that pass on either side of the epiglottis and into the upper esophagus, and the soft palate is pulled downward to assist in moving the bolus
- The soft palate is pulled down, the rima glottidis (space between the vocal folds) closes, and once the bolus is safely in the esophagus, all structures return to their starting positions

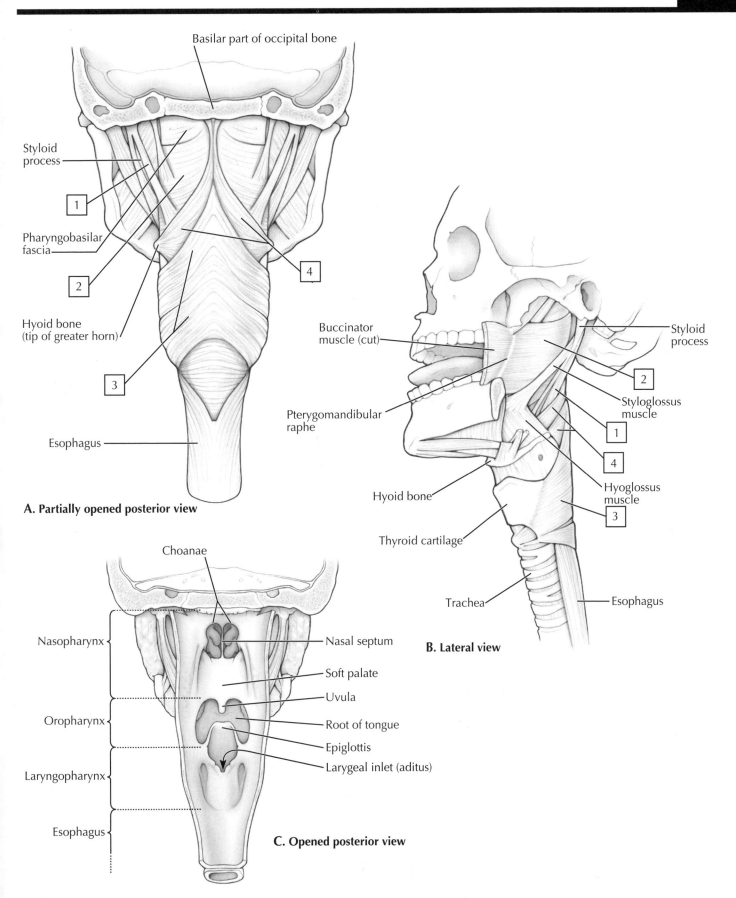

Basilar part of occipital bone

Styloid process

1

Pharyngobasilar fascia

2

Hyoid bone (tip of greater horn)

3

Esophagus

4

A. Partially opened posterior view

Buccinator muscle (cut)

Pterygomandibular raphe

Hyoid bone

Thyroid cartilage

Trachea

Styloid process

2

Styloglossus muscle

1

4

Hyoglossus muscle

3

Esophagus

B. Lateral view

Choanae

Nasopharynx

Oropharynx

Laryngopharynx

Esophagus

Nasal septum

Soft palate

Uvula

Root of tongue

Epiglottis

Larygeal inlet (aditus)

C. Opened posterior view

The intrinsic muscles of the larynx attach to the **cartilages of the larynx**, so these will be reviewed first. The larynx lies at the C3 to C6 vertebral level, just superior to the trachea, and consists of nine cartilages joined by ligaments and membranes. The nine cartilages are summarized in the table below.

CARTILAGE	DESCRIPTION
Thyroid	Two hyaline laminae and the laryngeal prominence (Adam's apple)
Cricoid	Signet ring–shaped hyaline cartilage just inferior to thyroid
Epiglottis	Spoon-shaped elastic cartilage plate attached to thyroid
Arytenoid	Paired pyramidal cartilages that rotate on cricoid cartilage
Corniculate	Paired cartilages that lie on apex of arytenoid cartilages
Cuneiform	Paired cartilages in ary-epiglottic folds that have no articulations

COLOR the following cartilages of the larynx, using a different color for each cartilage:

☐ **1. Epiglottis**

☐ **2. Thyroid**

☐ **3. Cricoid**

☐ **4. Arytenoid**

The **intrinsic muscles of the larynx** act largely to adjust the tension on the vocal cords (ligaments), opening or closing the **rima glottidis** (space between the vocal cords) and opening and closing the **rima vestibuli**, the opening above the **vestibular**

folds (false folds). This action is important during swallowing but also adjusts the size of the vestibule during phonation to add quality to the sound. All of these intrinsic muscles are innervated by the vagus nerve (CN X) and its branches.

The **vocal folds** (vocal ligaments covered by mucosa) control phonation much like the reed instrument. Vibrations of the folds produce sounds as air passes through the rima glottidis. The posterior crico-arytenoid muscles are important because they are the only laryngeal muscles that abduct the vocal folds and maintain the opening between the vocal cords. The vestibular folds are protective in function.

COLOR the following intrinsic muscles of the larynx, using a different color for each muscle:

☐ **5. Posterior crico-arytenoid: the only pair of muscles that abduct the vocal folds**

☐ **6. Arytenoid muscle: composed of transverse and oblique fibers, this muscle adducts the vocal folds and narrows the rima vestibuli**

☐ **7. Cricothyroid: pulls the thyroid cartilage anteroinferiorly on the cricoid cartilage and tenses the vocal folds by stretching them**

Clinical Note:
Hoarseness can be due to any condition that results in improper vibration or coaptation of the vocal folds. Inflammation and edema (swelling) are commonly the cause for hoarseness and can be induced by smoking, overuse of the voice, gastroesophageal reflux disease, cough, and infections. Surgical scarring, nodules or cysts, and cancer also may cause hoarseness.

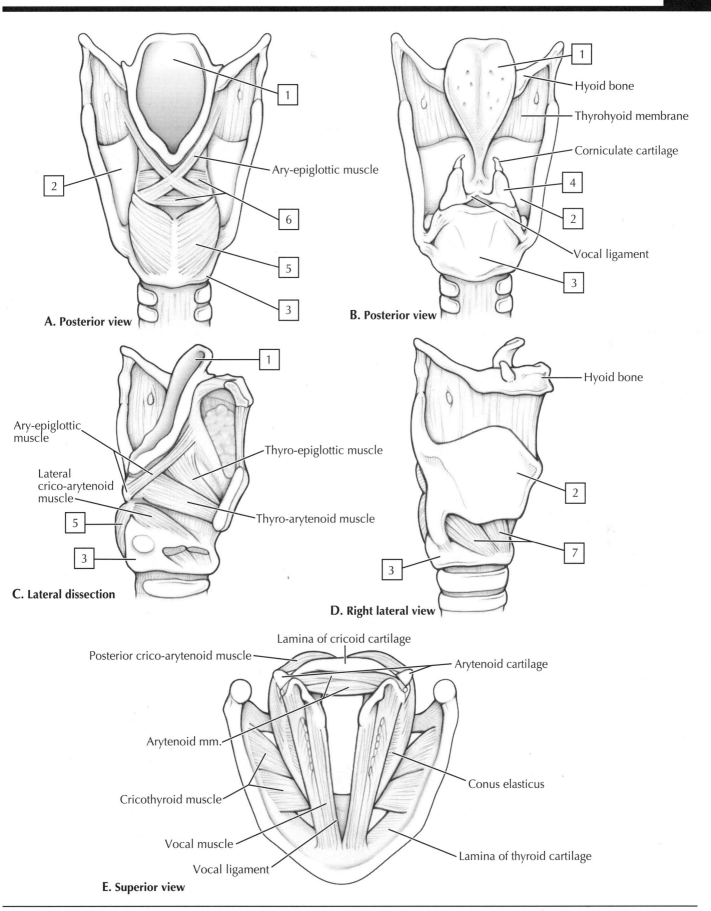

A. Posterior view

Ary-epiglottic muscle

B. Posterior view

Hyoid bone

Thyrohyoid membrane

Corniculate cartilage

Vocal ligament

C. Lateral dissection

Ary-epiglottic muscle

Lateral crico-arytenoid muscle

Thyro-epiglottic muscle

Thyro-arytenoid muscle

D. Right lateral view

Hyoid bone

Posterior crico-arytenoid muscle

Lamina of cricoid cartilage

Arytenoid cartilage

Arytenoid mm.

Conus elasticus

Cricothyroid muscle

Vocal muscle

Vocal ligament

Lamina of thyroid cartilage

E. Superior view

Muscles of the neck divide the neck into several descriptive "triangles" that are used by surgeons to identify key structures within these regions.

COLOR each of these triangles, using a different color to outline the boundaries of each triangle (color over the demarcated outline):

☐ 1. **Posterior: between the trapezius and sternocleidomastoid muscles, this triangle is not subdivided further**

Anterior, which is further subdivided into the triangles listed below:

☐ 2. **Submandibular: contains the submandibular salivary gland**

☐ 3. **Submental: lies beneath the chin**

☐ 4. **Muscular: lies anteriorly in the neck below the hyoid bone**

☐ 5. **Carotid: contains the carotid artery**

In general, the muscles of the neck position the larynx during swallowing, stabilize the hyoid bone, move the head and upper limb, or are postural muscles attached to the head and/or vertebrae. The key muscles are summarized in the table below. The muscles below the hyoid bone are called "infrahyoid" or "strap" muscles, whereas those above the hyoid bone are called "suprahyoid" muscles.

COLOR each of the following muscles, using a different color for each muscle:

☐ 6. **Stylohyoid**

☐ 7. **Posterior belly of the digastric**

☐ 8. **Sternocleidomastoid**

☐ 9. **Anterior belly of the digastric**

☐ 10. **Thyrohyoid**

☐ 11. **Sternohyoid**

☐ 12. **Sternothyroid**

☐ 13. **Omohyoid**

Clinical Note:
The neck provides a conduit that connects the head to the thorax. The muscles, vessels, and visceral structures (trachea and esophagus) are all tightly bound within **three fascial layers** that create compartments within the neck. Infections or masses (tumors) in one or another of these tight spaces can compress softer structures and cause significant pain. The fascial layers themselves also can limit the spread of infection between compartments. On the labeled diagram of the neck in transverse section, color the three fascial layers to highlight their extent. The three fascial layers include the:

• Investing layer of the deep cervical fascia: surrounds the neck and invests the trapezius and sternocleidomastoid muscles

• Pretracheal fascia: limited to the anterior neck, it invests the infrahyoid muscles, thyroid gland, trachea, and esophagus

• Prevertebral fascia: a tubular sheath, it invests the prevertebral muscles and vertebral column

The **carotid sheath** blends with these fascial layers but is distinct and contains the common carotid artery, internal jugular vein, and the vagus nerve.

MUSCLE	ORIGIN	INSERTION	INNERVATION	MAIN ACTIONS
Sternocleido-mastoid	*Sternal head:* manubrium *Clavicular head:* medial third of clavicle	Mastoid process and lateral half of superior nuchal line	Spinal root of cranial nerve (CN) XI and C2-C3	Tilts head to one side, i.e., laterally flexes and rotates head so face is turned superiorly toward opposite side; acting together, muscles flex neck
Digastric	*Anterior belly:* digastric fossa of mandible *Posterior belly:* mastoid notch	Intermediate tendon to hyoid bone	*Anterior belly:* mylohyoid nerve (V₃), a branch of inferior alveolar nerve *Posterior belly:* facial nerve (CN VII)	Depresses mandible; raises hyoid bone and steadies it during swallowing and speaking
Sternohyoid	Manubrium of sternum and medial end of clavicle	Body of hyoid bone	C1-C3 from ansa cervicalis	Depresses hyoid bone after swallowing
Sternothyroid	Posterior surface of manubrium	Oblique line of thyroid lamina	C2 and C3 from ansa cervicalis	Depresses larynx after swallowing
Thyrohyoid	Oblique line of thyroid cartilage	Body and greater horn of hyoid bone	C1 via hypoglossal nerve	Depresses hyoid bone and elevates larynx when hyoid bone is fixed
Omohyoid	Superior border of scapula near suprascapular notch	Inferior border of hyoid bone	C1-C3 from ansa cervicalis	Depresses, retracts, and fixes hyoid bone
Mylohyoid	Mylohyoid line of mandible	Raphe and body of hyoid bone	Mylohyoid nerve, a branch of inferior alveolar nerve of V₃	Elevates hyoid bone, floor of mouth, and tongue during swallowing and speaking
Stylohyoid	Styloid process	Body of hyoid bone	Facial nerve	Elevates and retracts hyoid bone

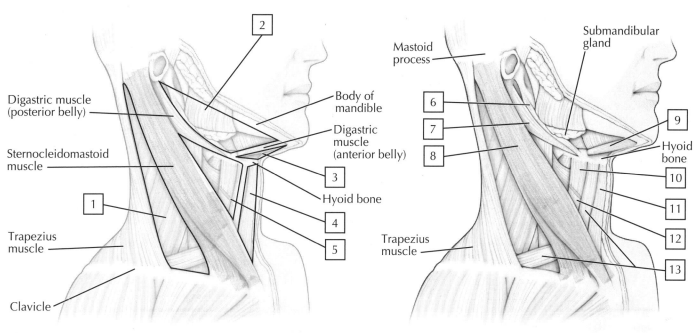

Digastric muscle
(posterior belly)

Sternocleidomastoid
muscle

Trapezius
muscle

Clavicle

2

Body of
mandible

Digastric
muscle
(anterior belly)

Hyoid bone

1

3

4

5

A. Lateral view

Mastoid
process

Submandibular
gland

6

7

8

Trapezius
muscle

9

Hyoid
bone

10

11

12

13

B. Lateral view

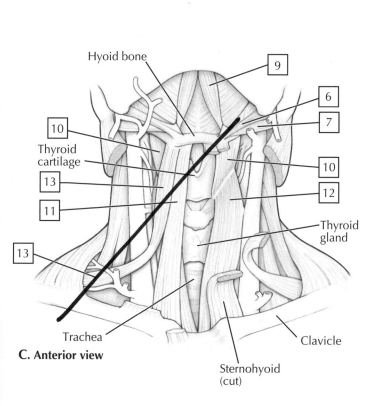

Hyoid bone

9

6

7

10

Thyroid
cartilage

13

11

10

12

Thyroid
gland

13

Trachea

Clavicle

C. Anterior view

Sternohyoid
(cut)

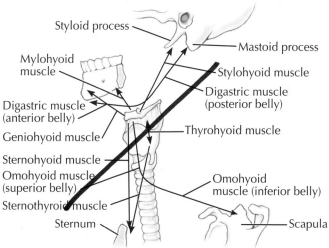

Styloid process

Mastoid process

Mylohyoid
muscle

Stylohyoid muscle

Digastric muscle
(anterior belly)

Digastric muscle
(posterior belly)

Geniohyoid muscle

Thyrohyoid muscle

Sternohyoid muscle

Omohyoid muscle
(superior belly)

Omohyoid
muscle (inferior belly)

Sternothyroid muscle

Scapula

Sternum

D. Infrahyoidal and suprahyoidal muscles and their actions

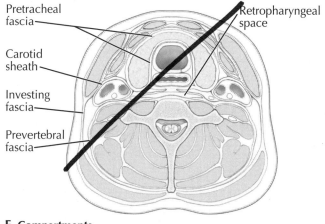

Pretracheal
fascia

Retropharyngeal
space

Carotid
sheath

Investing
fascia

Prevertebral
fascia

E. Compartments

The prevertebral fascia of the neck encloses many of the prevertebral muscles, which lie anterior to the vertebral column and are muscles that move the head and/or act as postural muscles supporting the head and neck. This group of muscles includes the scalene muscles (anterior, middle, and posterior) that attach to the upper ribs and also are accessory muscles of respiration. They help raise the thoracic cage during deep inspiration. The prevertebral muscles are summarized in the table below.

COLOR the following prevertebral muscles, using a different color for each muscle:

- [ ] 1. **Longus capitis (capitis refers to the head)**
- [ ] 2. **Longus colli (colli refers to the neck)**
- [ ] 3. **Anterior scalene (note that the subclavian vein passes anterior to this muscle)**
- [ ] 4. **Middle scalene (note that the subclavian artery passes between this muscle and the anterior scalene muscle)**
- [ ] 5. **Posterior scalene**

MUSCLE	INFERIOR ATTACHMENT	SUPERIOR ATTACHMENT	INNERVATION	MAIN ACTIONS
Longus colli	Body of T1-T3 with attachments to bodies of C4-C7 and transverse processes of C3-C6	Anterior tubercle of C1 (atlas), transverse processes of C4-C6, and bodies of C2-C6	C2-C6 spinal nerves	Flexes cervical vertebrae; allows slight rotation
Longus capitis	Anterior tubercles of C3-C6 transverse processes	Basilar part of occipital bone	C2-C3 spinal nerves	Flexes head
Rectus capitis anterior	Lateral mass of C1 (atlas)	Base of occipital bone, anterior to occipital condyle	C1-C2 spinal nerves	Flexes head
Rectus capitis lateralis	Transverse process of C1 (atlas)	Jugular process of occipital bone	C1-C2 spinal nerves	Flexes and helps stabilize head
Posterior scalene	Posterior tubercles of transverse processes of C4-C6	Second rib	C6-C8	Flexes neck laterally; elevates second rib
Middle scalene	Posterior tubercles of transverse processes of C2-C7	First rib	C3-C8	Flexes neck laterally; elevates first rib
Anterior scalene	Anterior tubercles of transverse processes of C3-C6	First rib	C5-C7	Flexes neck laterally; elevates first rib

Clinical Note:

Looking at the cross section of the neck and the fascial layers in the illustration on the previous page (Plate 3-7), note that there is a space between the pretracheal and prevertebral fascia called the **retropharyngeal space**. Infections and abscesses can gain access to this space and spread anywhere from the base of the skull to the upper portion of the thoracic cavity (superior mediastinum). For this reason, clinicians sometimes refer to this space as the "danger" space.

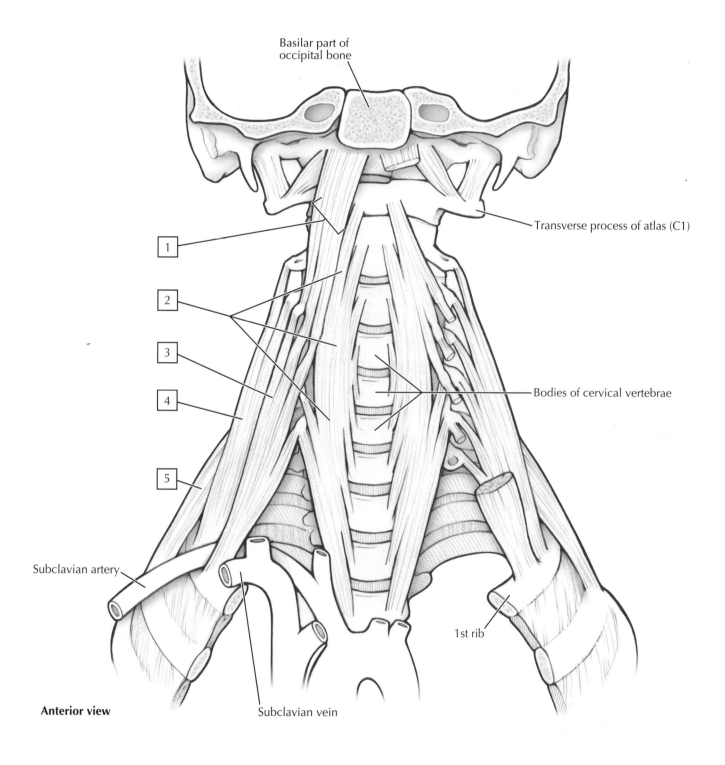

Basilar part of occipital bone

Transverse process of atlas (C1)

1

2

3

4

5

Bodies of cervical vertebrae

Subclavian artery

1st rib

Anterior view

Subclavian vein

The muscles of the back are divided functionally into three groups: superficial, intermediate, and deep.

Superficial muscles, which are superficially located, control movements of the upper limbs, largely by acting on the scapulae.

COLOR the following superficial muscles, using a different color for each:

☐ 1. **Trapezius: this muscle and the sternocleidomastoid are the only two muscles innervated by the accessory nerve (CN XI)**

☐ 2. **Latissimus dorsi**

Intermediate muscles, just deep to the superficial layer, are accessory muscles of respiration and have attachments to ribs. The trapezius and latissimus dorsi are removed from the right side of the plate so that you can see this group of muscles.

COLOR the following intermediate muscles, using a different color for each:

☐ 3. **Levator scapulae**

☐ 4. **Serratus posterior superior: intermediate group of muscles; have respiratory function**

☐ 5. **Rhomboid major (muscle cut to reveal deeper muscles)**

☐ 6. **Serratus posterior inferior: intermediate group of muscles; have respiratory function**

These groups of back muscles are summarized in the table below.

MUSCLE	PROXIMAL ATTACHMENT (ORIGIN)	DISTAL ATTACH-MENT (INSERTION)	INNERVATION	MAIN ACTIONS
Trapezius	Superior nuchal line, external occipital protuberance, nuchal ligament, and spinous processes of C7-T12	Lateral third of clavicle, acromion, and spine of scapula	Accessory nerve (cranial nerve XI) and C3-C4 (proprioception)	Elevates, retracts, and rotates scapula; lower fibers depress scapula
Latissimus dorsi	Spinous processes of T7-T12, thoracolumbar fascia, iliac crest, and last 3-4 ribs	Humerus (intertubercular sulcus)	Thoracodorsal nerve (C6-C8)	Extends, adducts, and medially rotates humerus
Levator scapulae	Transverse processes of C1-C4	Medial border of scapula	C3-C4 and dorsal scapular (C5) nerve	Elevates scapula and tilts glenoid cavity inferiorly
Rhomboid minor and major	*Minor*: nuchal ligament and spinous processes of C7-T1 *Major*: spinous processes of T2-T5	Medial border of scapula	Dorsal scapular nerve (C4-C5)	Retract scapula, rotate it to depress glenoid cavity, and fix scapula to thoracic wall
Serratus posterior superior	Ligamentum nuchae, spinous processes of C7-T3	Superior aspect of ribs 2-4	T1-T4	Elevates ribs
Serratus posterior inferior	Spinous processes of T11-L2	Inferior aspect of ribs 9-12	T9-T12	Depresses ribs

The superficial and intermediate groups of back muscles are segmentally innervated by ventral primary rami of spinal nerves (except the trapezius). The superficial group migrates onto the back during development of the embryo, although they function as muscles of the upper limb.

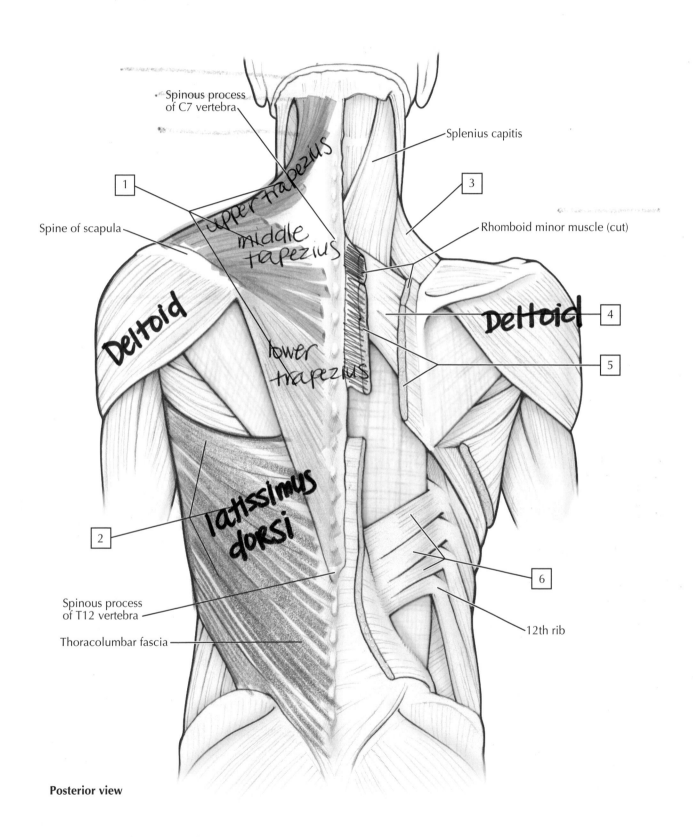

Spinous process
of C7 vertebra

Splenius capitis

1

3

Spine of scapula

Rhomboid minor muscle (cut)

upper trapezius

middle trapezius

Deltoid

Deltoid

4

lower trapezius

5

latissimus dorsi

2

6

Spinous process
of T12 vertebra

12th rib

Thoracolumbar fascia

Posterior view

The deep, or intrinsic, back muscles are beneath the intermediate layer. They participate in movement of the head and neck or postural control of the vertebral column. They are composed of **superficial** (splenius muscles), **intermediate** (erector spinae), and **deep layers** (transversospinal). They support the spine, permit movements of the spine, and are innervated by dorsal rami of spinal nerves. Additionally, the muscles of the back of the neck are transversospinal muscles that comprise the suboccipital region. The muscles are summarized in the table below.

- [ ] 3. **Longissimus** (erector spinae group, just lateral to the semispinalis muscles)
- [ ] 4. **Spinalis** (erector spinae group, found most medially in the back)
- [ ] 5. Rectus capitis posterior major (suboccipital region)
- [ ] 6. Obliquus capitis inferior (suboccipital region; muscles 5-7 in this list form the "suboccipital triangle")
- [ ] 7. Obliquus capitis superior (suboccipital region)

COLOR each of the following intrinsic muscles, using a different color for each muscle:

- [ ] 1. Splenius capitis
- [ ] 2. **Iliocostalis** (erector spinae group, just lateral to the longissimus muscles)

MUSCLE	PROXIMAL ATTACHMENT (ORIGIN)	DISTAL ATTACHMENT (INSERTION)	INNERVATION*	MAIN ACTIONS
Superficial Layer				
Splenius capitis	Nuchal ligament, spinous process C7-T3	Mastoid process of temporal bone and lateral third of superior nuchal line	Middle cervical nerves	*Bilaterally:* extends head *Unilaterally:* laterally bends (flexes) and rotates face to same side
Splenius cervicis	Spinous process T3-T6	Transverse process (C1-C3)	Lower cervical nerves	*Bilaterally:* extends neck *Unilaterally:* laterally bends (flexes) and rotates neck toward same side
Intermediate Layer				
Erector spinae	Posterior sacrum, iliac crest, sacrospinous ligament, supraspinous ligament, and spinous processes of lower lumbar and sacral vertebrae	*Iliocostalis:* angles of lower ribs and cervical transverse processes *Longissimus:* between tubercles and angles of ribs, transverse processes of thoracic and cervical vertebrae, and mastoid process *Spinalis:* spinous processes of upper thoracic and midcervical vertebrae	Respective spinal nerves of each region	Extends and laterally bends vertebral column and head
Semispinalis	Transverse processes C4-T12	Spinous processes of cervical and thoracic regions	Respective spinal nerves of each region	Extends head, neck, and thorax and rotates them to opposite side
Multifidi	Sacrum, ilium, and transverse processes of T1-T12, and articular processes of C4-C7	Spinous processes of vertebrae above, spanning two to four segments	Respective spinal nerves of each region	Stabilize spine
Rotatores	Transverse processes	Lamina and transverse process or spine above, spanning one or two segments	Respective spinal nerves of each region	Stabilize, extend, and rotate spine
Deep Layer				
Rectus capitis posterior major	Spine of axis	Lateral inferior nuchal line	Suboccipital nerve (C1)	Extends head and rotates to same side
Rectus capitis posterior minor	Tubercle of posterior arch of atlas	Median inferior nuchal line	Suboccipital nerve (C1)	Extends head
Obliquus capitis superior	Transverse process of atlas	Occipital bone	Suboccipital nerve (C1)	Extends head and bends it laterally
Obliquus capitis inferior	Spine of axis	Atlas transverse process	Suboccipital nerve (C1)	Rotates atlas to turn face to same side

*Dorsal rami of spinal nerves.

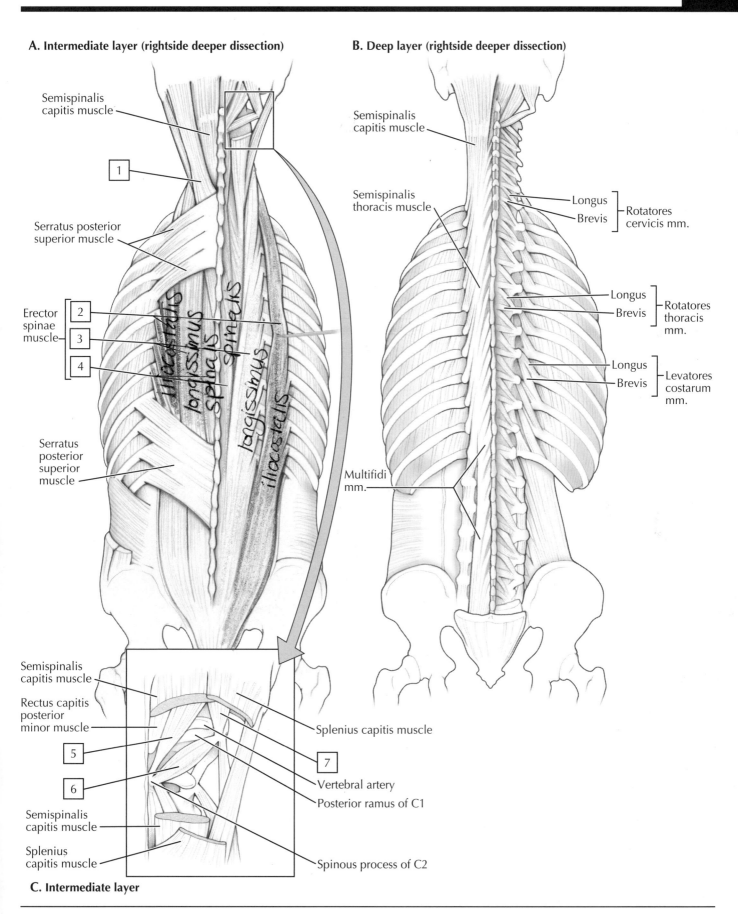

A. Intermediate layer (rightside deeper dissection)

Semispinalis capitis muscle

1

Serratus posterior superior muscle

Erector spinae muscle

2

3

4

Serratus posterior superior muscle

iliocostalis *longissimus* *spinalis* *spinalis* *longissimus* *iliocostalis*

B. Deep layer (rightside deeper dissection)

Semispinalis capitis muscle

Semispinalis thoracis muscle

Longus
Brevis } Rotatores cervicis mm.

Longus
Brevis } Rotatores thoracis mm.

Longus
Brevis } Levatores costarum mm.

Multifidi mm.

C. Intermediate layer

Semispinalis capitis muscle

Rectus capitis posterior minor muscle

5

6

Semispinalis capitis muscle

Splenius capitis muscle

Splenius capitis muscle

7

Vertebral artery

Posterior ramus of C1

Spinous process of C2

Muscles of the thoracic wall fill the spaces between adjacent ribs, or have attachments to the sternum or vertebrae and then attach to ribs or costal cartilages. Functionally, the muscles of the thoracic wall keep the intercostal spaces rigid, thereby preventing them from bulging out during expiration or being sucked in during inspiration. The exact role of individual intercostal muscles on the movements of the ribs is difficult to interpret despite many electromyographic studies.

On the anterior chest wall, the pectoralis major and minor muscles overlie the intercostal muscles, but these two muscles really act on the upper limb and will be discussed later. Segmental intercostal nerves and vessels travel between the internal and innermost intercostal muscles, as seen in the cross section of the thoracic wall.

COLOR each of the following muscles, using a different color for each muscle:

1. **External intercostals:** outermost layer of the three intercostal muscles; fibers run from superolateral to inferomedial
2. **Internal intercostals:** middle layer of intercostals; fibers tend to run from superomedial to inferolateral
3. **Innermost intercostals:** fibers almost parallel those of the internal intercostals and may sometimes be fused to this muscle
4. **Transversus thoracis**

MUSCLE	SUPERIOR ATTACHMENT (ORIGIN)	INFERIOR ATTACHMENT (INSERTION)	INNERVATION	MAIN ACTIONS
External intercostal	Inferior border of rib	Superior border of rib below	Intercostal nerve	Elevates ribs
Internal intercostal	Inferior border of rib	Superior border of rib below	Intercostal nerve	Elevates ribs (upper four and five); others depress ribs
Innermost intercostal	Inferior border of rib	Superior border of rib below	Intercostal nerve	Acts similar to internal intercostals
Transversus thoracis	Internal surface of costal cartilages 2-6	Posterior surface of lower sternum	Intercostal nerve	Depresses ribs and costal cartilages
Subcostal	Internal surface of lower rib near their angles	Superior borders of second or third ribs below	Intercostal nerve	Depresses ribs
Levator costarum	Transverse processes of C7 and T1-T11	Subjacent ribs between tubercle and angle	Dorsal primary rami of C8-T11	Elevates ribs

Clinical Note:

Sometimes it is necessary to introduce a needle or catheter through the chest wall into the underlying pleural cavity, usually to drain off fluids (blood or extracellular fluid and pus) or air that accumulates in this space and could potentially collapse the lung. Careful positioning of the needle or catheter is necessary to avoid impaling the intercostal nerve and vessels, which pass inferior to each rib in the costal groove.

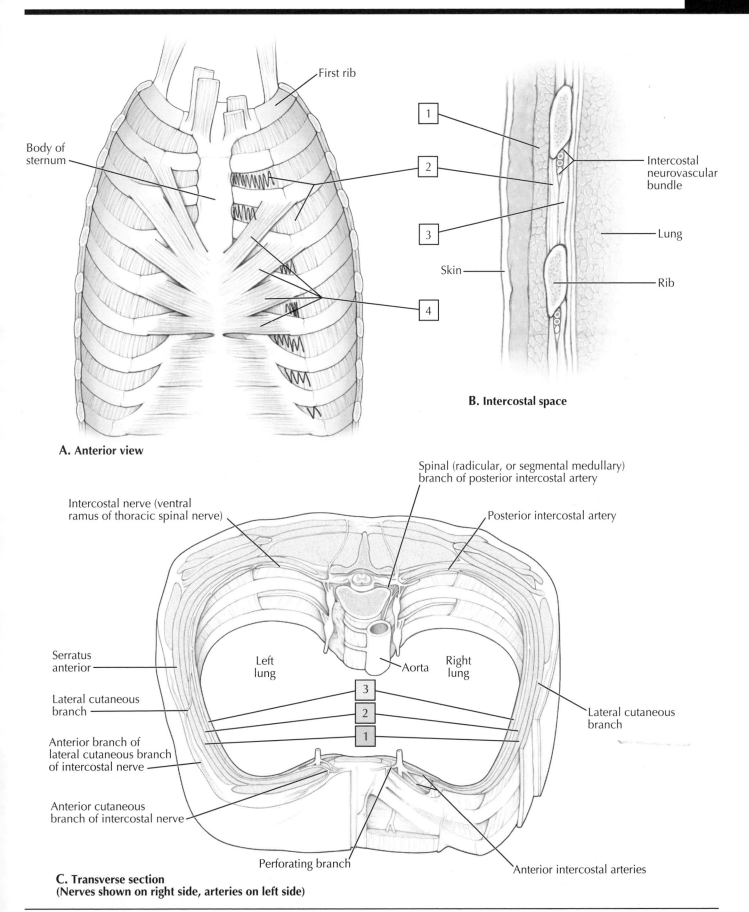

First rib

Body of sternum

1

2

3

4

Intercostal neurovascular bundle

Skin

Lung

Rib

B. Intercostal space

A. Anterior view

Intercostal nerve (ventral ramus of thoracic spinal nerve)

Spinal (radicular, or segmental medullary) branch of posterior intercostal artery

Posterior intercostal artery

Serratus anterior

Left lung

Aorta

Right lung

Lateral cutaneous branch

3

2

1

Lateral cutaneous branch

Anterior branch of lateral cutaneous branch of intercostal nerve

Anterior cutaneous branch of intercostal nerve

Perforating branch

Anterior intercostal arteries

C. Transverse section
(Nerves shown on right side, arteries on left side)

Anterior Abdominal Wall Muscles

Three muscles (external abdominal oblique, internal abdominal oblique, and transversus abdominis) wrap around the abdominal wall and are direct continuations of the three muscle layers found in the thoracic wall, where they lie between the ribs and comprise the intercostal muscles.

The functions of these anterior abdominal muscles include:
- Compressing the abdominal wall and increase intra-abdominal pressure, especially when lifting and during urination, defecation, and childbirth
- Assisting the diaphragm during forced expiration (this occurs unexpectedly when a blow is administered to the anterior abdominal wall and the "wind is knocked out of you")
- Helping flex and rotate the trunk
- Tensing the abdominal wall

COLOR these three labeled muscles using a different color for each. Work from the superficial to the deeper layer and note the direction of the muscle fibers as your color:

☐ **1. External abdominal oblique**

☐ **2. Internal abdominal oblique**

☐ **3. Transversus abdominis**

MUSCLE	PROXIMAL ATTACHMENT (ORIGIN)	DISTAL ATTACHMENT (INSERTION)	INNERVATION	MAIN ACTIONS
External oblique	External surfaces of 5th to 12th ribs	Linea alba, pubic tubercle, and anterior half of iliac crest	Inferior seven thoracic nerves	Compresses and supports abdominal viscera; flexes and rotates trunk
Internal oblique	Thoracolumbar fascia, anterior two thirds of iliac crest, and lateral two thirds of inguinal ligament	Inferior borders of 10th to 12th ribs, linea alba, and pubis via conjoint tendon	Ventral rami of inferior six thoracic and 1st lumbar nerves	Compresses and supports abdominal viscera; flexes and rotates trunk
Transversus abdominis	Internal surfaces of 7-12 costal cartilages, thoracolumbar fascia, iliac crest, and lateral third of inguinal ligament	Linea alba with aponeurosis of internal oblique, pubic crest, and pecten pubis via conjoint tendon	Ventral rami of inferior six thoracic and 1st lumbar nerves	Compresses and supports abdominal viscera
Rectus abdominis	Pubic symphysis and pubic crest	Xiphoid process and costal cartilages 5-7	Ventral rami of inferior six thoracic nerves	Flexes trunk and compresses abdominal viscera

Two midline muscles (rectus abdominis and pyramidalis) lie within the rectus sheath, a tendinous sheath composed of the aponeurotic layers of the three abdominal muscles colored (1-3). The layers (lamina) that compose the sheath are deficient below the arcuate line (in the lower quarter) of the rectus sheath, where only the transversalis fascia lies in contact with the rectus abdominis.

LAYER	COMMENT
Anterior lamina above arcuate line	Formed by fused aponeuroses of external and internal abdominal oblique muscles
Posterior lamina above arcuate line	Formed by fused aponeuroses of internal abdominal oblique and transversus abdominis muscles
Below arcuate line	All three muscle aponeuroses fuse to form anterior lamina, with rectus abdominis in contact only with transversalis fascia posteriorly

COLOR the midline muscles of the anterior abdominal wall, using a different color from those used previously:

☑ **4. Rectus abdominis (note the three tendinous intersections—the infamous "six-pack abs")**

☐ ~~5. Pyramidalis~~

COLOR the aponeurosis extending from the muscle to form the layers of the rectus sheath. Use a color different from the muscle colors, but note the relationship to the muscles.

☐ **1A. Aponeurosis of external oblique muscle**

☐ **2A. Aponeurosis of internal oblique muscle**

☐ **3A. Aponeurosis transverse abdominis muscle**

Clinical Note:

Hernias, abnormal outpouchings of underlying structures due to a weakness of the wall, can occur on the anterior abdominal wall. The most common types include:
- Umbilical hernias—usually seen up to age 3 years or after the age of 40
- Linea alba hernias—often occur in the epigastric region along the midline linea alba
- Incisional hernias—occur at sites of previous abdominal surgical scars
- Inguinal hernias—related to the inguinal canal in the inguinal region (where abdomen and thigh meet)

Right side: deeper dissection

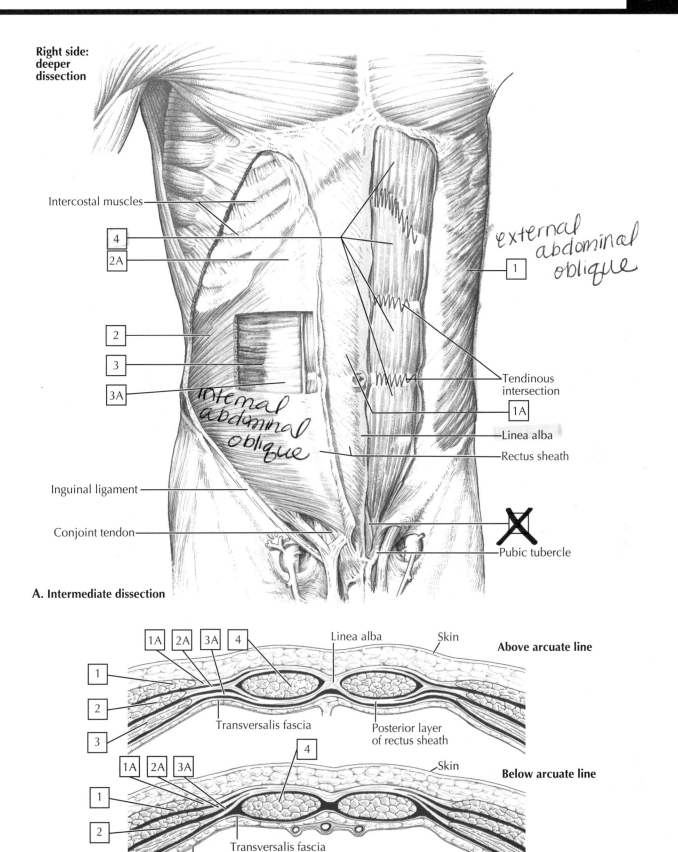

Intercostal muscles

4
2A

external abdominal oblique 1

2

3

3A

internal abdominal oblique

Tendinous intersection

1A

Linea alba

Rectus sheath

Inguinal ligament

Conjoint tendon

Pubic tubercle

A. Intermediate dissection

1A 2A 3A 4

Linea alba   Skin   **Above arcuate line**

1

2

3

Transversalis fascia

Posterior layer of rectus sheath

1A 2A 3A

4

Skin   **Below arcuate line**

1

2

3

Transversalis fascia

Peritoneum

B. Rectus sheath cross section

The muscles of the male and female inguinal region are similar. However, the presence of the spermatic cord in the inguinal canal and the descent of the testis during fetal development render this region clinically unique in males and predispose males to inguinal hernias.

During development, the testis descends from its site of embryological origin in the posterior abdominal region through the inguinal canal (an oblique, lateral-to-medial passageway through the lower anterior abdominal wall) and into the scrotum. Each testis is tethered by its **spermatic cord**, which among other structures contains the ductus (vas) deferens, which will provide a passageway for sperm to re-enter the body cavity and join with the prostatic urethra during sexual arousal.

As the **spermatic cord** runs in the inguinal canal, it picks up spermatic fascial layers derived from the abdominal wall structures as the testis descends. These derivatives include the:
- **External spermatic fascia**: derived from the external abdominal oblique muscle
- **Middle (cremasteric) fascia**: derived from the internal abdominal oblique muscle, this fascia really includes small skeletal muscle fibers of the cremaster muscle
- **Internal spermatic fascia**: derived from the transversalis fascia

The spermatic cord contains the following structures:
- Ductus (vas) deferens
- Testicular and cremasteric arteries, and the artery of the ductus deferens
- Pampiniform plexus of veins
- Autonomic nerve fibers
- Genital branch of the genitofemoral nerve (innervates the cremasteric muscle)
- Lymphatics

The **inguinal canal** itself is a small passageway through the abdominal musculature that is demarcated at both ends by inguinal rings, the deep ring opening in the abdomen and the superficial ring opening externally just lateral to the pubic tubercle. The features of the inguinal canal are noted in the table below.

COLOR the following features of the inguinal region and spermatic cord, using a different color for each feature:
- [ ] 1. Ductus deferens
- [ ] 2. External oblique muscle and aponeurosis
- [ ] 3. Internal oblique muscle
- [ ] 4. Transversus abdominis muscle
- [ ] 5. Transversalis fascia
- [ ] 6. External spermatic fascia (covering the spermatic cord)
- [ ] 7. Cremasteric fascia (muscle)
- [ ] 8. Internal spermatic fascia

Clinical Note:
Inguinal hernias are of two types:
- Indirect: 75% of inguinal hernias, they occur lateral to the inferior epigastric vessels, pass through the deep inguinal ring and inguinal canal in a protrusion of peritoneum within the spermatic cord (covered by all three layers of the spermatic cord)
- Direct: 25% of hernias, they occur medial to the inferior epigastric vessels and pass through the posterior wall of the inguinal canal; they are separate from the spermatic cord
- Inguinal hernias are much more frequent in males than females, probably related to the descent of the testes in males

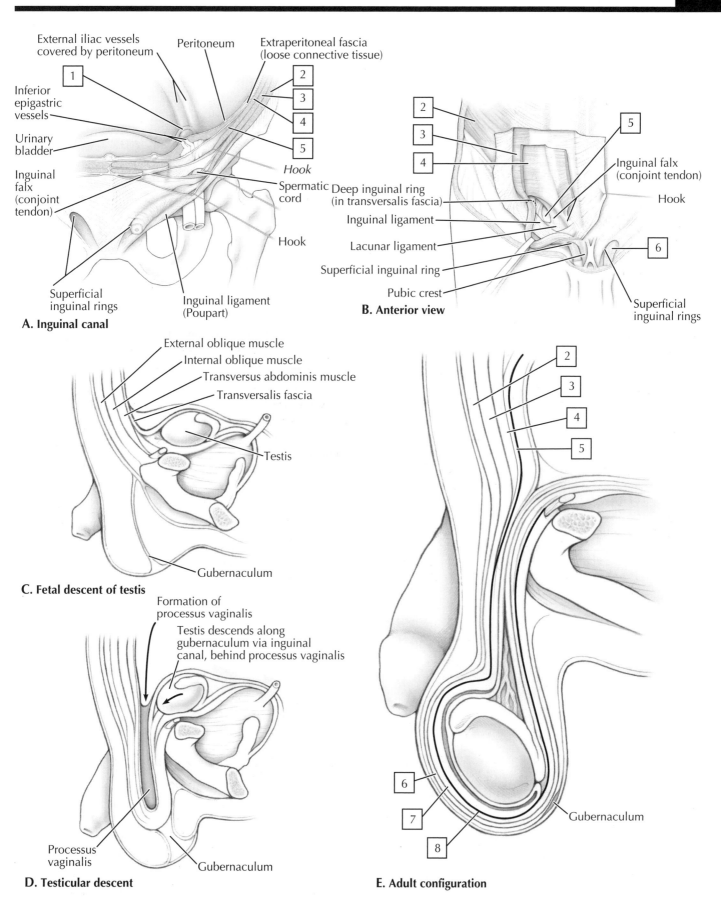

External iliac vessels covered by peritoneum

Peritoneum

Extraperitoneal fascia (loose connective tissue)

| 1 |

| 2 |
| 3 |
| 4 |
| 5 |

Inferior epigastric vessels

Urinary bladder

Inguinal falx (conjoint tendon)

Hook

Spermatic cord

Hook

Superficial inguinal rings

Inguinal ligament (Poupart)

A. Inguinal canal

| 2 |
| 3 |
| 4 |

| 5 |

Inguinal falx (conjoint tendon)

Hook

Deep inguinal ring (in transversalis fascia)

Inguinal ligament

Lacunar ligament

Superficial inguinal ring

Pubic crest

| 6 |

Superficial inguinal rings

B. Anterior view

External oblique muscle
Internal oblique muscle
Transversus abdominis muscle
Transversalis fascia

Testis

| 2 |
| 3 |
| 4 |
| 5 |

Gubernaculum

C. Fetal descent of testis

Formation of processus vaginalis

Testis descends along gubernaculum via inguinal canal, behind processus vaginalis

| 6 |
| 7 |
| 8 |

Gubernaculum

Processus vaginalis

Gubernaculum

D. Testicular descent

E. Adult configuration

Muscles of the Posterior Abdominal Wall

The muscles of the posterior abdominal wall lie behind the peritoneal cavity and their anterior surface is separated from this cavity by the following:
- Transversalis fascia
- A layer of extraperitoneal fat of variable thickness
- Parietal peritoneum lining the peritoneal cavity

These muscles fill in the space between the lower edge of the rib cage and line the abdominopelvic cavity to the level of the true pelvis. Often the **abdominal diaphragm** is included with these muscles, and its superior extent rises almost to the level of the 8th thoracic vertebral body. Contraction of the diaphragm pulls the central tendon inferiorly and this action increases the volume of the thoracic cavity, causing a drop in pressure slightly below that of the ambient pressure outside of the body. As a result, the air passively passes into the trachea and lungs. Relaxation of the diaphragm and the elastic recoil of the lungs expels the air during normal expiration. These muscles are summarized in the table below.

COLOR the following muscles of the posterior abdominal wall, using a different color for each muscle:

☐ 1. **Diaphragm (leave the central tendon uncolored)**
☐ 2. **Quadratus lumborum**
☐ 3. **Psoas major**
☐ 4. **Iliacus: this muscle and the psoas fuse to function as one muscle, the iliopsoas**

The psoas minor muscle is not always present but does act as a weak flexor of the lumbar vertebral column.

MUSCLE	SUPERIOR ATTACHMENT (ORIGIN)	INFERIOR ATTACHMENT (INSERTION)	INNERVATION	ACTIONS
Psoas major	Transverse processes of lumbar vertebrae; sides of bodies of T12-L5 vertebrae, and intervening intervertebral discs	Lesser trochanter of femur	Lumbar plexus via ventral branches of L1-L4 nerves	Acting superiorly with iliacus, flexes hip; acting inferiorly, flexes vertebral column laterally; used to balance trunk in sitting position; acting inferiorly with iliacus, flexes trunk
Iliacus	Superior two thirds of iliac fossa, ala of sacrum, and anterior sacro-iliac ligaments	Lesser trochanter of femur and shaft inferior to it, and to psoas major tendon	Femoral nerve (L2-L4)	Flexes hip and stabilizes hip joint; acts with psoas major
Quadratus lumborum	Medial half of inferior border of 12th rib and tips of lumbar transverse processes	Iliolumbar ligament and internal lip of iliac crest	Ventral branches of T12 and L1-L4 nerves	Extends and laterally flexes vertebral column; fixes 12th rib during inspiration
Diaphragm	Xiphoid process, lower six costal cartilages, L1-L3 vertebrae	Converge into central tendon	Phrenic nerve (C3-C5)	Draws central tendon down and forward during inspiration

Clinical Note:
An infection of an intervertebral disc at the level of the psoas major muscle can lead to a **psoas abscess**, which first appears at the superior origin of the muscle. This infection can spread beneath the psoas fascial sheath that covers this muscle and even extend inferior to the inguinal ligament.

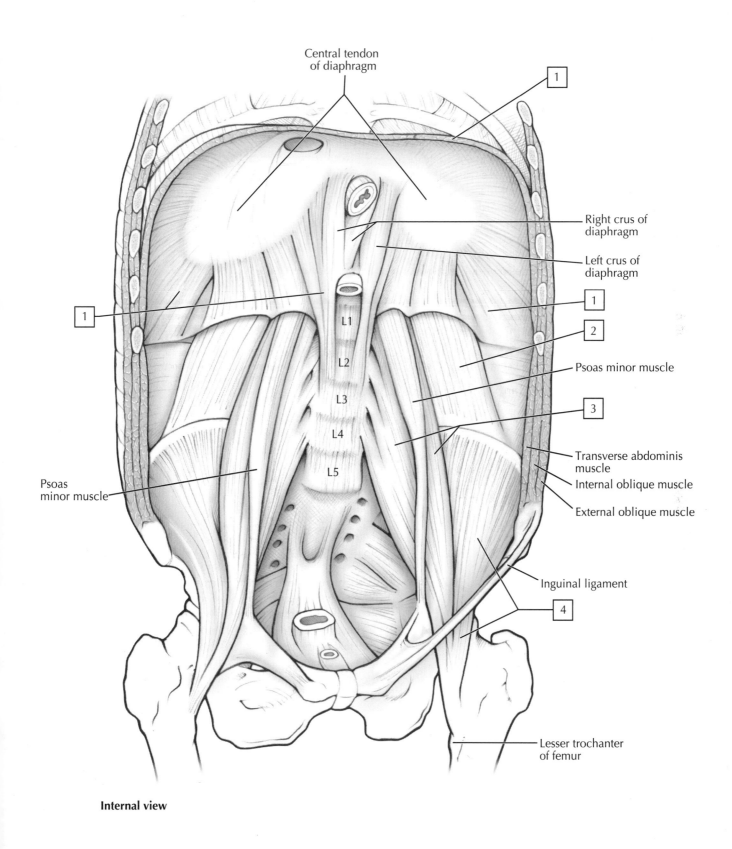

Central tendon of diaphragm

1

Right crus of diaphragm

Left crus of diaphragm

1

2

Psoas minor muscle

3

Transverse abdominis muscle

Internal oblique muscle

External oblique muscle

Inguinal ligament

4

Lesser trochanter of femur

1

L1

L2

L3

L4

L5

Psoas minor muscle

Internal view

The muscles of the pelvis line the lateral pelvic walls (obturator internus and piriformis) and attach to the femur (thigh bone) or cover the floor of the pelvis (levator ani and coccygeus) and form a "**pelvic diaphragm**." The two muscles that form our pelvic diaphragm are really muscles that we've co-opted for a different use than they were originally intended in most land-dwelling vertebrates. Most land-dwelling mammals, for example, are quadrupeds, whereas we are bipeds and exhibit an upright posture. Bipedalism places greater pressure on our lower pelvic floor as it supports our abdominopelvic viscera. Thus, in us, muscles that are used to tuck the tail between the hind legs (coccygeus) or used to wag the tail (levator ani), now subserve a support function in us because we've lost our tail! The levator ani muscle is really a fusion of three separate muscles: the pubococcygeus, puborectalis, and iliococcygeus muscles. The pelvic muscles are summarized in the table below.

COLOR the following muscles of the pelvis, using a different color for each muscle:

☐ 1. **Levator ani: really composed of three fused muscles, it is our old "tail-wagging" muscle**

☐ 2. **Obturator internus**

☐ 3. **Coccygeus: often partially fibrous, it is our old "tail-tucking" muscle**

☐ 4. **Piriformis: a pear-shaped muscle; wider on one end than the other, like a pear**

MUSCLE	PROXIMAL ATTACHMENT (ORIGIN)	DISTAL ATTACHMENT (INSERTION)	INNERVATION	MAIN ACTIONS
Obturator internus	Pelvic aspect of obturator membrane and pelvic bones	Greater trochanter of femur	Nerve to obturator internus	Rotates extended thigh laterally; abducts flexed thigh at hip
Piriformis	Anterior surface of 2nd to 4th sacral segments and sacrotuberous ligament	Greater trochanter of femur	Ventral rami of S1-S2	Rotates extended thigh laterally; abducts flexed thigh; stabilizes hip joint
Levator ani	Body of pubis, tendinous arch of obturator fascia, and ischial spine	Perineal body, coccyx, ano-coccygeal raphe, walls of prostate or vagina, rectum, and anal canal	Ventral rami of S3-S4, perineal nerve of the pudendal nerve	Supports pelvic viscera; raises pelvic floor
Coccygeus (ischiococcygeus)	Ischial spine and sacrospinous ligament	Inferior sacrum and coccyx	Ventral rami of S4-S5	Supports pelvic viscera; draws coccyx forward

Clinical Note:

During **defecation**, the levator ani, especially those muscle fibers around the rectum, relax to allow the anorectal (rectum and anal canal) region to straighten and facilitate evacuation. The normal angle between the rectum above and the anal canal below is about 90 degrees (this helps to close off the anorectal junction), but during defecation this angle increases about 40 to 50 degrees (the anal canal swings forward). This relaxation, along with relaxation of the anal sphincters (not shown), opens the anal canal.

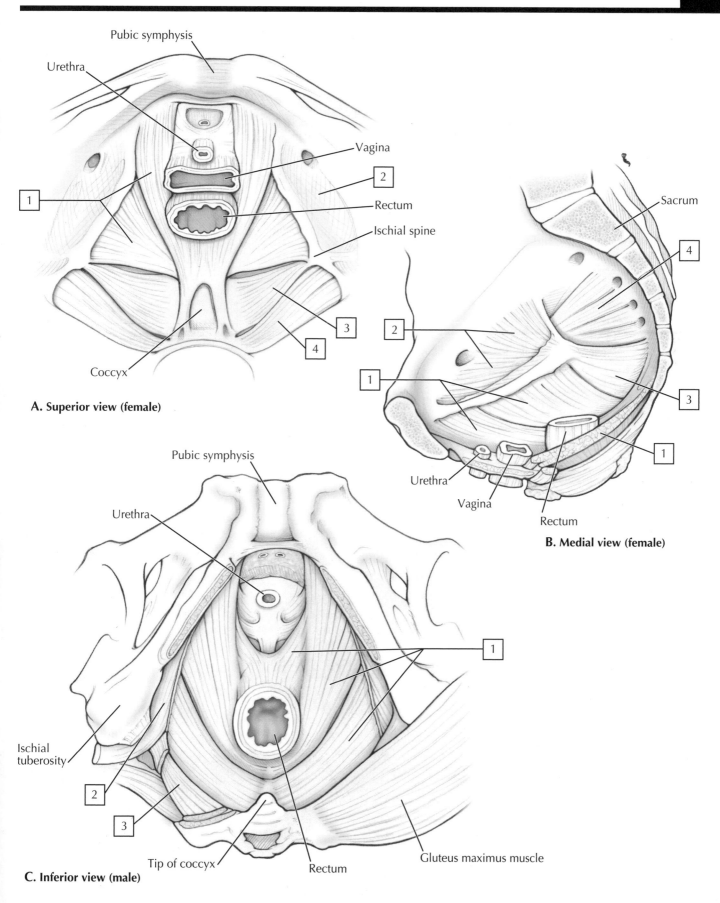

Pubic symphysis

Urethra

Vagina

2

1

Rectum

Ischial spine

3

4

Coccyx

A. Superior view (female)

Sacrum

4

2

1

3

1

1

Urethra

Vagina

Rectum

B. Medial view (female)

Pubic symphysis

Urethra

1

Ischial tuberosity

2

3

Tip of coccyx

Rectum

Gluteus maximus muscle

C. Inferior view (male)

The perineum is a diamond-shaped region between the thighs. It can be divided into an anterior **urogenital** (UG) triangle and a posterior **anal triangle** by an imaginary horizontal line connecting the two ischial tuberosities. Boundaries of the perineum include the:

- Pubic symphysis anteriorly
- Ischial tuberosities laterally
- Coccyx posteriorly

The muscles of the superficial perineal space are skeletal muscles and include the:

- **Ischiocavernosus**: paired muscles that surround the corpus cavernosum (erectile tissue) in males or the crus of the clitoris (also erectile tissue) in females
- **Bulbospongiosus**: a midline muscle that surrounds the bulb of the penis in males or splits to surround the bulbs of the vestibule in females; these also are erectile tissue structures
- **Superficial transverse perineal**: paired muscle that stabilizes the central tendon of the perineum (this muscle is often very small and difficult to identify)
- **External anal sphincter**: closes off the anal canal and rests upon the underlying levator ani muscle

The **central tendon of the perineum** is an important anchoring structure for the perineum. The bulbospongiosus, superficial transverse perineal, levator ani, and external anal sphincter all have attachments to the central tendon. The **UG triangle** contains the external genitalia of both sexes, whereas the **anal triangle** (the space is called the ischio-anal fossa) is largely filled with fat and fibrous tissue.

Deep to the muscles of the UG triangle lies the external urethral sphincter in males (closes the membranous urethra except when passing urine, or during orgasm and ejaculation of semen). In females, the urethral sphincter blends with the compressor urethrae and sphincter urethrovaginalis muscles in the deep perineal space. All of these muscles, in both sexes, are under voluntary control and innervated by the pudendal (means "shameful") nerve (S2-S4) from the sacral plexus (ventral rami).

COLOR the muscles of the perineum, using a different color for each muscle:

- [ ] 1. **Bulbocavernosus**
- [ ] 2. **Ischiocavernosus**
- [ ] 3. **External urethral sphincter (in male)**
- [ ] 4. **Urethral sphincter (in female)**
- [ ] 5. **Compressor urethrae (in female)**
- [ ] 6. **External anal sphincter**

Clinical Note:

During childbirth, it may become necessary to enlarge the birth opening to prevent extensive stretching or tearing of the perineum. An incision, called an **episiotomy**, can be made in the posterior midline (median episiotomy) or posterolaterally to the vaginal opening to facilitate delivery of the child. It is important to suture the episiotomy carefully so that the integrity of the central tendon of the perineum is preserved, because this is an important support structure for the muscles of the perineum.

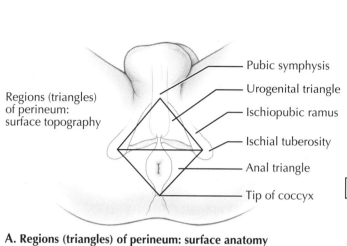

Regions (triangles) of perineum: surface topography

Pubic symphysis

Urogenital triangle

Ischiopubic ramus

Ischial tuberosity

Anal triangle

Tip of coccyx

A. Regions (triangles) of perineum: surface anatomy

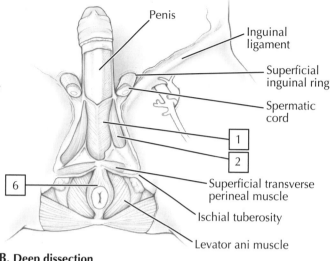

Penis

Inguinal ligament

Superficial inguinal ring

Spermatic cord

1

2

Superficial transverse perineal muscle

Ischial tuberosity

Levator ani muscle

B. Deep dissection

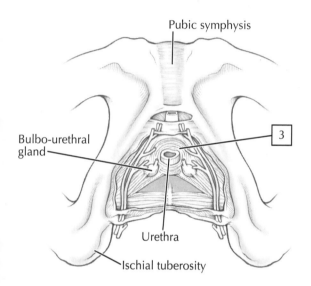

Pubic symphysis

Bulbo-urethral gland

3

Urethra

Ischial tuberosity

C. Male: inferior view

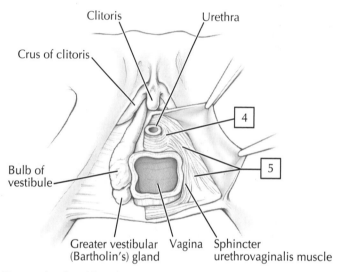

Clitoris

Urethra

Crus of clitoris

4

5

Bulb of vestibule

Greater vestibular (Bartholin's) gland

Vagina

Sphincter urethrovaginalis muscle

D. Female: deep dissection

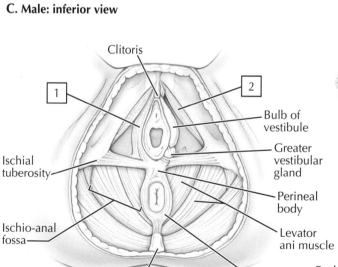

Clitoris

1

2

Bulb of vestibule

Greater vestibular gland

Perineal body

Levator ani muscle

Ischial tuberosity

Ischio-anal fossa

Coccyx

6

E. Female: deep perineum

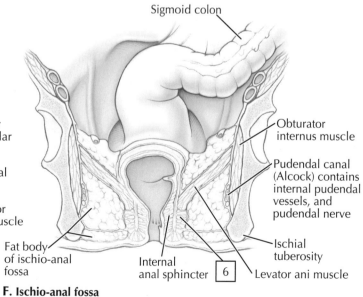

Sigmoid colon

Obturator internus muscle

Pudendal canal (Alcock) contains internal pudendal vessels, and pudendal nerve

Ischial tuberosity

Levator ani muscle

Fat body of ischio-anal fossa

Internal anal sphincter

6

F. Ischio-anal fossa

Muscles of the posterior shoulder have attachments to the scapula (the latissimus dorsi may or may not have a slight attachment to the inferior angle) and help in movements of the scapula and shoulder joint. Realize that when your arm is abducted above 20 degrees (angle between your armpit and your body as your arm is abducted), your scapula begins to rotate with the inferior angle swinging laterally (this tilts the glenoid fossa upward). These muscles largely elevate the scapula, facilitate its rotation, or bring it back into its resting position (arm adducted against the body). These muscles are summarized in the table below.

Among these muscles, four play a unique role in stabilizing the shallow ball-and-socket joint of the shoulder (shallow to provide for extensive mobility) and are called the **rotator cuff muscles.** They include the:

- Supraspinatus
- Infraspinatus
- Teres minor
- Subscapularis: lies on the anterior aspect of the scapula in the subscapular fossa

MUSCLE	PROXIMAL ATTACHMENT (ORIGIN)	DISTAL ATTACHMENT (INSERTION)	INNERVATION	MAIN ACTIONS
Trapezius	Medial third of superior nuchal line; external occipital protuberance, ligamentum nuchae, and spinous processes of C7-T12	Lateral third of clavicle, acromion, and spine of scapula	Accessory nerve (CN XI) and cervical nerves (C3 and C4)	Elevates, retracts, and rotates scapula; superior fibers elevate, middle fibers retract, and inferior fibers depress scapula
Latissimus dorsi	Spinous processes of T7-T12, thoracolumbar fascia, iliac crest, and inferior three or four ribs	Intertubercular groove of humerus	Thoracodorsal nerve (C6-C8)	Extends, adducts, and medially rotates humerus at shoulder
Levator scapulae	Transverse processes of C1-C4	Superomedial border of scapula	Dorsal scapular and cervical (C3-C4) nerves	Elevates scapula and tilts its glenoid cavity inferiorly by rotating scapula
Rhomboid minor and major	*Minor:* ligamentum nuchae and spinous processes of C7 and T1 *Major:* spinous processes of T2-T5	Medial border of scapula from level of spine to inferior angle	Dorsal scapular nerve (C4-C5)	Retracts scapula and rotates it to depress glenoid cavity; fixes scapula to thoracic wall
Supraspinatus (rotator cuff muscle)	Supraspinous fossa of scapula	Superior facet on greater tubercle of humerus	Suprascapular nerve (C5-C6)	Helps deltoid abduct arm at shoulder and acts with rotator cuff muscles
Infraspinatus (rotator cuff muscle)	Infraspinous fossa of scapula	Middle facet on greater tubercle of humerus	Suprascapular nerve (C5-C6)	Laterally rotates arm at shoulder; helps hold head in glenoid cavity
Teres minor (rotator cuff muscle)	Lateral border of scapula	Inferior facet on greater tubercle	Axillary nerve (C5-C6)	Laterally rotates arm at shoulder; helps hold head in glenoid cavity
Teres major	Dorsal surface of inferior angle of scapula	Medial lip of intertubercular groove of humerus	Lower subscapular nerve (C5-C6)	Extends arm and medially rotates shoulder
Subscapularis (rotator cuff muscle)	Subscapular fossa of scapula	Lesser tubercle of humerus	Upper and lower subscapular nerves (C5-C6)	Medially rotates arm at shoulder and adducts it; helps hold humeral head in glenoid cavity

 the following muscles, using a different color for each muscle:

1. Trapezius
2. Levator scapulae
3. Supraspinatus
4. Infraspinatus
5. Teres minor (may blend with the infraspinatus muscle)
6. Teres major
7. Subscapularis (on the anterior surface of the scapula)

Clinical Note:

The musculotendinous **rotator cuff** strengthens the shoulder joint on its superior, posterior, and anterior aspects, hence about 95% of shoulder dislocations occur in an anteroinferior direction. Repetitive abduction, extension, lateral (external) rotation, and flexion of the arm at the shoulder, the motion used in throwing a ball, places stress on the elements of the rotator cuff, especially the tendon of the supraspinatus muscle as it rubs on the acromion and coraco-acromial ligament. Tears or rupture of this tendon are relatively common athletic injuries.

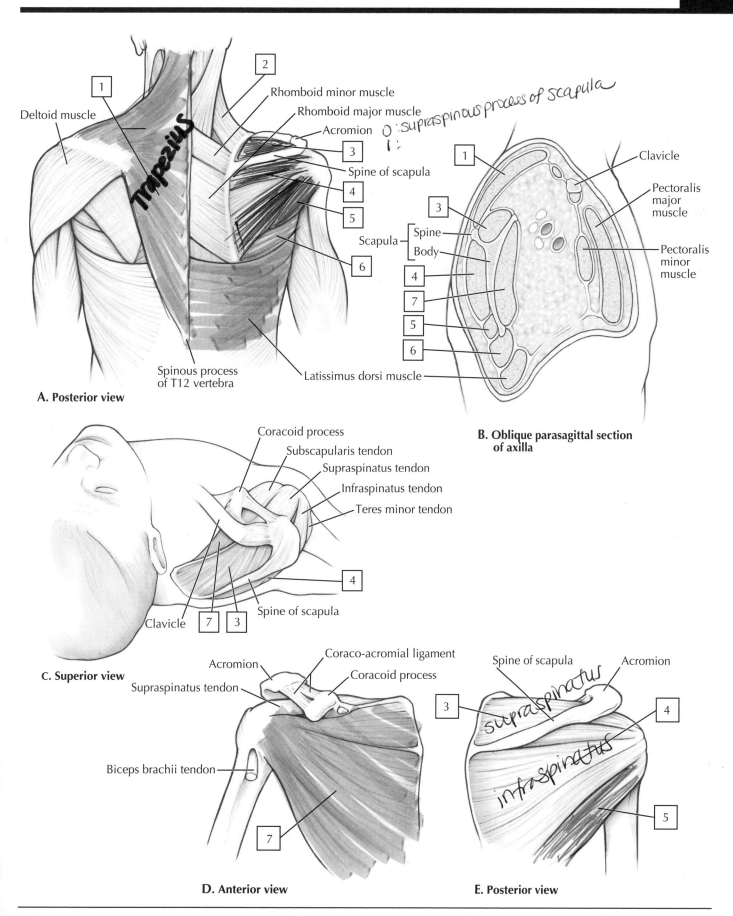

A. Posterior view

Deltoid muscle

1

2

Rhomboid minor muscle

Rhomboid major muscle

Acromion

3

Spine of scapula

4

5

6

Spinous process
of T12 vertebra

Latissimus dorsi muscle

O : supraspinous process of scapula

1

3

Scapula {
Spine
Body

4

7

5

6

Clavicle

Pectoralis
major
muscle

Pectoralis
minor
muscle

**B. Oblique parasagittal section
of axilla**

C. Superior view

Coracoid process

Subscapularis tendon

Supraspinatus tendon

Infraspinatus tendon

Teres minor tendon

4

Spine of scapula

Clavicle   7   3

D. Anterior view

Acromion

Coraco-acromial ligament

Coracoid process

Supraspinatus tendon

Biceps brachii tendon

7

E. Posterior view

Spine of scapula

Acromion

3

supraspinatus

infraspinatus

4

5

Muscles of the anterior shoulder have attachments to the pectoral girdle (scapula and clavicle) or the humerus, and assist in movements of the pectoral girdle and shoulder. These muscles "cap" the shoulder (deltoid muscle) or arise from the anterior or lateral thoracic wall, and are summarized in the table below.

COLOR the following muscles, using a different color for each muscle:

1. Deltoid
2. Pectoralis major
3. Serratus anterior
4. Subclavius
5. Pectoralis minor

The anterior and posterior muscles define the "axilla" (armpit) region, a pyramid-shaped area containing important neurovascular structures that pass through the shoulder region. The six boundaries of the axilla include the:

- **Base**: axillary fascia and skin of the armpit
- **Apex**: bounded by the 1st rib, clavicle, and superior part of the scapula; a passageway for structures entering or leaving the shoulder and arm
- **Anterior wall**: pectoralis major and minor muscles
- **Posterior wall**: subscapularis, teres major, and latissimus dorsi muscles
- **Medial wall**: upper rib cage, intercostal and serratus anterior muscles
- **Lateral wall**: proximal humerus (intertubercular groove)

MUSCLE	PROXIMAL ATTACHMENT (ORIGIN)	DISTAL ATTACHMENT (INSERTION)	INNERVATION	MAIN ACTIONS
Pectoralis major	Medial half of clavicle; sternum; superior six costal cartilages; aponeurosis of external abdominal oblique	Intertubercular groove of humerus	Lateral (C5-C7) and medial pectoral nerves (C8-T1)	Flexes, adducts, and medially rotates arm at shoulder; extension of flexed arm
Pectoralis minor	3rd to 5th ribs	Coracoid process of scapula	Medial pectoral nerve (C8-T1)	Depresses scapula and stabilizes it
Serratus anterior	Upper eight ribs	Medial border of scapula	Long thoracic nerve (C5-C7)	Rotates scapula upward and pulls it anterior toward thoracic wall
Subclavius	Junction of 1st rib and costal cartilage	Inferior surface of clavicle	Nerve to subclavius (C5-C6)	Depresses clavicle
Deltoid	Lateral third of clavicle, acromion, and spine of scapula	Deltoid tuberosity of humerus	Axillary nerve (C5-C6)	*Anterior part*: flexes and medially rotates arm at shoulder *Middle part*: abducts arm at shoulder *Posterior part*: extends and laterally rotates arm at shoulder

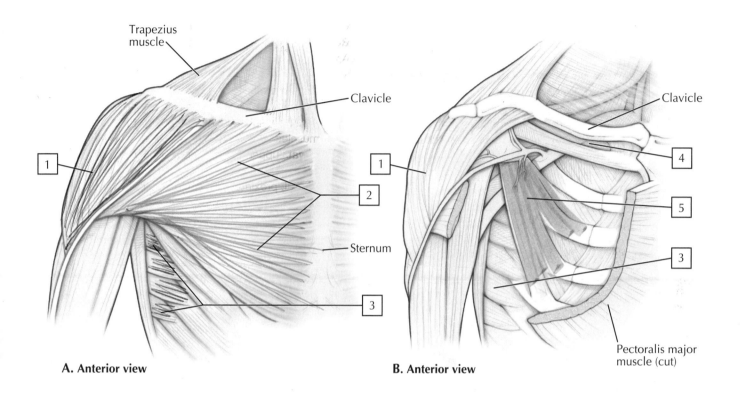

Trapezius
muscle

Clavicle

1

2

Sternum

3

A. Anterior view

Clavicle

1

4

5

3

Pectoralis major
muscle (cut)

B. Anterior view

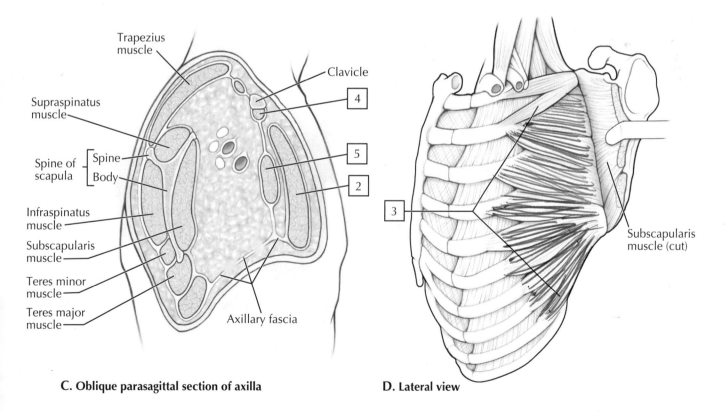

Trapezius
muscle

Clavicle

4

Supraspinatus
muscle

Spine of
scapula {
Spine
Body

5

2

Infraspinatus
muscle

Subscapularis
muscle

3

Teres minor
muscle

Subscapularis
muscle (cut)

Teres major
muscle

Axillary fascia

C. Oblique parasagittal section of axilla

D. Lateral view

The arm (region between the shoulder and elbow) is divided by a connective tissue intermuscular septum into two compartments:

- **Anterior**: contains muscles that primarily flex the elbow and/or the shoulder
- **Posterior**: contains muscles that primarily extend the elbow

Additionally, the biceps is a powerful supinator of the flexed forearm, used when turning a screw into wood, if right-handed, or for removing a screw, if left-handed. Of the arm flexors, the brachialis is the most powerful flexor of the forearm at the elbow, not the biceps, although it is the biceps that most weight lifters focus on, because it is the more visible of the two muscles. The muscles of the anterior and posterior compartments are summarized in the table below.

COLOR the following muscles, using a different color for each muscle:

- ▨ 1. **Biceps brachii (has a long and a short head)**
- ▨ 2. **Coracobrachialis**
- ▨ 3. **Brachialis**
- ☐ 4. **Triceps: has three components; its medial head lies deep to the overlying long and lateral heads**
- ☐ 5. **Anconeus: sometimes grouped with the forearm extensor muscles**

MUSCLE	PROXIMAL ATTACHMENT (ORIGIN)	DISTAL ATTACHMENT (INSERTION)	INNERVATION	MAIN ACTIONS
Biceps brachii	*Short head:* apex of coracoid process of scapula *Long head:* supraglenoid tubercle of scapula	Tuberosity of radius and fascia of forearm via bicipital aponeurosis	Musculocutaneous nerve (C5, C6, C7)	Supinates flexed forearm; flexes forearm at elbow; weak arm flexor
Brachialis	Distal half of anterior humerus	Coronoid process and tuberosity of ulna	Musculocutaneous nerve (C5, C6, C7)	Flexes forearm at elbow in all positions
Coracobrachialis	Tip of coracoid process of scapula	Middle third of medial surface of humerus	Musculocutaneous nerve (C5, C6, C7)	Helps flex and adduct arm at shoulder
Triceps brachii	*Long head:* infraglenoid tubercle of scapula *Lateral head:* posterior humerus *Medial head:* posterior surface of humerus, inferior to radial groove	Proximal end of olecranon of ulna and fascia of forearm	Radial nerve (C6, C7, C8)	Extends forearm at elbow; is chief extensor of elbow; steadies head of abducted humerus (long head)
Anconeus	Lateral epicondyle of humerus	Lateral surface of olecranon and superior part of posterior surface of ulna	Radial nerve (C5, C6, C7)	Assists triceps in extending elbow; abducts ulna during pronation

Clinical Note:

Rupture of the biceps brachii may occur at the proximal tendon or, rarely, the muscle belly. The biceps tendon has the highest rate of spontaneous rupture of any tendon in the body. It is seen most commonly in people older than 40 years, in association with rotator cuff injuries and with repetitive lifting (weight lifters). Rupture of the tendon of the long head of the biceps is most common.

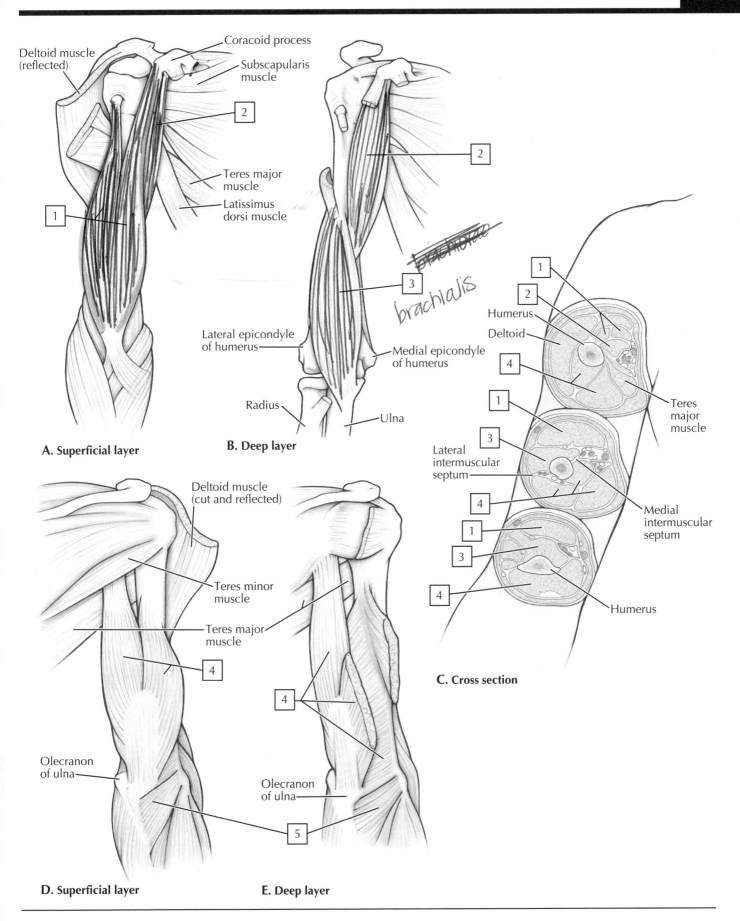

Deltoid muscle (reflected)

Coracoid process

Subscapularis muscle

2

Teres major muscle

Latissimus dorsi muscle

1

A. Superficial layer

2

~~BRACHIALIS~~

3

brachialis

Lateral epicondyle of humerus

Medial epicondyle of humerus

Radius

Ulna

B. Deep layer

1

2

Humerus

Deltoid

4

1

3

Lateral intermuscular septum

4

1

3

4

Teres major muscle

Medial intermuscular septum

Humerus

C. Cross section

Deltoid muscle (cut and reflected)

Teres minor muscle

Teres major muscle

4

Olecranon of ulna

D. Superficial layer

4

Olecranon of ulna

5

E. Deep layer

Two muscles pronate and two muscles supinate the radio-ulnar joints. The forearm in "anatomical position," with the palm facing forward, is **supinated** and the radius and ulna lie side by side in the forearm. Rotation of the palm medially so it faces backwards, or toward the ground if the elbow is flexed 90 degrees, is **pronation**.

The **pronator muscles** lie in the forearm; one is more superficial and lies near the elbow (pronator teres) and the other lies deep beneath other forearm muscles distally near the wrist (pronator quadratus). The word *teres* refers to "round earth" (in pronation of the flexed forearm at 90 degrees, the hand faces the ground or earth), whereas the word *quadratus* refers to the quadrangular shape of the wrist pronator. When the pronators contract, they wrap or pull the radius across the stable ulna, proximally by the pronator teres and distally by the pronator quadratus. The ulna is stabilized by its articulation at the elbow with the distal end of the humerus and moves very little.

The **supinator muscles** include the biceps brachii of the arm, which is a powerful supinator with the elbow flexed, but with the forearm straight, the supinator, a muscle of the extensor compartment of the forearm executes supination. From the illustrations on the facing page, note that when the supinator contracts, it unwraps the crossed radius and brings it back into alignment with the medially placed ulna.

COLOR the following muscles, using a different color for each muscle:

1. Supinator
2. Pronator teres
3. Pronator quadratus
4. Biceps brachii

Clinical Note:

When the **radius is fractured**, the muscles attaching to the bone deform the normal alignment of the radius and ulna. If the fracture of the radius is above the insertion of the pronator teres, the proximal fragment will be flexed and supinated by the action and pull of the biceps brachii and supinator muscles. The distal fragment will be pronated by the pronator teres and quadratus muscles (part *D*).

In fractures of the middle or distal radius that are distal to the insertion of the pronator teres, the supinator and pronator teres will keep the proximal bone fragment of the radius in the neutral position. The distal fragment, however, will be pronated by the pronator quadratus muscle, because it is unopposed by either supinator muscle (part *E*).

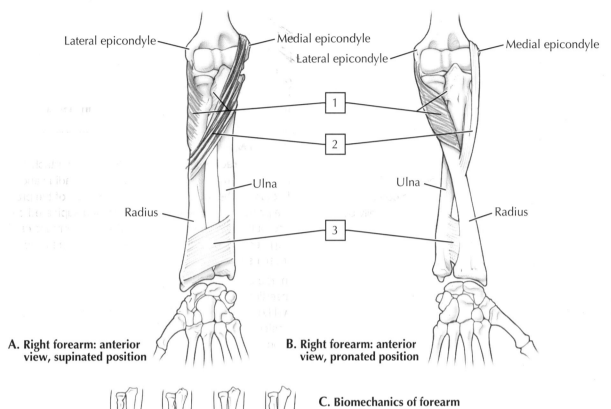

Lateral epicondyle

Medial epicondyle

Lateral epicondyle

Medial epicondyle

1

2

Ulna

Ulna

Radius

Radius

3

A. Right forearm: anterior view, supinated position

B. Right forearm: anterior view, pronated position

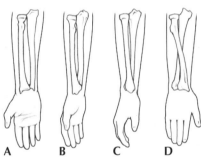

A B C D

C. Biomechanics of forearm

Tuberosity of radius useful indicator of degree of pronation or supination of radius

A. In full supination, tuberosity directed toward ulna
B. In about 40° supination, tuberosity primarily posterior
C. In neutral position, tuberosity directly posterior
D. In full pronation, tuberosity directed laterally

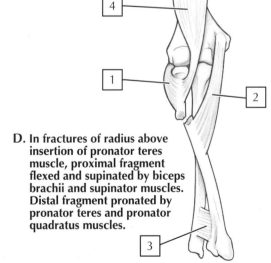

4

1

2

3

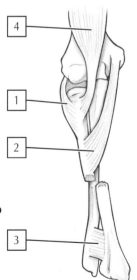

4

1

2

3

D. In fractures of radius above insertion of pronator teres muscle, proximal fragment flexed and supinated by biceps brachii and supinator muscles. Distal fragment pronated by pronator teres and pronator quadratus muscles.

E. In fractures of middle or distal radius that are distal to insertion of pronator teres muscle, supinator and pronator teres muscles keep proximal fragment in neutral position. Distal fragment pronated by pronator quadratus muscle.

3 | Anterior Forearm Muscles

The forearm is divided into two muscle compartments by a connective tissue intermuscular septum. The anterior compartment contains muscles that primarily flex the wrist and fingers. In the anterior compartment, a superficial layer of muscles arises from the medial epicondyle of the humerus, whereas a deep layer of muscles arises from the bones (radius and ulna) of the forearm or the interosseous membrane connecting these bones. If you squeeze your hand very tightly to make a fist and flex your wrist, you will note the contraction of these muscles in your own anterior forearm. These muscles are summarized in the table below.

COLOR each of the following muscles, using a different color for each muscle:

- ☑ 1. **Pronator teres**
- ☑ 2. **Flexor carpi radialis (also abducts the wrist)**
- ☑ 3. **Palmaris longus: absent in about 10% of humans, this muscle is of little importance in us but is the muscle in cats that allows them to retract their claws**
- ☐ 4. **Flexor carpi ulnaris (also adducts the wrist)**
- ☐ 5. **Flexor digitorum superficialis**
- ☐ 6. **Flexor digitorum profundus: "profundus" means deep, as in a profound comment**
- ☐ 7. **Flexor pollicis longus: "pollicis" refers to the thumb**

MUSCLE	PROXIMAL ATTACHMENT (ORIGIN)	DISTAL ATTACHMENT (INSERTION)	INNERVATION	MAIN ACTIONS
Pronator teres	Medial epicondyle of humerus and coronoid process of ulna	Middle of lateral surface of radius	Median nerve (C6-C7)	Pronates forearm and flexes elbow
Flexor carpi radialis	Medial epicondyle of humerus	Base of 2nd metacarpal bone	Median nerve (C6-C7)	Flexes hand at wrist and abducts it
Palmaris longus	Medial epicondyle of humerus	Distal half of flexor retinaculum and palmar aponeurosis	Median nerve (C7-C8)	Flexes hand at wrist and tightens palmar aponeurosis
Flexor carpi ulnaris	*Humeral head:* medial epicondyle of humerus *Ulnar head:* olecranon and posterior border of ulna	Pisiform bone, hook of hamate bone, and 5th metacarpal bone	Ulnar nerve (C7-C8 and T1)	Flexes hand at wrist and adducts it
Flexor digitorum superficialis	*Humero-ulnar head:* medial epicondyle of humerus, ulnar collateral ligament, and coronoid process of ulna *Radial head:* superior half of anterior radius	Bodies of middle phalanges of medial four digits on the palmar aspect	Median nerve (C8-T1)	Flexes middle phalanges of medial four digits; also weakly flexes proximal phalanges, forearm, and wrist
Flexor digitorum profundus	Proximal three fourths of medial and anterior surfaces of ulna and interosseous membrane	Bases of distal phalanges of medial four digits on the palmar aspect	*Medial part:* ulnar nerve (C8-T1) *Lateral part:* median nerve (C8-T1)	Flexes distal phalanges of medial four digits; assists with flexion of wrist
Flexus pollicis longus	Anterior surface of radius and adjacent interosseous membrane	Base of distal phalanx of thumb on the palmar aspect	Median nerve (anterior interosseous) (C7-C8)	Flexes phalanges of 1st digit (thumb)
Pronator quadratus	Distal fourth of anterior surface of ulna	Distal fourth of anterior surface of radius	Median nerve (anterior interosseous) (C7-C8)	Pronates forearm

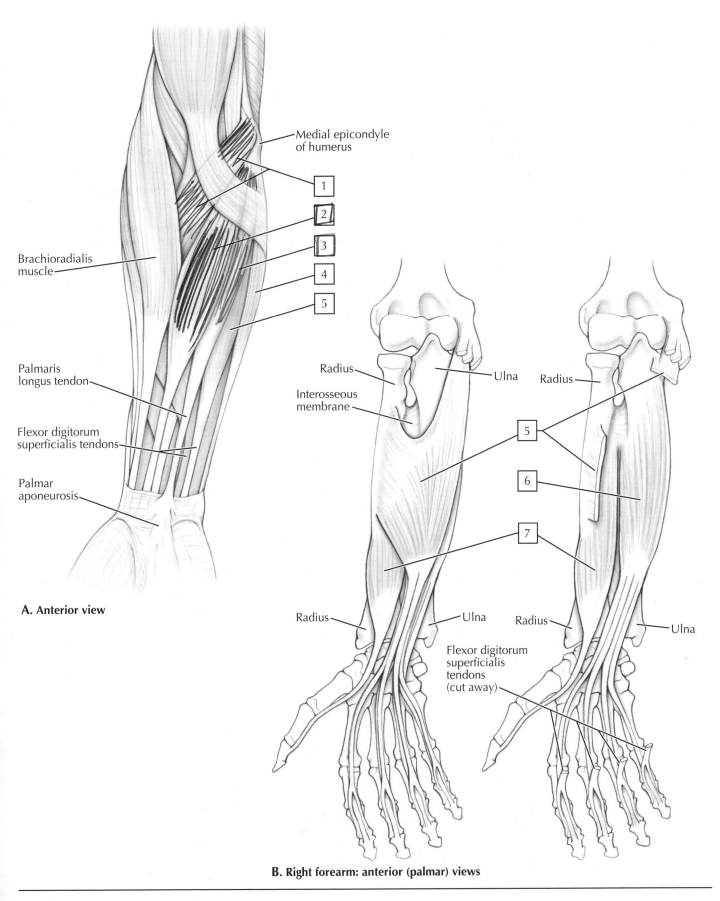

Medial epicondyle
of humerus

1

2

3

4

5

Brachioradialis
muscle

Palmaris
longus tendon

Flexor digitorum
superficialis tendons

Palmar
aponeurosis

A. Anterior view

Radius

Interosseous
membrane

Ulna

Radius

5

6

7

Radius

Ulna

Radius

Ulna

Flexor digitorum
superficialis
tendons
(cut away)

B. Right forearm: anterior (palmar) views

The forearm is divided into two muscle compartments by a connective tissue intermuscular septum. The posterior compartment contains muscles that primarily extend the wrist and fingers. In the posterior compartment, a superficial layer of muscles arises largely from the lateral epicondyle of the humerus, whereas a deep layer of muscles arises from the bones of the forearm (radius and ulna) or the interosseous membrane connecting these bones. If you hyperextend your fingers and wrist and pronate your forearm, you will note the contraction of these muscles in your own posterior forearm. Extending the wrist when gripping an object adds extra strength to our grip (the power grip). These muscles are summarized in the table below.

MUSCLE	PROXIMAL ATTACHMENT (ORIGIN)	DISTAL ATTACHMENT (INSERTION)	INNERVATION	MAIN ACTIONS
Brachioradialis	Proximal two thirds of lateral supracondylar ridge of humerus	Lateral surface of distal end of radius	Radial nerve (C5-C6)	Flexes forearm at elbow, especially in midpronation
Extensor carpi radialis longus	Lateral supracondylar ridge of humerus	Base of second metacarpal bone	Radial nerve (C6-C7)	Extends and abducts hand at wrist
Extensor carpi radialis brevis	Lateral epicondyle of humerus	Base of 3rd metacarpal bone	Radial nerve (deep branch) (C7-C8)	Extends and abducts hand at wrist
Extensor digitorum	Lateral epicondyle of humerus	Extensor expansions of medial four digits	Radial nerve (posterior interosseous) (C7-C8)	Extends medial four digits at metacarpophalangeal joints; extends hand at wrist joint
Extensor digiti minimi	Lateral epicondyle of humerus	Extensor expansion of 5th digit	Radial nerve (posterior interosseous) (C7-C8)	Extends 5th digit at metacarpophalangeal and interphalangeal joints
Extensor carpi ulnaris	Lateral epicondyle of humerus and posterior border of ulna	Base of 5th metacarpal bone	Radial nerve (posterior interosseous) (C7-C8)	Extends and adducts hand at wrist
Supinator	Lateral epicondyle of humerus; radial collateral, and anular ligaments; supinator fossa; and crest of ulna	Lateral, posterior, and anterior surfaces of proximal third of radius	Radial nerve (deep branch) (C6-C7)	Supinates forearm
Abductor pollicis longus	Posterior surfaces of ulna, radius, and interosseous membrane	Base of 1st metacarpal bone on the lateral aspect	Radial nerve (posterior interosseous) (C7-C8)	Abducts thumb and extends it at carpometacarpal joint
Extensor pollicis brevis	Posterior surfaces of radius and interosseous membrane	Base of proximal phalanx of thumb on the dorsal aspect	Radial nerve (posterior interosseous) (C7-C8)	Extends proximal phalanx of thumb at carpometacarpal joint
Extensor pollicis longus	Posterior surface of middle third of ulna and interosseous membrane	Base of distal phalanx of thumb on the dorsal aspect	Radial nerve (posterior interosseous) (C7-C8)	Extends distal phalanx of thumb at metacarpophalangeal and interphalangeal joints
Extensor indicis	Posterior surface of ulna and interosseous membrane	Extensor expansion of second digit	Radial nerve (posterior interosseous) (C7-C8)	Extends second digit and helps extend hand at wrist

COLOR each of the following muscles, using a different color for each muscle:

1. **Extensor carpi ulnaris (also adducts the wrist)**
2. **Extensor digiti minimi ("minimi" refers to the little finger)**
3. **Brachioradialis: lumped with the posterior forearm muscles because of its innervation, it actually flexes the forearm at the elbow**
4. **Extensor carpi radialis longus (also abducts the wrist; important in power grip)**
5. **Extensor carpi radialis brevis (also abducts the wrist; important in power grip)**
6. **Extensor digitorum**
7. **Abductor pollicis longus ("pollicis" refers to the thumb)**
8. **Extensor pollicis brevis**
9. **Extensor pollicis longus**
10. **Extensor indicis ("indicis" refers to the index finger)**

Clinical Note:

"Tennis elbow" is a condition that clinicians call lateral epicondylitis, which itself is a somewhat misleading diagnosis because the problem really involves a tendinosis of the extensor carpi radialis brevis (probably the most important wrist extensor), which arises just proximal to this epicondyle. Moreover, most sufferers are not tennis players! The elbow pain experienced in tennis elbow occurs just distal and posterior to the lateral epicondyle and is exacerbated during wrist extension, especially against resistance. The pain may be due to the muscle, its innervating nerve, and/or something within the elbow joint itself.

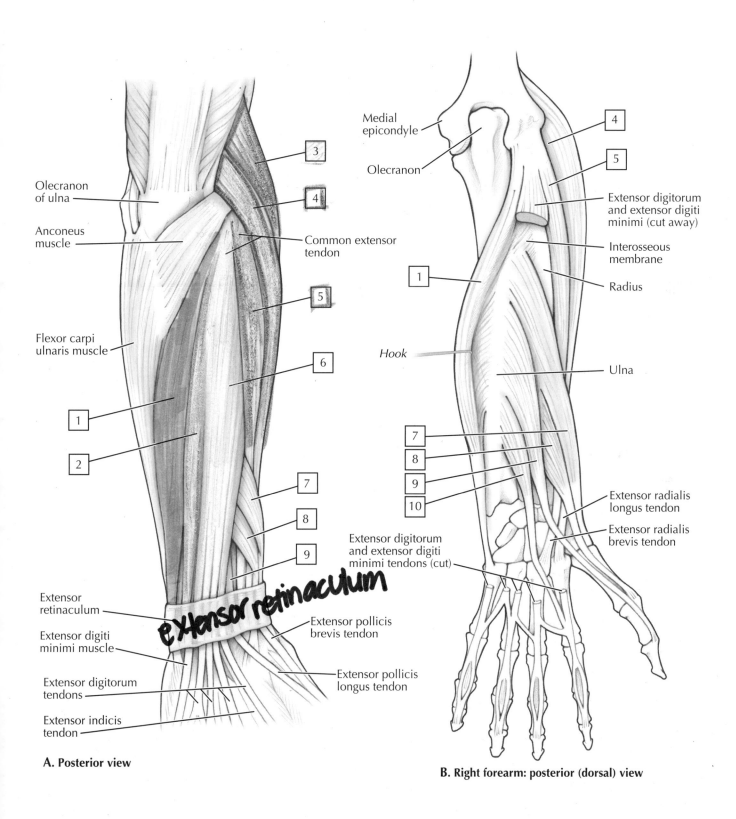

Olecranon
of ulna

Anconeus
muscle

Flexor carpi
ulnaris muscle

Extensor
retinaculum

Extensor digiti
minimi muscle

Extensor digitorum
tendons

Extensor indicis
tendon

3

4

Common extensor
tendon

5

6

7

8

9

extensor retinaculum

Extensor pollicis
brevis tendon

Extensor pollicis
longus tendon

1

2

A. Posterior view

Medial
epicondyle

Olecranon

4

5

Extensor digitorum
and extensor digiti
minimi (cut away)

Interosseous
membrane

Radius

1

Hook

Ulna

7

8

9

10

Extensor digitorum
and extensor digiti
minimi tendons (cut)

Extensor radialis
longus tendon

Extensor radialis
brevis tendon

B. Right forearm: posterior (dorsal) view

The intrinsic hand muscles move the fingers, complementing the long flexor and extensor forearm muscles that also move the fingers. Two groups of muscle lie most superficial:

- **Thenar eminence**: a cone of three thenar muscles at the base of the thumb
- **Hypothenar eminence**: a cone of three hypothenar muscles at the base of the little finger

Deeper intrinsic muscles include the:

- **Adductor pollicis**: deep in the palm, it adducts the thumb
- **Lumbricals**: four small muscles attached to the flexor digitorum profundus tendons
- **Interossei**: three palmar and four dorsal interosseous muscles between the metacarpals; palmar interossei adduct the digits (**PAD**) and dorsal interossei abduct the digits (**DAB**)

These intrinsic muscles are summarized in the table below.

COLOR each of the following muscles, using a different color for each muscle:

- [ ] 1. **Opponens pollicis (thenar muscle)**
- [ ] 2. **Abductor pollicis brevis (thenar muscle)**
- [ ] 3. **Flexor pollicis brevis (thenar muscle)**
- [ ] 4. **Adductor pollicis**
- [ ] 5. **Abductor digiti minimi (hypothenar muscle)**
- [ ] 6. **Flexor digiti minimi (hypothenar muscle)**
- [ ] 7. **Opponens digiti minimi (hypothenar muscle)**
- [ ] 8. **Dorsal interossei**
- [ ] 9. **Palmar interossei**

MUSCLE	PROXIMAL ATTACHMENT (ORIGIN)	DISTAL ATTACHMENT (INSERTION)	INNERVATION	MAIN ACTIONS
Abductor pollicis brevis	Flexor retinaculum and tubercles of scaphoid and trapezium	Lateral side of base of proximal phalanx of thumb	Median nerve (recurrent branch) (C8-T1)	Abducts thumb at metacarpophalangeal joint
Flexor pollicis brevis	Flexor retinaculum and tubercle of trapezium	Lateral side of base of proximal phalanx of thumb	Median nerve (recurrent branch) (C8-T1)	Flexes proximal phalanx of thumb
Opponens pollicis	Flexor retinaculum and tubercle of trapezium	Lateral side of first metacarpal bone	Median nerve (recurrent branch) (C8-T1)	Opposes thumb toward center of palm and rotates it medially
Adductor pollicis	Oblique head: bases of 2nd and 3rd metacarpals and capitate; Transverse head: anterior surface of body of 3rd metacarpal bone	Medial side of base of proximal phalanx of thumb	Ulnar nerve (deep branch) (C8-T1)	Adducts thumb toward middle digit
Abductor digiti minimi	Pisiform and tendon of flexor carpi ulnaris	Medial side of base of proximal phalanx of 5th digit	Ulnar nerve (deep branch) (C8-T1)	Abducts 5th digit
Flexor digiti minimi brevis	Hook of hamate and flexor retinaculum	Medial side of base of proximal phalanx of 5th digit	Ulnar nerve (deep branch) (C8-T1)	Flexes proximal phalanx of 5th digit
Opponens digiti minimi	Hook of hamate and flexor retinaculum	Palmar surface of 5th metacarpal bone	Ulnar nerve (deep branch) (C8-T1)	Draws 5th metacarpal bone anteriorly and rotates it, bringing it into opposition with thumb
Lumbricals 1 and 2	Lateral two tendons of flexor digitorum profundus	Lateral sides of extensor expansions of 2nd to 5th digits	Median nerve (C8-T1)	Flex digits at metacarpophalangeal joints and extend interphalangeal joints
Lumbricals 3 and 4	Medial three tendons of flexor digitorum profundus	Lateral sides of extensor expansions of 2nd to 5th digits	Ulnar nerve (deep branch) (C8-T1)	Flex digits at metacarpophalangeal joints and extend interphalangeal joints
Dorsal interossei	Adjacent sides of two metacarpal bones	Extensor expansions and bases of proximal phalanges of 2nd to 4th digits	Ulnar nerve (deep branch) (C8-T1)	Dorsal interossei abduct digits; flex digits at metacarpophalangeal joint and extend interphalangeal joints
Palmar interossei	Palmar surfaces of 2nd, 4th, and 5th metacarpal bones	Extensor expansions of digits and bases of proximal phalanges of 2nd, 4th, and 5th digits	Ulnar nerve (deep branch) (C8-T1)	Palmar interossei adduct digits; flex digits at metacarpophalangeal joint and extend interphalangeal joints

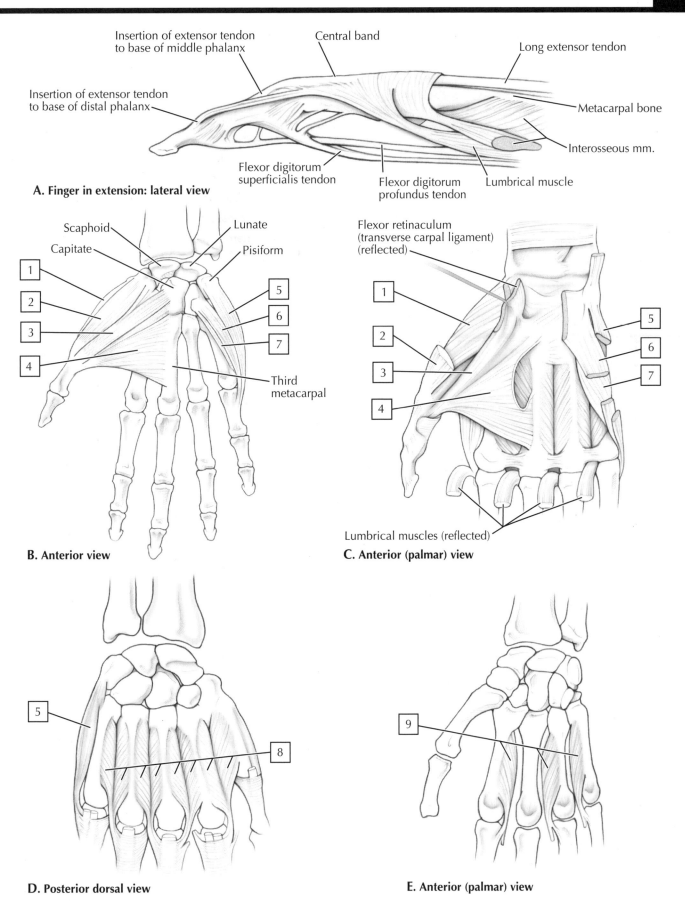

A. Finger in extension: lateral view

Insertion of extensor tendon to base of middle phalanx

Central band

Long extensor tendon

Insertion of extensor tendon to base of distal phalanx

Flexor digitorum superficialis tendon

Flexor digitorum profundus tendon

Lumbrical muscle

Metacarpal bone

Interosseous mm.

Scaphoid

Capitate

Lunate

Pisiform

Third metacarpal

B. Anterior view

Flexor retinaculum (transverse carpal ligament) (reflected)

Lumbrical muscles (reflected)

C. Anterior (palmar) view

D. Posterior dorsal view

E. Anterior (palmar) view

Summary of Upper Limb Muscles

It is best to learn the action of the muscles by knowing which **compartment** (anterior or posterior) they reside in and then knowing the primary action of the muscles in that compartment. Few muscles act in isolation; more often, they act as a group. In general, muscles of the upper back and anterior chest wall primarily act on the shoulder, muscles of the arm primarily act on the elbow (with some shoulder movement), and muscles of the forearm act primarily on the wrist and fingers. The table below summarizes some of the major muscles acting on the joints of the upper limb (this table is not comprehensive, but highlights the major muscles*).

COLOR the following muscles, using a different color for each muscle:

- ☐ 1. **Biceps brachii**
- ☐ 2. **Brachialis**
- ☐ 3. **Triceps**
- ☐ 4. **Brachioradialis**
- ☐ 5. **Extensor carpi radialis longus**
- ☐ 6. **Extensor digitorum**
- ☐ 7. **Extensor digiti minimi**
- ☐ 8. **Flexor carpi radialis**
- ☐ 9. **Flexor carpi ulnaris**
- ☐ 10. **Flexor digitorum superficialis**

SCAPULA	SHOULDER
Elevate: levator scapulae, trapezius **Depress:** pectoralis minor **Protrude:** serratus anterior **Depress glenoid:** rhomboids **Elevate glenoid:** serratus anterior, trapezius **Retract:** rhomboids, trapezius	**Flex:** pectoralis major, coracobrachialis **Extend:** latissimus dorsi, teres major **Abduct:** deltoid, supraspinatus **Adduct:** pectoralis major, latissimus dorsi **Rotate medially:** subscapularis, teres major, pectoralis major, latissimus dorsi **Rotate laterally:** infraspinatus, teres minor
ELBOW	**RADIO-ULNAR**
Flex: brachialis, biceps **Extend:** triceps, anconeus	**Pronate:** pronators (teres and quadratus) **Supinate:** supinator, biceps brachii
WRIST	**METACARPOPHALANGEAL**
Flex: flexor carpi radialis, ulnaris **Extend:** all extensor carpi muscles **Abduct:** flexor/extensor carpi radialis muscles **Adduct:** flexor and extensor carpi ulnaris **Circumduct:** combination of all movements	**Flex:** interossei and lumbricals **Extend:** extensor digitorum **Abduct:** dorsal interossei **Adduct:** palmar interossei **Circumduct:** combination of all movements
INTERPHALANGEAL-PROXIMAL	**INTERPHALANGEAL-DISTAL**
Flex: flexor digitorum superficialis **Extend:** interossei and lumbricals	**Flex:** flexor digitorum profundus **Extend:** interossei and lumbricals

*Accessory actions of muscles are detailed in the muscle tables.

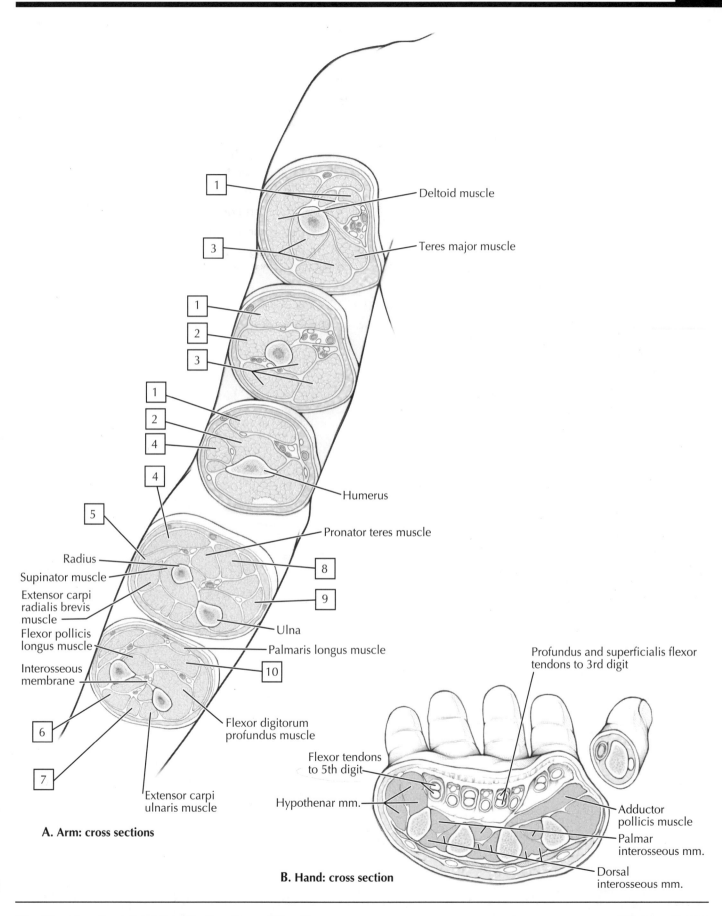

A. Arm: cross sections

Deltoid muscle

Teres major muscle

Humerus

Pronator teres muscle

Radius

Supinator muscle

Extensor carpi radialis brevis muscle

Flexor pollicis longus muscle

Interosseous membrane

Ulna

Palmaris longus muscle

Flexor digitorum profundus muscle

Extensor carpi ulnaris muscle

Profundus and superficialis flexor tendons to 3rd digit

Flexor tendons to 5th digit

Hypothenar mm.

Adductor pollicis muscle

Palmar interosseous mm.

Dorsal interosseous mm.

B. Hand: cross section

The gluteal muscles (muscles of the buttock) extend, abduct, and laterally rotate the femur (thigh bone) at the hip joint. The gluteus maximus is the strongest muscle, in total strength, in the body and is especially important in extension, where it is used to rise from a sitting position or to climb stairs (exercising this muscle on a Stairmaster exercise unit will give you "buns of steel!"). A number of other gluteal muscles lie deep to the maximus and are summarized in the table below.

COLOR the following muscles, using a different color for each muscle:

- 1. **Gluteus medius**
- 2. **Gluteus maximus**
- 3. **Gluteus minimus**
- 4. **Piriformis: arises from inside the pelvic wall off of the anterior sacrum and sacrotuberous ligament**
- 5. **Obturator internus: also arises from inside the pelvic cavity**
- 6. **Gemelli: superior and inferior heads; "Gemini" refers to these twin muscles; separated by the tendon of the obturator internus**
- 7. **Quadratus femoris**

MUSCLE	PROXIMAL ATTACHMENT (ORIGIN)	DISTAL ATTACHMENT (INSERTION)	INNERVATION	MAIN ACTIONS
Gluteus maximus	Ilium posterior to posterior gluteal line, dorsal surface of sacrum and coccyx, and sacrotuberous ligament	Most fibers end in iliotibial tract that inserts into lateral condyle of tibia; some fibers insert on gluteal tuberosity of femur	Inferior gluteal nerve (L5-S2)	Extends thigh at the hip and assists in its lateral rotation; steadies thigh and assists in raising trunk from flexed position
Gluteus medius	External surface of ilium	Lateral surface of greater trochanter	Superior gluteal nerve (L4-L5 and S1)	Abducts and medially rotates thigh at hip; steadies pelvis on limb when opposite limb is raised
Gluteus minimus	External surface of ilium	Anterior surface of greater trochanter	Superior gluteal nerve (L4-L5 and S1)	Abducts and medially rotates thigh at hip; steadies pelvis on limb when opposite limb is raised
Piriformis	Anterior surface of sacrum and sacrotuberous ligament	Superior border of greater trochanter	Branches of ventral rami S1-S2	Laterally rotates extended thigh at hip and abducts flexed thigh at hip; steadies femoral head in acetabulum
Obturator internus	Pelvic surface of obturator membrane and surrounding bones	Medial aspect of greater trochanter	Nerve to obturator internus (L5-S1)	Laterally rotates extended thigh at hip and abducts flexed thigh at hip; steadies femoral head in acetabulum
Gemelli, superior and inferior	*Superior:* ischial spine *Inferior:* ischial tuberosity	Medial aspect of greater trochanter	Superior gemellus: same nerve supply as obturator internus; inferior gemellus: same nerve supply as quadratus femoris	Laterally rotate extended thigh at the hip and abduct flexed thigh at the hip; steady femoral head in acetabulum
Quadratus femoris	Lateral border of ischial tuberosity	Quadrate tubercle on intertrochanteric crest of femur	Nerve to quadratus femoris (L5-S1)	Laterally rotates thigh at hip; steadies femoral head in acetabulum

Clinical Note:

Weakness or paralysis of the gluteus medius and minimus muscles can lead to an unstable pelvis, because these muscles stabilize the pelvis while walking by abducting and keeping the pelvis level when the opposite foot is off the ground and in its swing phase. If weakened, the pelvis becomes unstable during walking and tilts to the unaffected side.

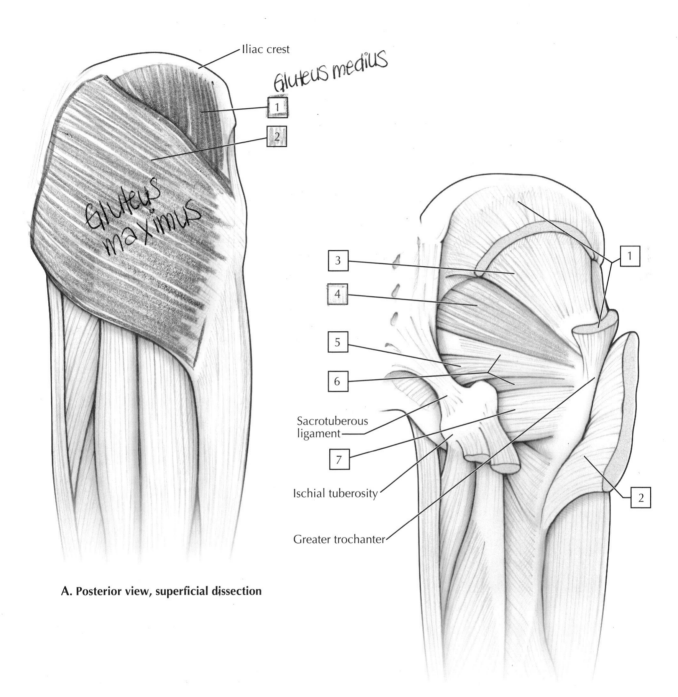

Iliac crest

Gluteus medius

1

2

Gluteus maximus

A. Posterior view, superficial dissection

3

4

5

6

Sacrotuberous ligament

7

Ischial tuberosity

Greater trochanter

1

2

B. Posterior view, deeper dissection

The thigh is divided into three muscle compartments by connective tissue intermuscular septae. The muscles of the posterior compartment primarily extend the hip and flex the knee. Three of the four muscles in this compartment comprise the hamstrings:

COLOR the following muscles, using a different color for each muscle:

- [ ] 1. **Semitendinosus**
- [ ] 2. **Semimembranosus**
- [ ] 3. **Biceps femoris, short head (not a hamstring muscle)**
- [ ] 4. **Biceps femoris, long head**

These muscles all arise from the ischial tuberosity, and both extend the hip and flex the knee. The short head of the biceps femoris is not a hamstring muscle and primarily flexes the knee. These muscles are summarized in the table below.

Clinical Note:

The **hamstrings** cross two joints, extending at the hip and flexing at the knee. Hence, it is important to warm these muscles up before rigorous exercise by stretching the muscles, getting adequate blood flow into the muscle tissue and activating the muscle fiber units.

MUSCLE	PROXIMAL ATTACHMENT (ORIGIN)	DISTAL ATTACHMENT (INSERTION)	INNERVATION	MAIN ACTIONS
Semitendinosus	Ischial tuberosity	Medial surface of superior part of tibia	Tibial division of sciatic nerve (L2-S2)	Extends thigh at hip; flexes leg at knee and rotates it medially; with flexed hip and knee, extends trunk
Semimembranosus	Ischial tuberosity	Posterior part of medial condyle of tibia	Tibial division of sciatic nerve (L5-S2)	Extends thigh at hip; flexes leg at knee and rotates it medially; with flexed hip and knee, extends trunk
Biceps femoris	*Long head:* ischial tuberosity *Short head:* linea aspera and lateral supracondylar line of femur	Lateral side of head of fibula; tendon at this site split by fibular collateral ligament of knee	*Long head:* tibial division of sciatic nerve (L5-S2) *Short head:* common fibular (peroneal) division of sciatic nerve (L5-S2)	Flexes leg at knee and rotates it laterally; extends thigh at hip e.g., when starting to walk (long head only)

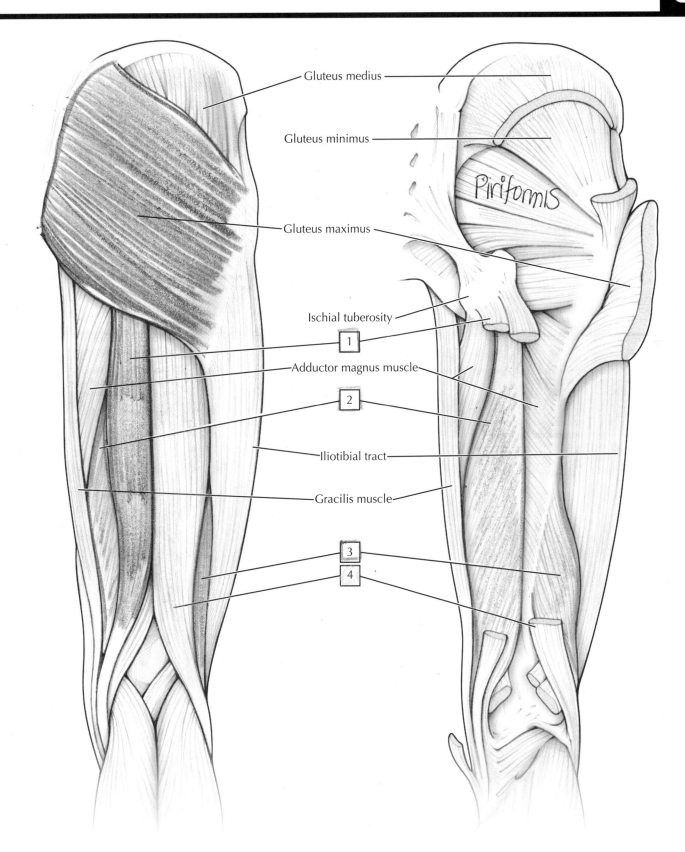

Gluteus medius

Gluteus minimus

Piriformis

Gluteus maximus

Ischial tuberosity

1

Adductor magnus muscle

2

Iliotibial tract

Gracilis muscle

3

4

A. Posterior view, superficial dissection

B. Posterior view, deeper dissection

The thigh is divided into three muscle compartments by connective tissue intermuscular septae. The muscles of the anterior compartment primarily extend the knee, although several muscles cross both the hip and knee and act on both joints. Additionally, two muscles of the posterior abdominal wall, the psoas and iliacus (iliopsoas) pass into the upper thigh and are the most powerful flexors of the hip joint (see Plate 3-14). The anterior thigh muscles are summarized in the table below.

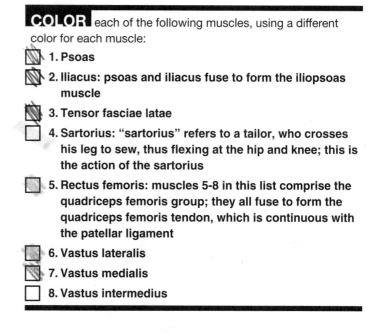

COLOR each of the following muscles, using a different color for each muscle:

1. **Psoas**
2. **Iliacus:** psoas and iliacus fuse to form the iliopsoas muscle
3. **Tensor fasciae latae**
4. **Sartorius:** "sartorius" refers to a tailor, who crosses his leg to sew, thus flexing at the hip and knee; this is the action of the sartorius
5. **Rectus femoris:** muscles 5-8 in this list comprise the quadriceps femoris group; they all fuse to form the quadriceps femoris tendon, which is continuous with the patellar ligament
6. **Vastus lateralis**
7. **Vastus medialis**
8. **Vastus intermedius**

MUSCLE	PROXIMAL ATTACHMENT (ORIGIN)	DISTAL ATTACHMENT (INSERTION)	INNERVATION	MAIN ACTIONS
Tensor fasciae latae	Anterior superior iliac spine and anterior iliac crest	Iliotibial tract that attaches to lateral condyle of tibia	Superior gluteal nerve (L4-S1)	Abducts, medially rotates, and flexes thigh at hip; helps keep knee extended
Sartorius	Anterior superior iliac spine and superior part of notch inferior to it	Superior part of medial surface of tibia	Femoral nerve (L2-L4)	Flexes, abducts, and laterally rotates thigh at hip joint; flexes knee joint
Quadriceps Femoris				
Rectus femoris	Anterior inferior iliac spine and ilium superior to acetabulum	Base of patella and by patellar ligament to tibial tuberosity	Femoral nerve (L2-L4)	Extends leg at knee joint; rectus femoris also steadies hip joint and helps iliopsoas flex thigh at hip
Vastus lateralis	Greater trochanter and lateral lip of linea aspera of femur	Base of patella and by patellar ligament to tibial tuberosity	Femoral nerve (L2-L4)	Extends leg at knee joint
Vastus medialis	Intertrochanteric line and medial lip of linea aspera of femur	Base of patella and by patellar ligament to tibial tuberosity	Femoral nerve (L2-L4)	Extends leg at the knee joint
Vastus intermedius	Anterior and lateral surfaces of femoral shaft	Base of patella and by patellar ligament to tibial tuberosity	Femoral nerve (L2-L4)	Extends the leg at knee joint

Clinical Note:

Tapping the patellar **ligament** with a reflex hammer elicits the patellar reflex, causing the flexed knee to jerk upward in extension. This maneuver tests the integrity of the muscle and its innervation by the femoral nerve.

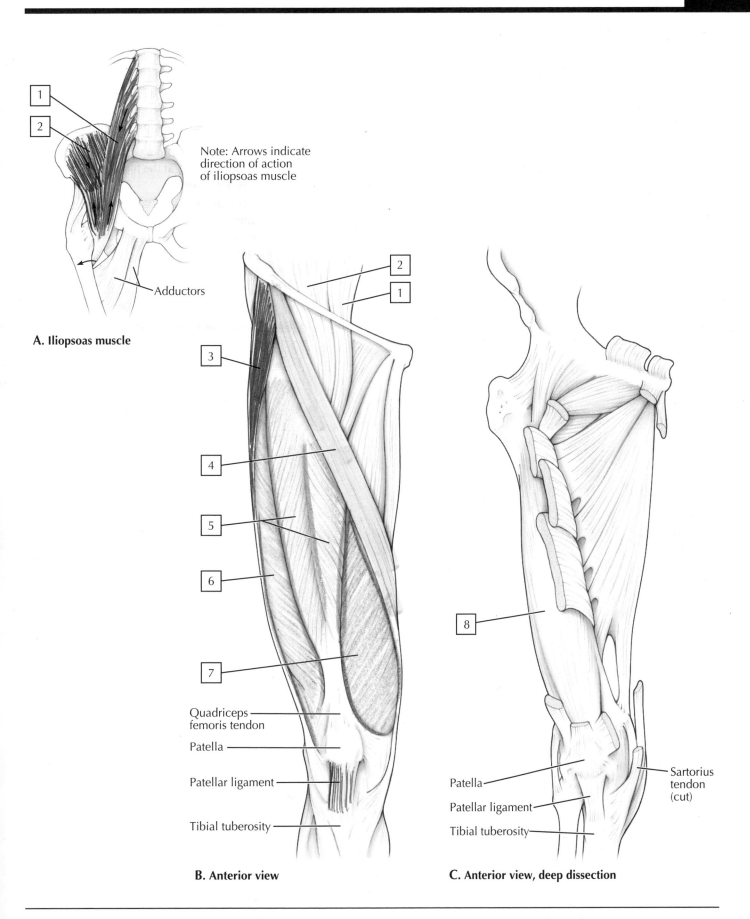

Note: Arrows indicate
direction of action
of iliopsoas muscle

Adductors

A. Iliopsoas muscle

Quadriceps
femoris tendon

Patella

Patellar ligament

Tibial tuberosity

B. Anterior view

Patella

Patellar ligament

Tibial tuberosity

Sartorius
tendon
(cut)

C. Anterior view, deep dissection

The thigh is divided into three muscle compartments by connective tissue intermuscular septae. The muscles of the medial compartment primarily adduct the lower limb at the hip. Several muscles cross both the hip and knee joints and act on both joints. These muscles are summarized in the table below.

COLOR the following muscles, using a different color for each muscle:

☐ 1. **Pectineus**

☐ 2. **Adductor longus**

☐ 3. **Gracilis**

☐ 4. **Adductor brevis:** lies deep to the adductor longus (cut in illustration)

☐ 5. **Obturator externus:** lies very deep in the thigh

☐ 6. **Adductor magnus:** the most powerful adductor of the hip

MUSCLE	PROXIMAL ATTACHMENT (ORIGIN)	DISTAL ATTACHMENT (INSERTION)	INNERVATION	MAIN ACTIONS
Pectineus	Superior ramus of pubis	Pectineal line of femur, just inferior to lesser trochanter	Femoral nerve; may receive a branch from obturator nerve (L2-L4)	Adducts and flexes thigh at hip; assists with medial rotation of thigh
Adductor longus	Body of pubis inferior to pubic crest	Middle third of linea aspera of femur	Obturator nerve (L2-L4)	Adducts and medially rotates thigh at hip
Adductor brevis	Body and inferior ramus of pubis	Pectineal line and proximal part of linea aspera of femur	Obturator nerve (L2-L4)	Adducts thigh at hip and to some extent flexes it
Adductor magnus	Inferior ramus of pubis, ramus of ischium, and ischial tuberosity	Gluteal tuberosity, linea aspera, medial supracondylar line (adductor part), and adductor tubercle of femur (hamstring part)	*Adductor part:* obturator nerve (L2-L4) *Hamstring part:* tibial part of sciatic nerve	Adducts thigh at hip; *Adductor part:* also flexes thigh at hip; *Hamstring part:* extends thigh
Gracilis	Body and inferior ramus of pubis	Superior part of medial surface of tibia	Obturator nerve (L2-L3)	Adducts thigh at hip, flexes leg at knee and helps rotate it medially
Obturator externus	Margins of obturator foramen and obturator membrane	Trochanteric fossa of femur	Obturator nerve (L3-L4)	Rotates thigh laterally at hip; steadies femoral head in acetabulum

Clinical Note:

A "**groin pull**" is a common athletic injury and is a stretching or tearing of one or more of the adductor muscles in the medial compartment of the thigh. The adductor longus and magnus are especially vulnerable.

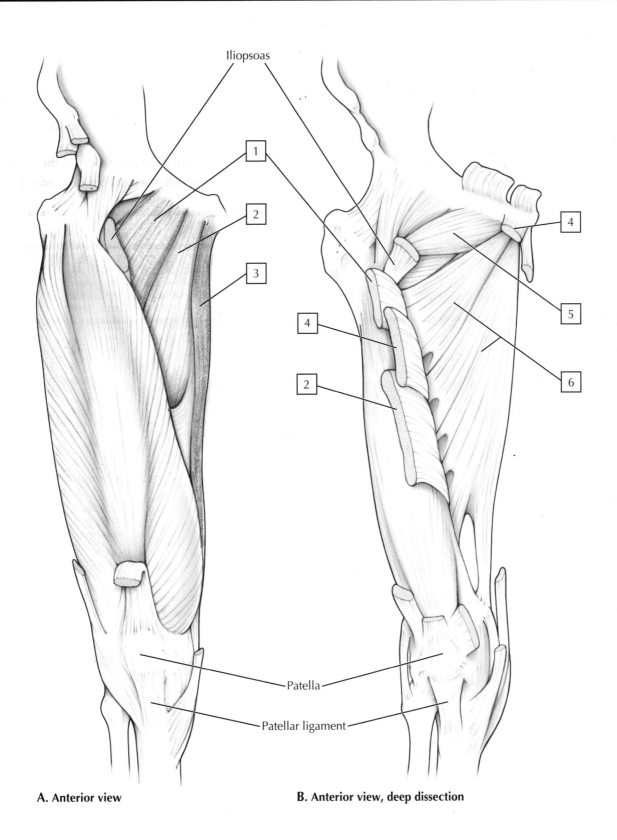

Iliopsoas

1

2

3

4

5

4

2

6

Patella

Patellar ligament

A. Anterior view

B. Anterior view, deep dissection

The leg is divided into three muscle compartments by connective tissue intermuscular septae. The muscles of the **anterior compartment:**

- Dorsiflex the foot at the ankle joint
- Extend the toes
- Invert (turn the sole inward) the foot

Realize that the muscles of the lower limb are just the reverse of the upper limb. Lower limb flexors are in the **posterior** compartments (anterior compartment in the upper limb) and extensors are in the **anterior** compartments (posterior compartment in the upper limb). This arrangement occurs because of the different way the limbs rotate during embryonic development.

The muscles of the **lateral compartment** primarily evert (turn the sole outward) the foot. The muscles of these two compartments are summarized in the table below.

COLOR the following muscles, using a different color for each muscle:

 1. **Fibularis longus:** the tendon crosses deep within the sole and inserts into the 1st metatarsal

 2. **Tibialis anterior**

 3. **Fibularis brevis:** the tendon inserts into the 5th metatarsal

 4. **Extensor digitorum longus**

☐ 5. **Extensor hallucis longus** ("hallucis" refers to the big toe)

☐ 6. **Fibularis tertius:** tendon only; muscle deep to extensor digitorum longus

MUSCLE	PROXIMAL ATTACHMENT (ORIGIN)	DISTAL ATTACHMENT (INSERTION)	INNERVATION	MAIN ACTIONS
Tibialis anterior	Lateral condyle and superior half of lateral surface of tibia	Medial and inferior surfaces of medial cuneiform and base of first metatarsal	Deep fibular (peroneal) nerve (L4-L5)	Dorsiflexes foot at ankle and inverts foot
Extensor hallucis longus	Middle part of anterior surface of fibula and interosseous membrane	Dorsal aspect of base of distal phalanx of great toe	Deep fibular (peroneal) nerve (L5-S1)	Extends great toe and dorsiflexes foot at ankle
Extensor digitorum longus	Lateral condyle of tibia and superior three fourths of anterior surface of interosseous membrane and fibula	Middle and distal phalanges of lateral four digits	Deep fibular (peroneal) nerve (L5-S1)	Extends lateral four digits and dorsiflexes foot at ankle
Fibularis (peroneus) tertius	Inferior third of anterior surface of fibula and interosseous membrane	Dorsum of base of 5th metatarsal	Deep fibular (peroneal) nerve (L5-S1)	Dorsiflexes foot at ankle and aids in eversion of foot
Fibularis (peroneus) longus	Head and superior two thirds of lateral surface of fibula	Base of first metatarsal and medial cuneiform	Superficial fibular (peroneal) nerve (L5-S2)	Everts foot and weakly plantarflexes foot at ankle
Fibularis (peroneus) brevis	Inferior two thirds of lateral surface of fibula	Dorsal aspect of tuberosity on lateral side of 5th metatarsal	Superficial fibular (peroneal) nerve (L5-S2)	Everts foot and weakly plantarflexes foot at ankle

Clinical Note:

Anterior compartment syndrome (sometimes called **anterior shin splints**) occurs from excessive contraction of anterior compartment muscles. The pain over these muscles radiates down the ankle and onto the dorsum of the foot overlying the extensor tendons. This condition is usually chronic and swelling of the muscle in the tightly ensheathed muscular compartment may lead to nerve and vascular compression. In the acute syndrome (rapid, unrelenting swelling), the compartment may have to be opened surgically (fasciotomy) to relieve the pressure.

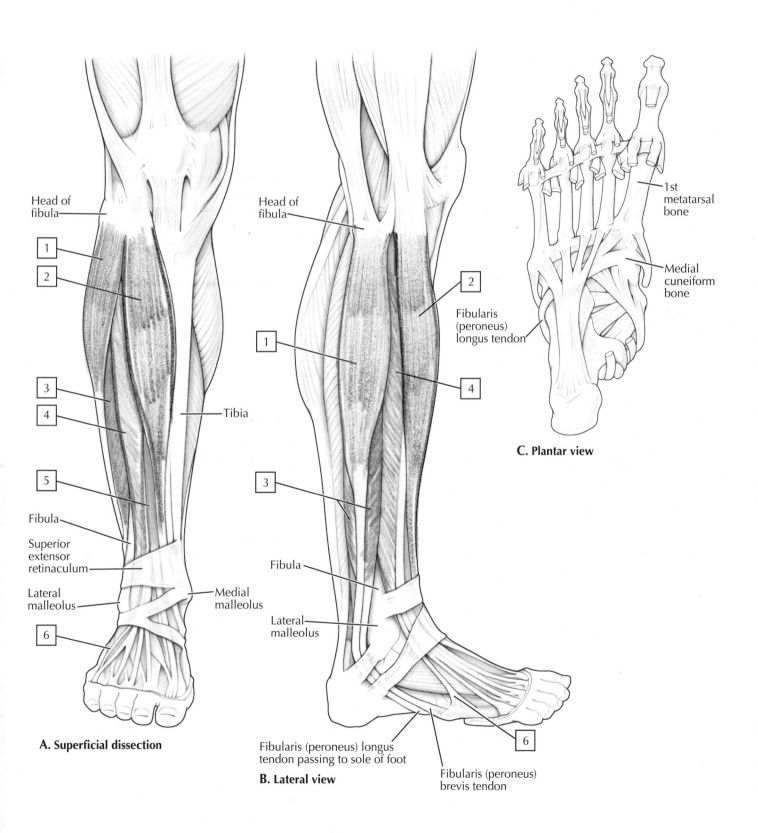

Head of
fibula

1

2

3

4

5

Fibula

Superior
extensor
retinaculum

Lateral
malleolus

6

A. Superficial dissection

Head of
fibula

2

1

Fibularis
(peroneus)
longus tendon

4

3

Fibula

Lateral
malleolus

6

Fibularis (peroneus) longus
tendon passing to sole of foot

B. Lateral view

Fibularis (peroneus)
brevis tendon

Tibia

Medial
malleolus

1st
metatarsal
bone

Medial
cuneiform
bone

C. Plantar view

The leg is divided into three muscle compartments by connective tissue intermuscular septae. The muscles of the posterior compartment:

- Plantarflex the foot at the ankle joint
- Flex the toes
- Invert (turn the sole inward) the foot

The muscles of the posterior compartment are arranged into a superficial and a deep group. The superficial group of muscles all merge their tendons of insertion into a strong calcaneal (Achilles) tendon that attaches to the heel (calcaneal tuberosity). These muscles are summarized in the table below.

COLOR the following muscles, using a different color for each muscle:

☐ 1. Plantaris (muscles 1-3 of this list comprise the superficial group)

☐ 2. Gastrocnemius: lateral and medial heads, the "calf" muscle

☐ 3. Soleus

☐ 4. Popliteus

☐ 5. Flexor digitorum longus

☐ 6. Tibialis posterior

☐ 7. Flexor hallucis longus ("hallucis" refers to the big toe)

MUSCLE	PROXIMAL ATTACHMENT (ORIGIN)	DISTAL ATTACHMENT (INSERTION)	INNERVATION	MAIN ACTIONS
Gastrocnemius	*Lateral head:* lateral aspect of lateral condyle of femur *Medial head:* popliteal surface of femur, superior to medial condyle	Posterior aspect of calcaneus via calcaneal tendon	Tibial nerve (S1-S2)	Plantarflexes foot at ankle; raises heel during walking; flexes leg at knee joint
Soleus	Posterior aspect of head of fibula, superior fourth of posterior surface of fibula, soleal line, and medial border or tibia	Posterior aspect of calcaneus via calcaneal tendon	Tibial nerve (S1-S2)	Plantarflexes foot at ankle; steadies leg on foot
Plantaris	Inferior end of lateral supracondylar line of femur and oblique popliteal ligament	Posterior aspect of calcaneus via calcaneal tendon (tendo calcaneus)	Tibial nerve (S1-S2)	Weakly assists gastrocnemius in plantarflexing foot at ankle and flexing knee
Popliteus	Lateral epicondyle of femur and lateral meniscus	Posterior surface of tibia, superior to soleal line	Tibial nerve (L4-S1)	Weakly flexes leg at knee and unlocks it
Flexor hallucis longus	Inferior two thirds of posterior surface of fibula and inferior interosseous membrane	Base of distal phalanx of great toe (big toe)	Tibial nerve (S2-S3)	Flexes great toe at all joints and weakly plantarflexes foot at ankle; supports longitudinal arches of foot
Flexor digitorum longus	Medial part of posterior surface of tibia inferior to soleal line, and from fascia covering tibialis posterior	Bases of distal phalanges of lateral four digits	Tibial nerve (S2-S3)	Flexes lateral four digits and plantarflexes foot at ankle; supports longitudinal arch of foot
Tibialis posterior	Interosseous membrane, posterior surface of tibia inferior to soleal line, and posterior surface of fibula	Tuberosity of navicular, cuneiform, and cuboid and bases of metatarsals 2, 3, and 4	Tibial nerve (L4-L5)	Plantarflexes foot at ankle and inverts foot

Clinical Note:
"Shin splints" refers to pain along the inner distal two thirds of the tibial shaft and is a common syndrome in athletes. The primary cause is repetitive pulling of the tibialis posterior tendon as one pushes off the foot during running.

Tendinitis of the calcaneal (Achilles) tendon is a painful inflammation that often occurs in runners who run on hills or uneven surfaces. Repetitive stress on the tendon occurs as the heel strikes the ground and when plantarflexion lifts the foot and toes. This is the strongest muscle tendon in the body. Rupture of the tendon is a serious injury, because the avascular tendon heals slowly. In general, most tendon injuries heal more slowly because of their avascular nature.

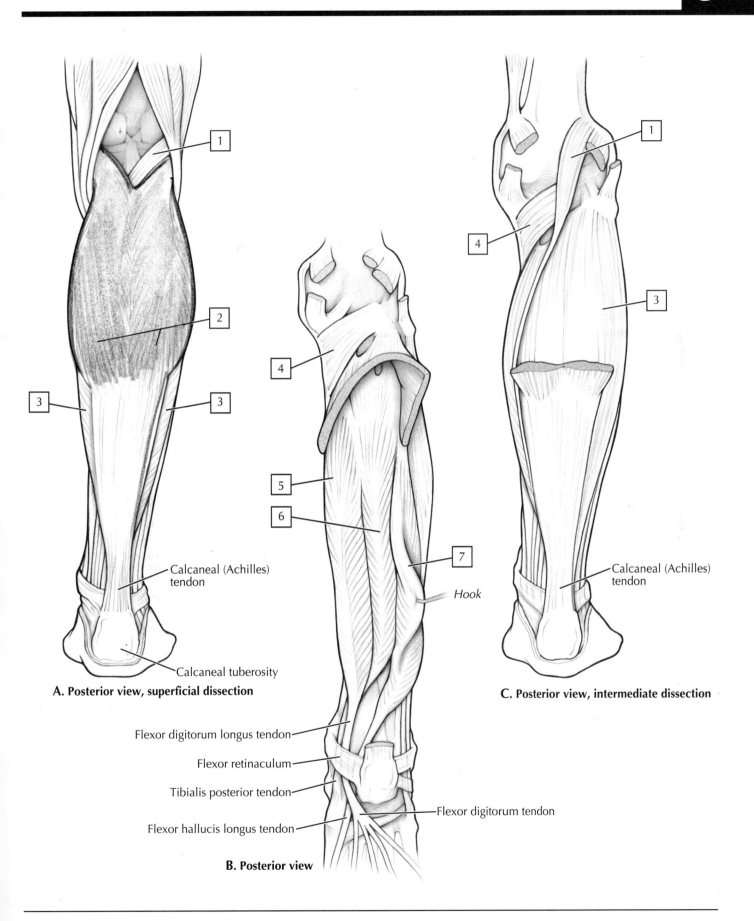

A. Posterior view, superficial dissection

Calcaneal (Achilles) tendon

Calcaneal tuberosity

B. Posterior view

Flexor digitorum longus tendon

Flexor retinaculum

Tibialis posterior tendon

Flexor hallucis longus tendon

Flexor digitorum tendon

Hook

C. Posterior view, intermediate dissection

Calcaneal (Achilles) tendon

Plate 3-30

The intrinsic muscles are arranged in four layers on the sole of the foot and complement the actions of the leg long flexor tendons as they pass into the foot. These muscles are summarized in the table below.

MUSCLE	PROXIMAL ATTACHMENT (ORIGIN)	DISTAL ATTACHMENT (INSERTION)	INNERVATION	MAIN ACTIONS
Abductor hallucis	Medial tubercle of tuberosity of calcaneus, flexor retinaculum, and plantar aponeurosis	Medial aspect of base of proximal phalanx of 1st digit	Medial plantar nerve (S1-S3)	Abducts and flexes great toe at metacarpophalangeal joint
Flexor digitorum brevis	Medial tubercle of tuberosity of calcaneus, plantar aponeurosis, and intermuscular septa	Both sides of middle phalanges of lateral four digits	Medial plantar nerve (S1-S3)	Flexes lateral four digits at interphalangeal joints
Abductor digiti minimi	Medial and lateral tubercles of tuberosity of calcaneus, plantar aponeurosis, and intermuscular septa	Lateral aspect of base of proximal phalanx of 5th digit	Lateral plantar nerve (S1-S3)	Abducts and flexes little toe
Quadratus plantae	Medial aspect and lateral margin of plantar surface of calcaneus	Posterolateral margin of tendon of flexor digitorum longus	Lateral plantar nerve (S1-S3)	Assists flexor digitorum longus in flexing lateral four digits
Lumbricals	Tendons of flexor digitorum longus	Medial aspect of expansion over lateral four digits	*Medial one:* medial plantar nerve *Lateral three:* lateral plantar nerve (S2-S3)	Flex proximal phalanges and extend middle and distal phalanges of lateral four digits
Flexor hallucis brevis	Plantar surfaces of cuboid and lateral cuneiforms	Both sides of base of proximal phalanx of 1st digit	Medial plantar nerve (S1-S2)	Flexes proximal phalanx of great toe
Adductor hallucis	*Oblique head:* bases of metatarsals 2-4 *Transverse head:* plantar ligaments of metatarsophalangeal joints	Tendons of both heads attach to lateral side of base of proximal phalanx of 1st digit	Deep branch of lateral plantar nerve (S2-S3)	Adducts great toe; assists in maintaining transverse arch of foot
Flexor digiti minimi brevis	Base of 5th metatarsal	Base of proximal phalanx of 5th digit	Superficial branch of lateral plantar nerve (S2-S3)	Flexes proximal phalanx of little toe, thereby assisting with its flexion
Plantar interossei (3 muscles)	Bases and medial sides of metatarsals 3-5	Medial sides of bases of proximal phalanges of digits 3-5	Lateral plantar nerve (S2-S3)	Adduct digits (2-4) and flex metatarsophalangeal joints
Dorsal interossei (4 muscles)	Adjacent sides of metatarsals 1-5	*First:* medial side of proximal phalanx of 2nd digit *Second to fourth:* lateral sides of digits 2-4	Lateral plantar nerve (S2-S3)	Abduct digits and flex metatarsophalangeal joints

COLOR the following muscles, using a different color for each muscle (the muscles of the sole are organized into several layers beneath a tough plantar aponeurosis, as seen in the illustrations):

☐ 1. **Flexor digiti minimi brevis**

☐ 2. **Abductor digiti minimi**

☐ 3. **Lumbricals: four small muscles that attach to the long flexor tendons**

☐ 4. **Flexor hallucis brevis: has two heads whose tendons contain two small sesamoid bones**

☐ 5. **Abductor hallucis**

☐ 6. **Flexor digitorum brevis**

☐ 7. **Quadratus plantae**

☐ 8. **Plantar interossei: three muscles that adduct the toes, PAD**

☐ 9. **Adductor hallucis: has two heads (transverse and oblique)**

☐ 10. **Dorsal interossei: four muscles that abduct the toes, DAB**

Clinical Note:
Just beneath the skin of the sole of the foot and overlying the superficial layer of intrinsic muscles lies the plantar aponeurosis, a broad, flat tendon that stretches from the heel to the toes. **Plantar fasciitis** is a common cause of heel pain, especially in joggers, and results from inflammation of the plantar aponeurosis at its point of attachment for the calcaneus, with pain often radiating distally toward the toes.

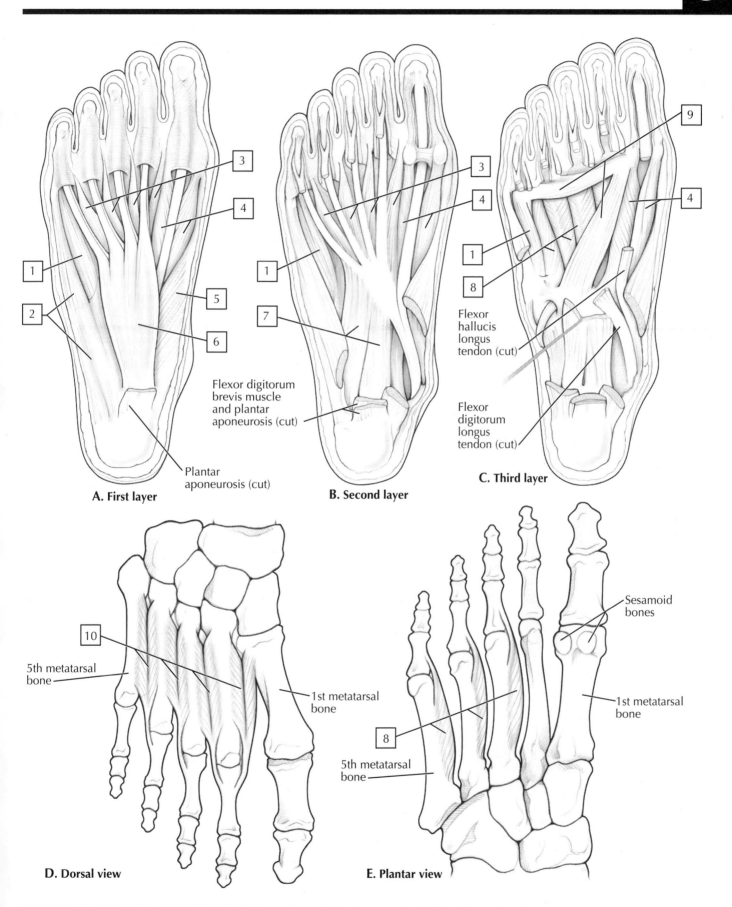

A. First layer

3

4

1

2

5

6

Plantar
aponeurosis (cut)

B. Second layer

3

4

1

7

Flexor digitorum
brevis muscle
and plantar
aponeurosis (cut)

C. Third layer

9

4

1

8

Flexor
hallucis
longus
tendon (cut)

Flexor
digitorum
longus
tendon (cut)

D. Dorsal view

10

5th metatarsal
bone

1st metatarsal
bone

E. Plantar view

Sesamoid
bones

1st metatarsal
bone

8

5th metatarsal
bone

It is best to learn the action of the muscles by knowing which **compartment** they reside in and then knowing the primary action of the muscles in that compartment. Few muscles act in isolation; more often, they act as a group. Generally, muscles of the gluteal region extend the hip, abduct the limb, and rotate it. Muscles of the anterior thigh act on the knee to extend it, whereas the muscles of the medial thigh adduct the limb at the hip. Muscles of the posterior thigh extend the hip and flex the knee. Muscles of the lateral leg evert the foot, muscles of the anterior leg dorsiflex the ankle and extend the toes, whereas muscles of the posterior leg plantarflex the ankle and flex the toes.

HIP	KNEE
Flex: iliopsoas, rectus femoris, sartorius	**Flex:** hamstrings, gracilis, sartorius, gastrocnemius
Extend: hamstrings, gluteus maximus	**Extend:** quadriceps femoris
Abduct: gluteus medius and minimus, tensor fasciae latae	**Rotate medially:** semitendinosus, semimembranosus
Rotate medially: gluteus medius and minimus	**Rotate laterally:** biceps femoris
Rotate laterally: obturator internus, gemelli, piriformis	
Adduct: adductor group of muscles	

ANKLE	METATARSOPHALANGEAL
Plantarflex: gastrocnemius, soleus, tibialis posterior, flexor digitorum longus, flexor hallucis longus	**Flex:** interossei and lumbricals
	Extend: extensor digitorum longus, brevis
Dorsiflex: tibialis anterior, extensor digitorum longus, extensor hallucis longus, fibularis tertius	**Abduct:** dorsal interossei
	Adduct: plantar interossei

INTERPHALANGEAL	INTERTARSAL
Flex: flexor digitorum longus, brevis	**Evert:** fibularis longus, brevis, tertius
Extend: extensor digitorum longus, brevis	**Invert:** tibialis anterior and posterior

COLOR the following muscles, using a different color for each muscle:

☐ 1. **Rectus femoris**
☐ 2. **Sartorius**
☐ 3. **Gracilis**
☐ 4. **Adductor magnus**
☐ 5. **Tibialis anterior**
☐ 6. **Soleus**
☐ 7. **Tibialis posterior**
☐ 8. **Fibularis longus**
☐ 9. **Adductor hallucis**
☐ 10. **Abductor digiti minimi**

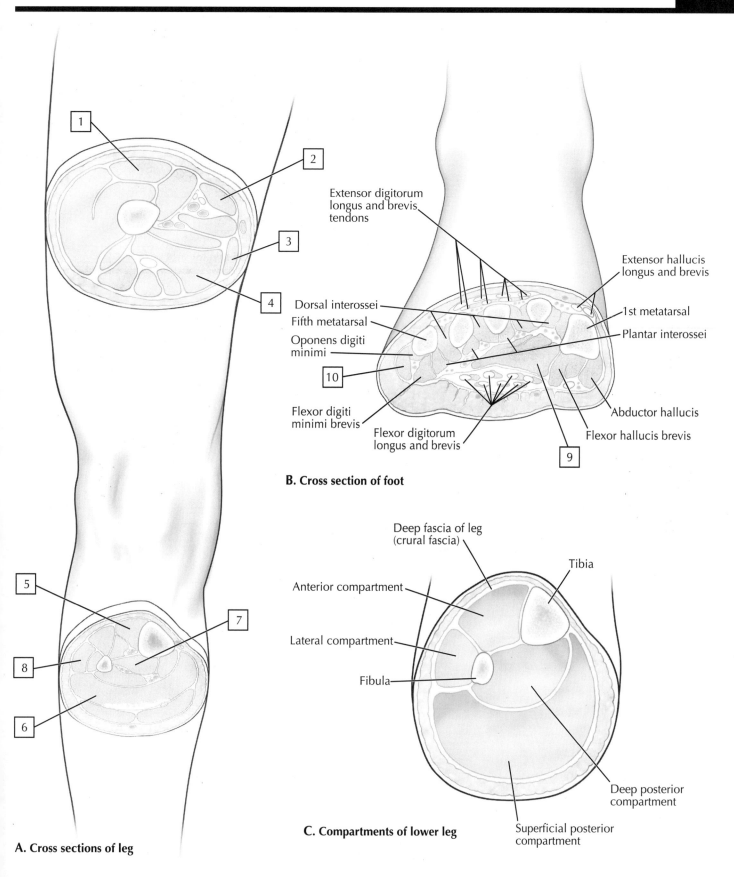

Extensor digitorum
longus and brevis
tendons

Extensor hallucis
longus and brevis

Dorsal interossei

Fifth metatarsal

1st metatarsal

Oponens digiti
minimi

Plantar interossei

Flexor digiti
minimi brevis

Abductor hallucis

Flexor digitorum
longus and brevis

Flexor hallucis brevis

B. Cross section of foot

Deep fascia of leg
(crural fascia)

Tibia

Anterior compartment

Lateral compartment

Fibula

Deep posterior
compartment

Superficial posterior
compartment

C. Compartments of lower leg

A. Cross sections of leg

1. Why might a patient with Bell's palsy (unilateral facial nerve inflammation) be unable to close his or her ipsilateral eye?
   _____

2. Which muscle might be paralyzed if, during an eye exam (clinical testing), an inability to adduct and depress the eyeball was demonstrated? _____

3. What are the three muscles that line the posterior wall of the pharynx and assist in swallowing? _____
   _____

4. The deep intrinsic muscles of the back innervated by a dorsal ramus of the spinal nerve include which of the following muscle groups?
   A. Erector spinae _____
   B. Latissimus dorsi _____
   C. Levator scapulae_____
   D. Rhomboid major_____
   E. Serratus posterior inferior _____

5. A hernia occurs in the groin region and a portion of bowel and mesentery descends into the scrotum. This patient most likely has which of the following types of hernias?
   A. Femoral _____
   B. Direct inguinal _____
   C. Hiatal _____
   D. Indirect inguinal _____
   E. Umbilical _____

6. An athlete suffers a rotator cuff injury. Which of the following muscles is most likely torn?
   A. Infraspinatus _____
   B. Subscapularis _____
   C. Supraspinatus _____
   D. Teres major _____
   E. Teres minor _____

7. A groin pull injury would most likely involve which of the following muscles?
   A. Adductor longus _____
   B. Rectus femoris _____
   C. Sartorius _____
   D. Semitendinosus _____
   E. Vastus medialis _____

Color each muscle described below:

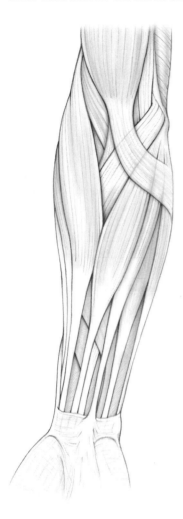

8. This muscle is absent in a small percentage of the population (color it red).

9. This muscle is innervated by the radial nerve (color it blue).

10. This muscle flexes the wrist and is innervated by the ulnar nerve (color it green).

7. A

8. Palmaris longus muscle

9. Brachioradialis muscle

10. Flexor carpi ulnaris muscle

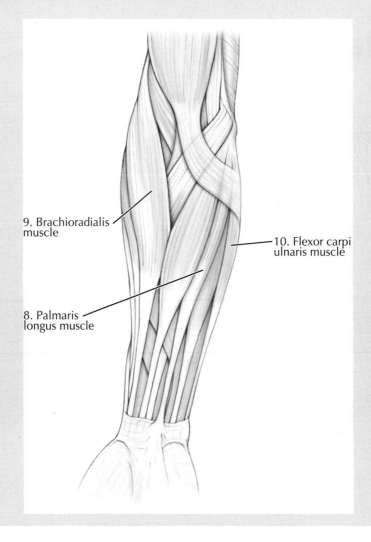

9. Brachioradialis
muscle

10. Flexor carpi
ulnaris muscle

8. Palmaris
longus muscle

Chapter 4 **Nervous System**

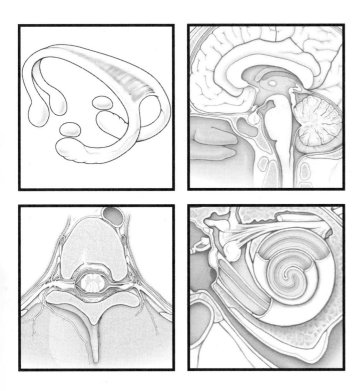

Nerve cells are called neurons and their structure reflects the functional characteristics of an individual neuron. Information comes to the neuron largely via processes called **axons**, which terminate on the neuron at specialized junctions called **synapses**. Synapses can occur on neuronal processes called **dendrites** or on the neuronal cell body, called a **soma** or **perikaryon**.

COLOR each of the following features of a neuron, using a different color for each feature:

☐ **1. Dendrites**

☐ **2. Axon**

☐ **3. Soma, or cell body of the neuron**

Neurons convey efferent information via action potentials that course along a single axon arising from the soma that then synapses on a selective target, usually another neuron or target cell, for example muscle cells. There are many different types of neurons, and some of the more common types include:

• **Unipolar (often called pseudounipolar)**: one axon that divides into two long processes; usually sensory neurons

• **Bipolar**: possesses one axon and one dendrite; rare, but found in the retina and olfactory epithelium

• **Multipolar**: possesses one axon and two or more dendrites; most common

COLOR each different type of neuron, using a different color for each type:

☐ **4. Unipolar (pseudounipolar)**

☐ **5. Bipolar**

☐ **6. Multipolar**

Although the human nervous system contains more than 10 billion neurons (a very rough estimate), they can be classified largely into one of three functional types:

• **Motor neurons**: convey efferent impulses from the central nervous system (CNS) or ganglia (collections of neurons outside the CNS) to target (effector) cells; somatic efferent axons target skeletal muscle, and visceral efferent axons target smooth muscle, cardiac muscle, and glands

• **Sensory neurons**: convey afferent impulses from receptors to the CNS; somatic afferent axons convey pain, temperature, touch, pressure, and proprioception (nonconscious) sensations, and visceral afferent axons convey pain and other sensations (e.g., nausea) from organs, glands, and smooth muscle to the CNS

• **Interneurons**: convey impulses between sensory and motor neurons, thus forming integrating networks between cells; interneurons probably comprise more than 99% of all neurons in the body

Neurons can vary considerably in size, ranging from several micrometers to over 100 μm in diameter. They may possess numerous branching dendrites, studded with **dendritic spines** that increase the receptive area of the neuron manyfold. The neuron's axon may be quite short or over a meter long, and the axonal diameter may vary, with axons that are larger than 1 to 2 μm in diameter being insulated by **myelin sheaths**. In the CNS, axons are myelinated by a special glial cell called an **oligodendrocyte**, whereas all the axons in the peripheral nervous system (PNS) are surrounded by a type of glia cell called **Schwann cells**. Schwann cells also myelinate many of the PNS axons they surround.

Plate 4-1   **Nervous System**

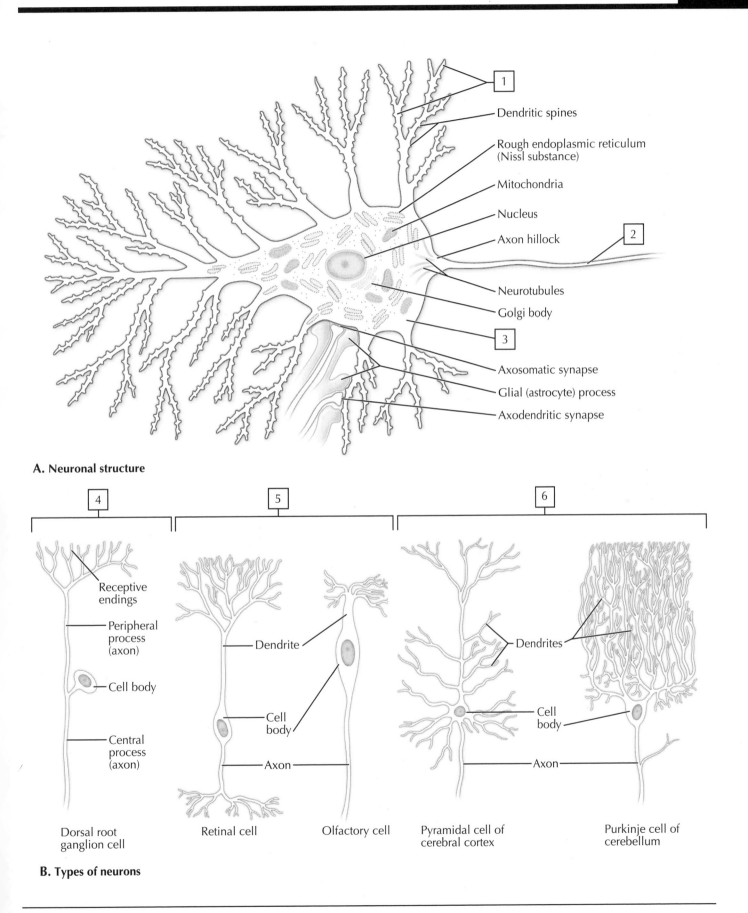

Dendritic spines

Rough endoplasmic reticulum (Nissl substance)

Mitochondria

Nucleus

Axon hillock

Neurotubules

Golgi body

Axosomatic synapse

Glial (astrocyte) process

Axodendritic synapse

A. Neuronal structure

Receptive endings

Peripheral process (axon)

Cell body

Central process (axon)

Dendrite

Cell body

Axon

Dendrites

Cell body

Axon

Dorsal root ganglion cell

Retinal cell

Olfactory cell

Pyramidal cell of cerebral cortex

Purkinje cell of cerebellum

B. Types of neurons

Glia are the cells that support neurons, both within the CNS (the neuroglia) and within the PNS. Glial cells far outnumber the neurons in the nervous system and, along with myelination of new axons, contribute to most of the postnatal growth seen in the CNS. Functionally, glia:

- Provide structural isolation of neurons and their synapses
- Sequester ions in the extracellular compartment
- Provide trophic support to the neurons and their processes
- Support growth and secrete growth factors
- Support some of the signaling functions of neurons
- Myelinate axons
- Phagocytize debris and participate in inflammatory responses
- Participate in the formation of the blood-brain barrier

The different types of glial cells include the:

- **Astrocytes**: the most numerous of the glial cells, they provide physical and metabolic support for CNS neurons, and contribute to the formation of the blood-brain barrier
- **Oligodendrocytes**: smaller glial cells that are responsible for the formation and maintenance of myelin in the CNS
- **Microglia**: smallest and most rare of the CNS glia (still more numerous than neurons in the CNS!), they are phagocytic cells and participate in inflammatory reactions
- **Ependymal cells**: line the ventricles of the brain and the central canal of the spinal cord that contain cerebrospinal fluid (CSF)
- **Schwann cells**: glial cells of the PNS, they surround all axons, myelinating many of them, and provide trophic support, facilitate regrowth of PNS axons, and clean away cellular debris

While ependymal cells line the brain's ventricles, the surface of the brain and spinal cord is lined by the pia mater.

COLOR each of the different types of CNS glia, using a different color for each glial cell:

- [ ] 1. Astrocytes
- [ ] 2. Oligodendrocyte (with myelinating processes)
- [ ] 3. Microglial cell
- [ ] 4. Ependymal cells

Clinical Note:

Multiple sclerosis, or MS, is a demyelination disease of the CNS where the myelin is progressively destroyed, leading to inflammation and axonal damage. MS is an autoimmune disease that can also destroy the oligodendrocytes that synthesize and maintain myelin. Common symptoms include:

- Visual impairment
- Loss of sensation over the skin
- Problems with balance and motor coordination
- Loss of bladder and bowel control

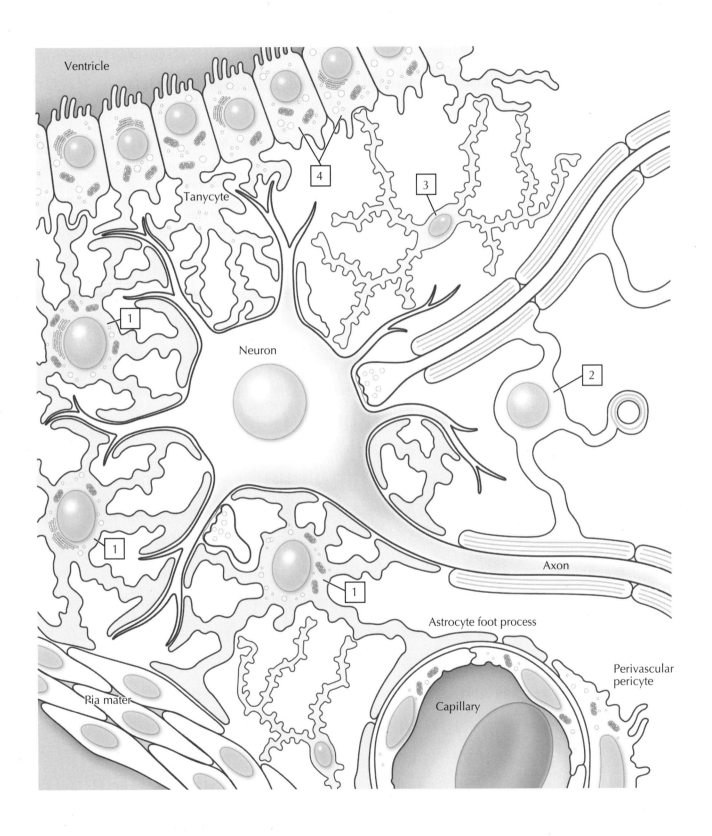

Ventricle

Tanycyte

4

3

2

Neuron

Axon

Astrocyte foot process

Perivascular pericyte

Pia mater

Capillary

The major form of communication in the nervous system is by synapses, discrete sites where the axon, or its extensive branching of axonal terminals, sometimes numbering in the thousands, abut another neuron or target cell. Typically, a neuron receives numerous synaptic contacts on its arborization of dendrites and dendritic spines or on the soma. As the axon approaches its target site, it loses its myelin sheath, often undergoes extensive branching, and then terminates on the target as **synaptic boutons**. Communication is by electrochemical transmission, triggering the release of neurotransmitter(s) into the **synaptic cleft**. The transmitter(s) bind to receptors on the postsynaptic membrane and initiate a graded excitatory or inhibitory response, or neuromodulatory effect, on the target cell.

COLOR the features of the typical synapse, using a different color for each feature:

☐ 1. **Synaptic vesicles: contain the neurotransmitter and/or neuromodulatory substance**

☐ 2. **Vesicle exocytosis: fusion of the synaptic vesicle membrane with the presynaptic membrane, thus releasing the transmitter**

☐ 3. **Postsynaptic membrane: thickened site where membrane postsynaptic receptors bind the neurotransmitter and initiate an appropriate graded response**

A variety of morphological synaptic types can be identified:
• Simple axodendritic or axosomatic (most common synapses)
• Dendritic spine
• Dendritic crest
• Simple synapse along with an axoaxonic synapse
• Combined axoaxonic and axodendritic
• Varicosities (*boutons en passant*)
• Dendrodendritic
• Reciprocal
• Serial

Synapses are dynamic structures and exhibit significant "plasticity." New synapses are formed continuously in many regions, and some are "pruned" or eliminated for any one of a variety of reasons, including lack of use, atrophy or loss of target cells, or degenerative processes due to normal aging or pathology.

Plate 4-3   **Nervous System**

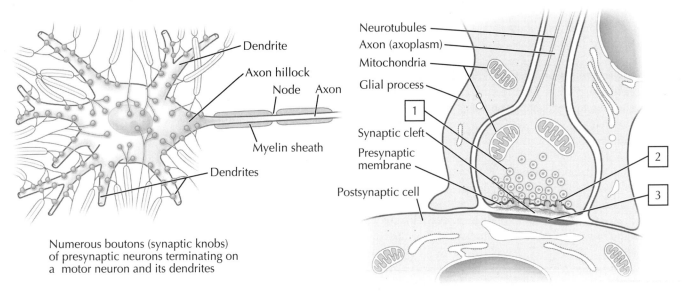

Numerous boutons (synaptic knobs) of presynaptic neurons terminating on a motor neuron and its dendrites

Dendrite

Axon hillock

Node   Axon

Myelin sheath

Dendrites

Neurotubules

Axon (axoplasm)

Mitochondria

Glial process

1

Synaptic cleft

Presynaptic membrane

Postsynaptic cell

2

3

A. Schematic of synaptic endings

B. Enlarged section of bouton

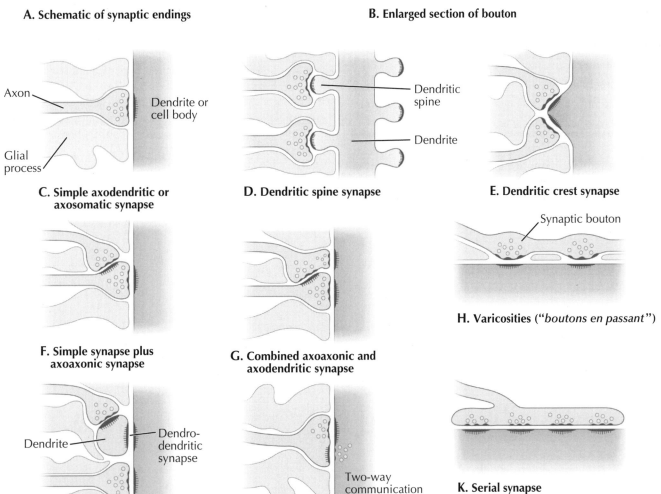

Axon

Dendrite or cell body

Glial process

C. Simple axodendritic or axosomatic synapse

Dendritic spine

Dendrite

D. Dendritic spine synapse

E. Dendritic crest synapse

F. Simple synapse plus axoaxonic synapse

G. Combined axoaxonic and axodendritic synapse

Synaptic bouton

H. Varicosities ("boutons en passant")

Dendrite

Dendro-dendritic synapse

I. Dendrodendritic synapse

Two-way communication

J. Reciprocal synapse

K. Serial synapse

As reviewed in Chapter 1, the human brain consists of the following parts:

- Cerebrum (cerebral cortex)
- Diencephalon (thalamus, hypothalamus, and pineal gland)
- Midbrain (also called the mesencephalon, a part of the brainstem)
- Pons (connects to the cerebellum and medulla and is part of the brainstem)
- Medulla oblongata (connects to the spinal cord and is part of the brainstem)
- Cerebellum

The cerebrum is divided into two large hemispheres and is characterized by its convoluted cerebral cortex, which significantly increases the surface area for neurons by folding the tissue into a compact volume. The cerebral cortex is divided into four visible lobes and one lobe that lies deep to the outer cortex.

COLOR the five lobes of the cerebral cortex, using a different color for each lobe:

- [ ] **1. Frontal lobe**
- [ ] **2. Parietal lobe**
- [ ] **3. Occipital lobe**
- [ ] **4. Temporal lobe**
- [ ] **5. Insula: a fifth, deep lobe lying medial to the temporal lobe**

Regions of the cerebral cortex are associated with specific functional attributes. Many of these areas overlap, and some may be more or less developed in individuals with specific talents or with specific deficits, either from congenital anomalies (birth defects) or from pathology, such as a stroke.

COLOR the following functional regions of the cerebral hemisphere, using a different color for each region:

- [ ] **6. Primary motor cortex (just anterior to the central sulcus)**
- [ ] **7. Primary somatosensory cortex (just posterior to the central sulcus)**
- [ ] **8. Primary visual cortex**
- [ ] **9. Primary auditory cortex**

The fold of cortical tissue just anterior to the central sulcus is the **precentral gyrus** of the frontal lobes. The primary motor cortex is located in this gyrus, and the human body is represented topographically over this cortical area. That is, the cortical neurons concerned with certain motor functions associated with a region of the human body, such as the thumb, can be identified in a particular region of the precentral gyrus. To represent this topographical relationship, a motor homunculus ("little man") is drawn over the motor cortex (see part E), and the size of each body part is representative of the portion of the cortex devoted to innervating this body part. Note that the motor cortex is disproportionately large for the face, oral cavity, and hand. The sensory cortex (see D) is especially large over the face and hand.

The **postcentral gyrus** of the parietal lobe is the primary sensory cortex and represents the cortical area devoted to sensory function. Similar to the motor cortex, a sensory homunculus can be represented over this cortical region.

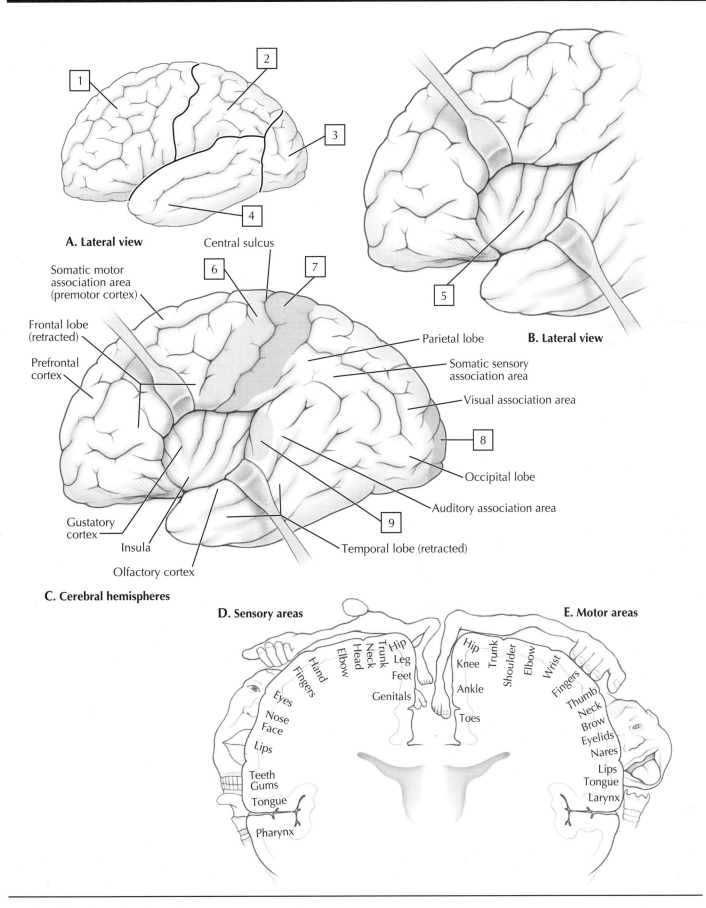

A. Lateral view

Central sulcus

Somatic motor
association area
(premotor cortex)

Frontal lobe
(retracted)

Prefrontal
cortex

B. Lateral view

Parietal lobe

Somatic sensory
association area

Visual association area

Occipital lobe

Auditory association area

Gustatory
cortex

Insula

Olfactory cortex

Temporal lobe (retracted)

C. Cerebral hemispheres

D. Sensory areas

E. Motor areas

Sensory areas labels: Hand, Fingers, Elbow, Head, Neck, Trunk, Hip, Leg, Feet, Genitals, Eyes, Nose, Face, Lips, Teeth, Gums, Tongue, Pharynx

Motor areas labels: Hip, Knee, Trunk, Shoulder, Elbow, Wrist, Fingers, Thumb, Neck, Brow, Eyelids, Nares, Lips, Tongue, Larynx, Ankle, Toes

The convoluted surface of the cerebral hemispheres containing the cortical neurons comprises the **gray matter** and lies above the deeper situated **white matter**, which comprises the fiber connections that course from deeper brain regions or the interconnections that permit communication between the two hemispheres. These fiber pathways are called white matter because they appear more white because of the myelin that insulates most of these fiber connections. The major white matter tracts forming these connections include the:

- **Corpus callosum**: commissural fibers that interconnect the two hemispheres
- **Association tracts**: connect cortical regions within the same hemisphere
- **Corona radiata**: two-way connections between the cortex and subcortical nuclei and the spinal cord; narrows into the **internal capsule** as it passes by the thalamus and basal ganglia

The major fiber pathway that interconnects the two hemispheres is called the **corpus callosum**. These commissural fibers provide important coordination of functional activity between the two separate hemispheres. The fibers interconnecting the frontal and occipital lobes in particular curve rostrally and caudally after they cross the midline. In essence, the corpus callosum forms a roof over the subcortical nuclei (*nucleus* in the CNS is a term used to describe collections of neurons that subserve similar functions).

Additionally, **association tracts** of fibers connect the anterior and posterior aspects of the cerebral cortex, and can exist as very long tracts connecting frontal lobe regions with the occipital lobes or as shorter tracts.

Finally, a fan-shaped white matter tract of fibers called the **corona radiata** provides a projection system that "radiates" inferiorly and caudally from the cortex and descends between the caudate nucleus and thalamus medially and the putamen, which lies lateral to this projection (at this point the radiation is called the **internal capsule**). The axons in this projection tract both ascend and descend from lower brainstem and spinal cord areas, providing connections to and from these regions to the cerebral cortex.

COLOR the following white matter fiber pathways, using a different color for each pathway:

- [ ] **1. Corpus callosum**
- [ ] **2. Corona radiata**
- [ ] **3. Internal capsule**

Plate 4-5   **Nervous System**

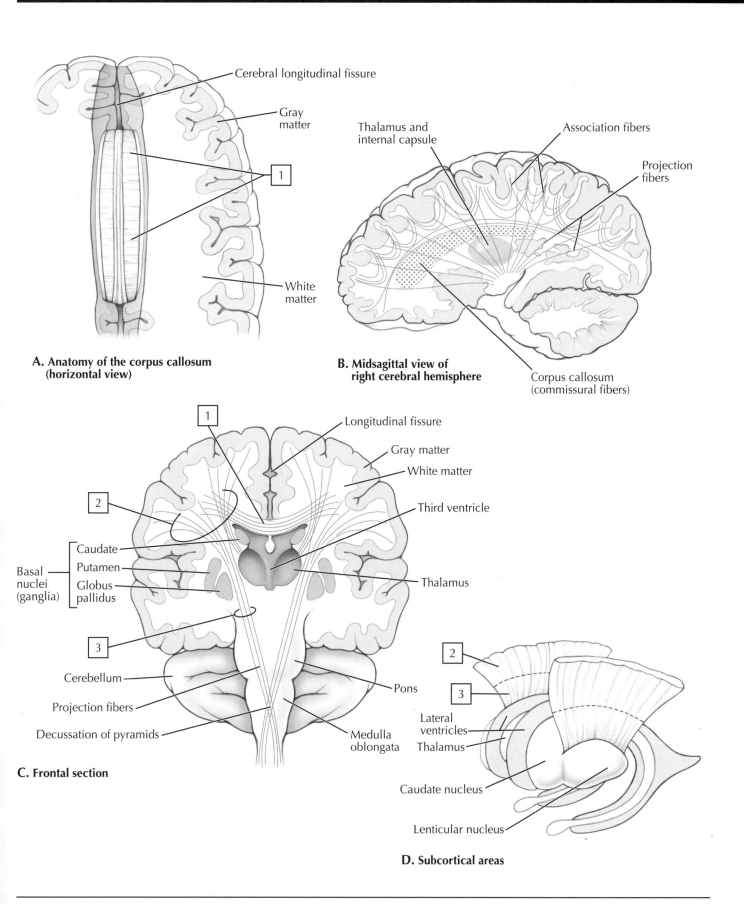

Cerebral longitudinal fissure

Gray matter

1

White matter

A. Anatomy of the corpus callosum (horizontal view)

Thalamus and internal capsule

Association fibers

Projection fibers

B. Midsagittal view of right cerebral hemisphere

Corpus callosum (commissural fibers)

1

Longitudinal fissure

Gray matter

White matter

2

Third ventricle

Caudate

Putamen

Basal nuclei (ganglia)

Globus pallidus

Thalamus

3

Cerebellum

Projection fibers

Decussation of pyramids

Pons

Medulla oblongata

C. Frontal section

2

3

Lateral ventricles

Thalamus

Caudate nucleus

Lenticular nucleus

D. Subcortical areas

Many of the deeper midline structures of the brain are visible if the brain is viewed in a midsagittal section between the cerebral hemispheres and through the diencephalon, midbrain, pons, medulla oblongata, and upper spinal cord. Likewise, basal views of the brain and isolated views of the brainstem help one to delineate the individual regions that comprise the brain below the level of the cerebrum.

First, note the prominent corpus callosum, the commissural connection between the two cerebral hemispheres. Its major parts include the:
- **Genu**: anterior portion
- **Body**: larger midsection
- **Splenium**: posterior portion

Just beneath the corpus callosum lie the diencephalic structures, including the:
- **Thalamus**: the "executive secretary" of the cortex, because it is reciprocally connected to the cortex and conveys motor, sensory, and autonomic information from the brainstem and spinal cord
- **Hypothalamus**: lies beneath the thalamus, and its connections with the pituitary gland reflect its important role in neuroendocrine function
- **Pineal gland**: an endocrine organ that secrets melatonin and is important is regulating circadian (day-night) rhythms

The **midbrain** contains fiber tracts that ascend and descend through the thalamus; it also includes the:
- **Colliculi (*colliculus*, "small hill")**: superior and inferior colliculi are sensory nuclei associated with visual reflexes and auditory reflexes, respectively
- **Cerebral peduncles (*pedunculus*, "little feet")**: convey descending motor fibers to the spinal cord and connections to the cerebellum

The **pons**, meaning "bridge," literally connects the cerebellum with the other portions of the brain and spinal cord. Some deep fiber tracts connect higher brain centers with the spinal cord, whereas more superficial tracts relay information between the cortex and cerebellum via three cerebellar peduncles.

The **medulla** links the brainstem with the spinal cord, and all of the ascending and descending fiber pathways pass through the medulla and/or synapse on sensory and motor nuclei within this region. Important regulatory cardiopulmonary centers also are located in the medulla oblongata.

COLOR each of the following features of the diencephalon, midbrain, pons, and medulla, using a different color for each feature:

- [ ] **1. Corpus callosum**
- [ ] **2. Pineal gland**
- [ ] **3. Colliculi of the midbrain (superior and inferior)**
- [ ] **4. Mammillary bodies of the hypothalamus**
- [ ] **5. Thalamus**
- [ ] **6. Cerebellar peduncles (superior, middle, and inferior)**
- [ ] **7. Medulla oblongata (often just called the medulla)**

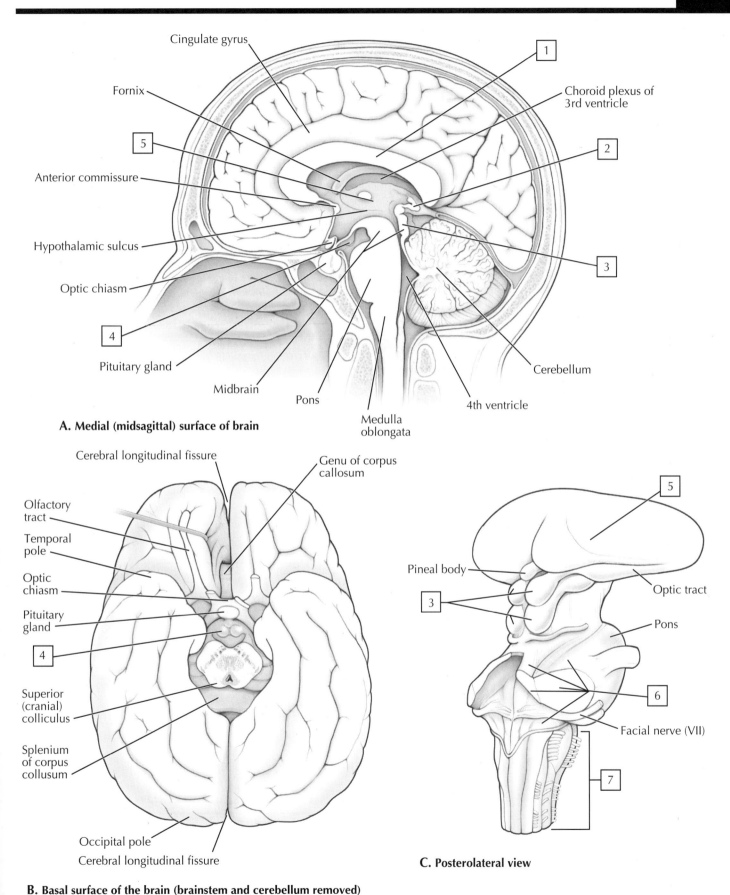

Cingulate gyrus

1

Choroid plexus of
3rd ventricle

Fornix

5

2

Anterior commissure

Hypothalamic sulcus

3

Optic chiasm

4

Cerebellum

Pituitary gland

Midbrain

Pons

4th ventricle

Medulla
oblongata

A. Medial (midsagittal) surface of brain

Cerebral longitudinal fissure

Genu of corpus
callosum

5

Olfactory
tract

Temporal
pole

Pineal body

Optic
chiasm

3

Optic tract

Pituitary
gland

Pons

4

6

Superior
(cranial)
colliculus

Facial nerve (VII)

Splenium
of corpus
collusum

7

Occipital pole

Cerebral longitudinal fissure

C. Posterolateral view

B. Basal surface of the brain (brainstem and cerebellum removed)

The basal ganglia (basal nuclei) provide subconscious control of skeletal muscle tone and coordination of learned movements. Once a voluntary movement is initiated cortically, the natural rhythm and patterns that we take for granted in walking or reaching for objects are controlled subconsciously by the basal ganglia. Additionally, they inhibit unnecessary movements. The interconnections of the basal ganglia are complex, involve both excitatory and inhibitory pathways, and use multiple transmitters (dopamine, glutamate, GABA, ACh, and 5HT; summarized in the diagram below). While it is probably not important to memorize this schematic diagram, it does illustrate the complexity of interconnections in this network.

The basal ganglia (nuclei) include the:
- **Caudate nucleus**: descriptively, it has a large head and a slender tail, which arches over the diencephalon
- **Putamen**: the putamen and globus pallidus together form the **lentiform nucleus**
- **Globus pallidus**: the putamen and globus pallidus together form the lentiform nucleus

COLOR the nuclei associated with the basal ganglia, using a different color for each nucleus:

☐ 1. **Caudate (head and tail)**
☐ 2. **Putamen**
☐ 3. **Globus pallidus**
☐ 4. **Lentiform nucleus**

Clinical Note:

Disorders affecting the basal ganglia involve either defects that result in too much movement or not enough movement. **Huntington's disease** results in a hereditary loss of basal ganglia and cortical neurons that leads to a hyperactive state of involuntary movements. The jerky movements of this disease almost resemble a dancer out of control, and the term **chorea** ("dance") aptly characterizes this fatal condition. In its late stages, mental deterioration is common.

A contrasting disease to Huntington's chorea is **Parkinson's disease**. Resulting from the degeneration of dopamine-secreting neurons of the substantia nigra, this progressive disease results in bradykinesia (slow movements), resting rhythmic muscular tremor, muscular rigidity, stooped posture, a masked or expressionless face, and a shuffling gait.

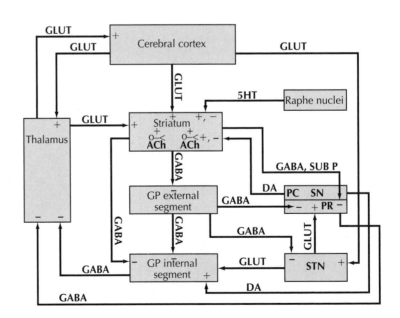

SN = Substantia nigra
STN = Subthalamic nucleus
GLUT = Glutamate
GABA = Gamma aminobutyric acid
DA = Dopamine

5HT = 5-Hydroxytryptamine (serotonin)
PC = Pars compacta
PR = Pars reticularis
ACh = Acetylcholine
GP = Globus pallidus
SUB P = Substance P

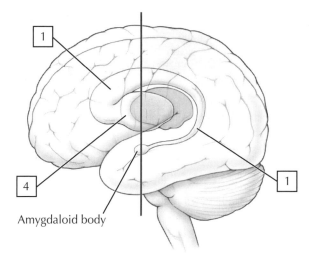

A. Level of section for C below

Amygdaloid body

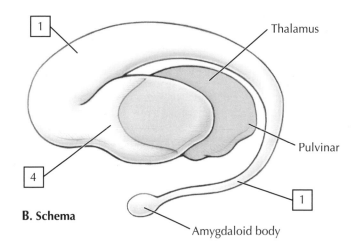

Thalamus

Pulvinar

Amygdaloid body

B. Schema

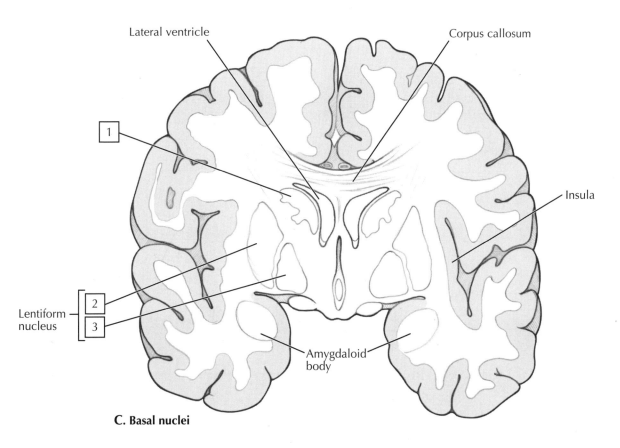

Lateral ventricle

Corpus callosum

Insula

Lentiform
nucleus

Amygdaloid
body

C. Basal nuclei

The limbic system is a functional group of structures that form a ring ("limbus") around the diencephalon. The limbic system participates in emotional behaviors (fear, rage, pleasure, and sexual arousal) and the interpretation of internal and external stimuli (linking conscious functions with autonomic functions, and aspects of memory and retrieval). Structural components of the limbic system (classification of which structures are part of the system or simply communicate with it vary) typically include the:

• Cingulate gyrus
• Parahippocampal gyrus
• Hippocampus (memory)
• Amygdala (and its axonal projection called the stria terminalis, which projects to the hypothalamus and basal forebrain structures)
• Septal nuclei: lies just rostral to the hippocampus; regulates emotions
• Hypothalamus (autonomic and neuroendocrine functions)
• Olfactory area (smell)

The limbic system forms extensive connections with cortical regions and the brainstem, allowing for extensive integration of stimuli, emotional states, and conscious behaviors linked to these stimuli and emotions.

COLOR the following structures associated with the limbic system, using a different color for each structure:

- [ ] 1. **Cingulate gyrus**
- [ ] 2. **Hippocampus**
- [ ] 3. **Amygdala and stria terminalis**
- [ ] 4. **Septal nuclei**
- [ ] 5. **Olfactory tract**

Clinical Note:

The **hypothalamus**, as a center for neuroendocrine and autonomic functioning, and as a processing center for smell and emotions along with other limbic structures, plays a key role in **psychosomatic illness.** Stress and its accompanying emotions can trigger autonomic visceral reactions that are the hallmark of psychosomatic, or emotion-driven, illnesses.

Plate 4-8   **Nervous System**

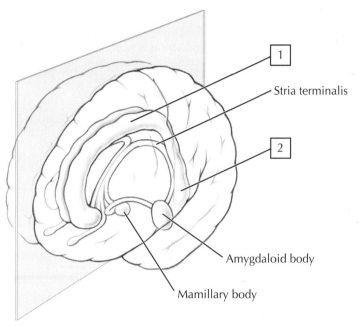

Stria terminalis

Amygdaloid body

Mamillary body

A. Anterolateral schematic

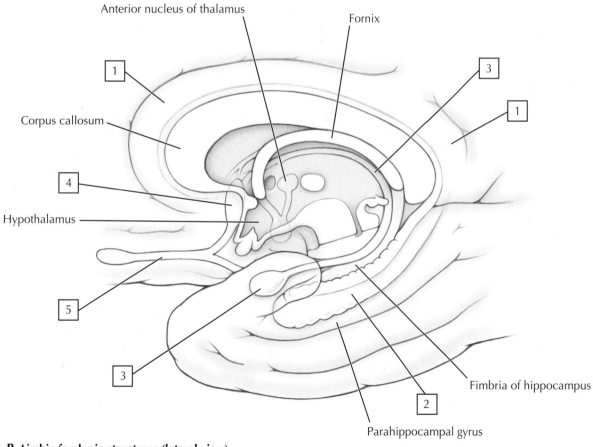

Anterior nucleus of thalamus

Fornix

Corpus callosum

Hypothalamus

Fimbria of hippocampus

Parahippocampal gyrus

B. Limbic forebrain structures (lateral view)

4 Hippocampus

The hippocampus extends from the amygdala and arches up and forward into the diencephalon in close association with the dentate gyrus. Its appearance resembles a sea horse (in coronal sections), which is what the term hippocampus actually means. It occupies a portion of the medial temporal lobes, lying just medial to the temporal pole of the lateral ventricles. The efferent fiber tract of the hippocampus is the **fornix**, which arches forward under the corpus callosum and toward the mammillary bodies of the hypothalamus, where many of its fibers terminate. The hippocampal formation (dentate gyrus, hippocampus proper, and subiculum) has many interconnections with the limbic system and cortical association areas.

Functionally, the hippocampus and amygdala are important in memory consolidation and access. Moreover, the hippocampus plays a role in spatial relationships, whereas the amygdala associates a variety of sensory memories and links them to our emotional responses, especially fear and aversion.

COLOR the following structures associated with the hippocampal formation, using a different color for each structure:

- ☐ **1. Body of the fornix**
- ☐ **2. Crura ("legs") of the fornix**
- ☐ **3. Dentate gyrus**
- ☐ **4. Hippocampus**

Clinical Note:
Alzheimer's disease is a common cause of dementia in the elderly and is characterized by the progressive degeneration of neurons, especially evident in the frontal, temporal, and parietal lobes. The neuronal degeneration leads to atrophy of the brain resulting in narrowed cerebral gyri and widening of the sulci of the cortex. The presence of neurofibrillary tangles (filamentous aggregates in the cytoplasm of neurons) is common in the cortex, hippocampus, basal forebrain, and some regions of the brainstem. Memory loss and cognitive impairments lead to progressive loss of orientation, language, and other higher cortical functions.

 See Netter: *Atlas of Human Anatomy,* 6th Edition, Plate 113

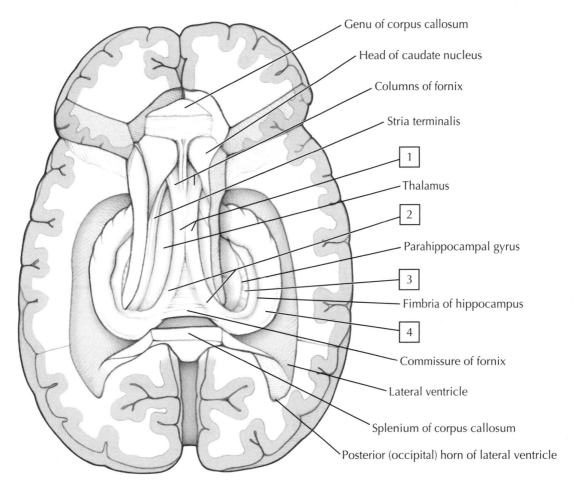

Genu of corpus callosum

Head of caudate nucleus

Columns of fornix

Stria terminalis

1

Thalamus

2

Parahippocampal gyrus

3

Fimbria of hippocampus

4

Commissure of fornix

Lateral ventricle

Splenium of corpus callosum

Posterior (occipital) horn of lateral ventricle

A. Dissection of the hippocampal formation and fornix

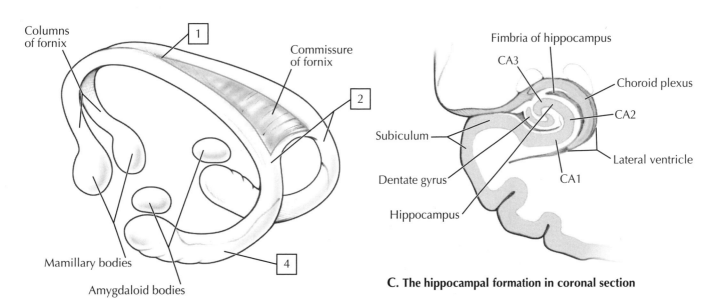

Columns of fornix

1

Commissure of fornix

2

4

Mamillary bodies

Amygdaloid bodies

B. 3-D reconstruction of the fornix

Fimbria of hippocampus

CA3

Choroid plexus

CA2

Subiculum

Lateral ventricle

CA1

Dentate gyrus

Hippocampus

C. The hippocampal formation in coronal section

The right and left thalamus ("inner room") are separated by the 3rd ventricle and form the major portion of the diencephalon (about 80%). The thalamic nuclei are consolidated into an ovoid mass and divided into three major groups:

• Anterior
• Medial
• Lateral

The central location of the thalamus is representative of its importance; essentially, no sensory information, except olfactory information, passes to the higher cortical regions without synapsing in the thalamus. Thus the thalamus has been characterized as the "**executive secretary**" of the brain because it sorts and edits information. Sensory, motor, and autonomic information from the spinal cord and brainstem is conveyed to the cortex via the thalamus. Likewise, the thalamic nuclei are reciprocally interconnected with the cortex. A white matter tract, the medullary laminae, runs through the thalamus and relays information to the cortex.

Inputs passing through the thalamus on their way to the cerebral cortex include those that:

• Regulate emotion and visceral functions from the hypothalamus
• Direct motor activity from the cerebellum and basal ganglia
• Integrate sensory function
• Relay visual and auditory information
• Participate in autonomic and limbic-related functions

In general, the thalamic nuclei project to the following cortical areas (many of these connections are reciprocal):

• **VPL**: primary sensory cortex (postcentral gyrus)
• **VPM**: primary sensory cortex and primary somesthetic cortex
• **VL**: primary motor cortex (precentral gyrus)
• **VI**: primary motor cortex (precentral gyrus)
• **VA**: premotor and supplementary motor cortex
• **Anterior**: cingulate gyrus
• **LD**: cingulate gyrus and precuneus
• **LP**: precuneus and superior parietal lobe
• **MD**: prefrontal cortex and frontal lobe
• **Pulvinar**: association areas of the parietal, temporal, and occipital lobes

COLOR the following thalamic nuclei, using a different color for each nucleus:

☐ **1. Medial dorsal**
☐ **2. Pulvinar**
☐ **3. Lateral posterior**
☐ **4. Ventral posterolateral**
☐ **5. Ventral posteromedial**
☐ **6. Anterior**

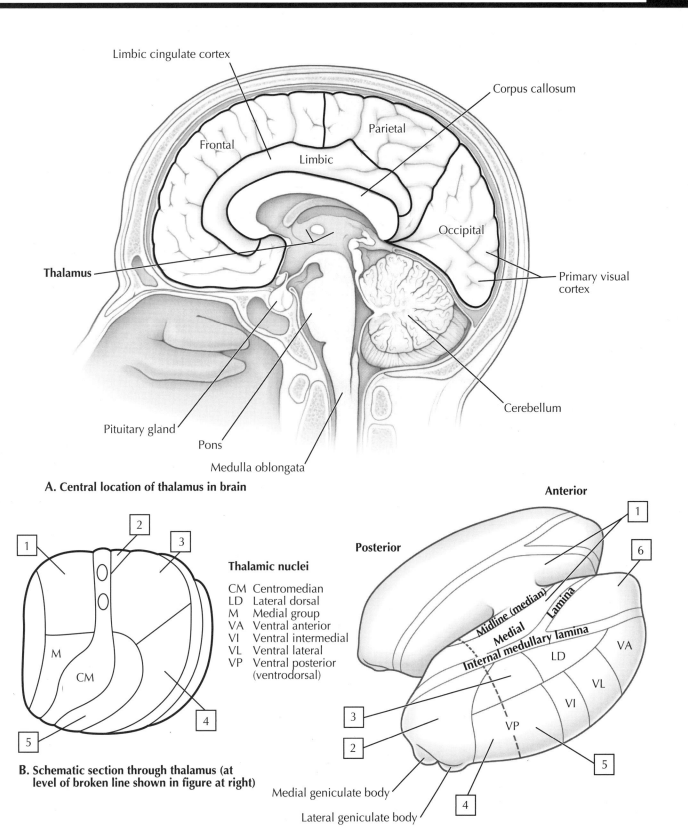

A. Central location of thalamus in brain

Limbic cingulate cortex

Corpus callosum

Frontal

Parietal

Limbic

Occipital

Thalamus

Primary visual cortex

Pituitary gland

Cerebellum

Pons

Medulla oblongata

Thalamic nuclei

CM Centromedian
LD Lateral dorsal
M   Medial group
VA Ventral anterior
VI Ventral intermedial
VL Ventral lateral
VP Ventral posterior
    (ventrodorsal)

B. Schematic section through thalamus (at level of broken line shown in figure at right)

Anterior

Posterior

Midline (median)

Medial

Internal medullary lamina

Lamina

Medial geniculate body

Lateral geniculate body

C. Schematic representation of thalamus (reticular nuclei and external medullary lamina removed)

The hypothalamus lies below the thalamus and the 3rd ventricle, comprising most of the remainder of the diencephalon besides the thalamus and the small epithalamus (pineal gland). The hypothalamic nuclei are grouped into three regions:
• **Anterior**: above the optic chiasm
• **Tuberal**: above the tuber cinereum (leads into the pituitary stalk and gland)
• **Posterior**: region above and including the mammillary bodies

Additionally, each side of the hypothalamus is divided into medial and lateral zones, making six regions on each side. There are seven principal nuclei of the hypothalamus.

COLOR each of the principal hypothalamic nuclei, using a different color for each nucleus:

☐ **1. Paraventricular**
☐ **2. Posterior**
☐ **3. Dorsomedial**
☐ **4. Supra-optic**
☐ **5. Ventromedial**
☐ **6. Arcuate (infundibular)**
☐ **7. Mammillary**

Functionally, the hypothalamus is very important in visceral control and homeostasis and possesses extensive connections with other brain regions (septal nuclei, hippocampus, amygdala, brainstem, and spinal cord). Specifically, its main functions include:
• Regulation of the autonomic nervous system (heart rate, blood pressure, respiration, and digestion)
• Expression and regulation of emotional responses
• Water balance and thirst
• Sleep and wakefulness related to our daily biological cycles
• Temperature regulation
• Food intake and appetite regulation
• Reproductive and sexual behaviors
• Endocrine control

MAJOR FUNCTIONS OF THE HYPOTHALAMUS	
HYPOTHALAMIC AREA	**MAJOR FUNCTIONS***
Preoptic and anterior	Heat loss center: cutaneous vasodilation and sweating
Posterior	Heat conservation center: cutaneous vasoconstriction and shivering
Lateral	Feeding center: eating behavior
Ventromedial	Satiety center: inhibits eating behavior
Supra-optic (subfornical organ and organum vasculosum)	ADH† and oxytocin secretion
Paraventricular	ADH† and oxytocin secretion
Periventricular	Secretion of releasing hormones for the anterior pituitary

*Stimulation of the center causes the responses listed.
†ADH, Antidiuretic hormone (vasopressin)

Clinical Note:
Because the hypothalamus has such far-reaching regulatory effects on so many functions, impairments to this brain region can have significant consequences. Disorders can include emotional imbalance, sexual dysfunction, obesity, sleep disturbances, body wasting, dehydration, and temperature disturbances, to name a few.

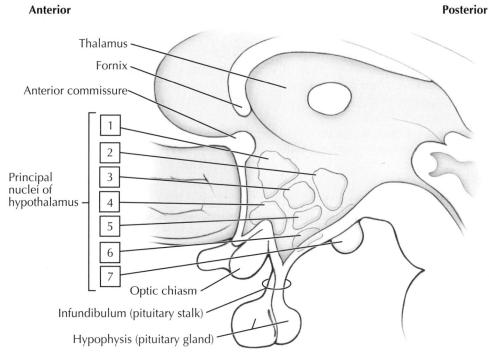

Anterior   Posterior

Thalamus

Fornix

Anterior commissure

1

2

3

Principal nuclei of hypothalamus

4

5

6

7

Optic chiasm

Infundibulum (pituitary stalk)

Hypophysis (pituitary gland)

A. Lateral view of hypothalamus and its major nuclei

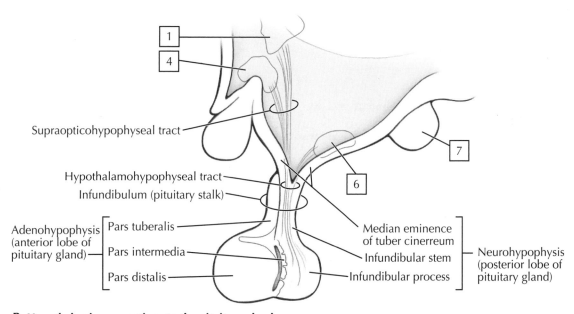

1

4

Supraopticohypophyseal tract

7

Hypothalamohypophyseal tract

6

Infundibulum (pituitary stalk)

Adenohypophysis (anterior lobe of pituitary gland) — Pars tuberalis

Pars intermedia

Pars distalis

Median eminence of tuber cinerreum

Infundibular stem

Infundibular process

Neurohypophysis (posterior lobe of pituitary gland)

B. Hypothalamic connections to the pituitary gland

The cerebellum consists of two hemispheres, connected in the middle by the **vermis**, with gray matter (neurons) on the surface, like the cerebral cortex. Deep nuclei also are embedded in the white matter, which forms an arborlike pattern when viewed grossly in section. The cerebellum overlies the pons and medulla and is connected to the diencephalon and brainstem by three cerebellar peduncles:

- **Superior (connects to the diencephalon)**: afferent and efferent fibers, with connections to the thalamus and then the cerebral motor cortex
- **Middle (connects to the pons)**: afferent fibers only from the pons to the cerebellum, conveying information about voluntary motor activities initiated by the cortex
- **Inferior (connects to the medulla)**: afferent and efferent fibers, with sensory information (proprioceptive) from the body and vestibular system

COLOR each of the three cerebellar anatomical lobes (on the right side only), using a different color for each lobe:

- ☐ 1. **Anterior lobe**
- ☐ 2. **Posterior lobe**
- ☐ 3. **Flocculonodular lobe**

Functionally, the cerebellum is organized in a vertical fashion, so that each hemisphere contains three functional zones.

COLOR each of the three functional zones of the cerebellum (on the left side only), using a different color for each zone:

- ☐ 4. **Lateral hemisphere: planning movements**
- ☐ 5. **Paravermis (intermediate) zone: adjust limb movements**
- ☐ 6. **Vermis (in the midline): postural adjustments and eye movements**

Each of these functional divisions is associated with specific deep nuclei.

Functionally, the deep cerebellar nuclei provide the course adjustment, upon which is layered the finer adjustment provided by the cerebellar cortex. Generally, the cerebellum functions to:

- Regulate the postural muscles of the body to maintain balance and stereotyped movements associated with walking
- Adjust limb movements initiated by the cerebral motor cortex
- Participate in the planning and programming of voluntary, learned, skilled movements
- Play a role in the eye movement
- Play a role in cognition

Clinical Note:
Malnutrition, often associated with chronic alcoholism, can lead to degeneration of the cerebellar cortex, often starting anteriorly **(anterior lobe syndrome)**. An uncoordinated or staggering gait may result and this is known as ataxia. Damage to the lateral hemisphere causes ataxia in both the upper and lower extremities and may affect speech as well. The nodule of the flocculonodular lobe overlies the 4th ventricle, where tumors called **medulloblastomas** arising from the roof of the ventricle can impinge on the nodule and affect balance, sometimes accompanied by problems associated with eye movements.

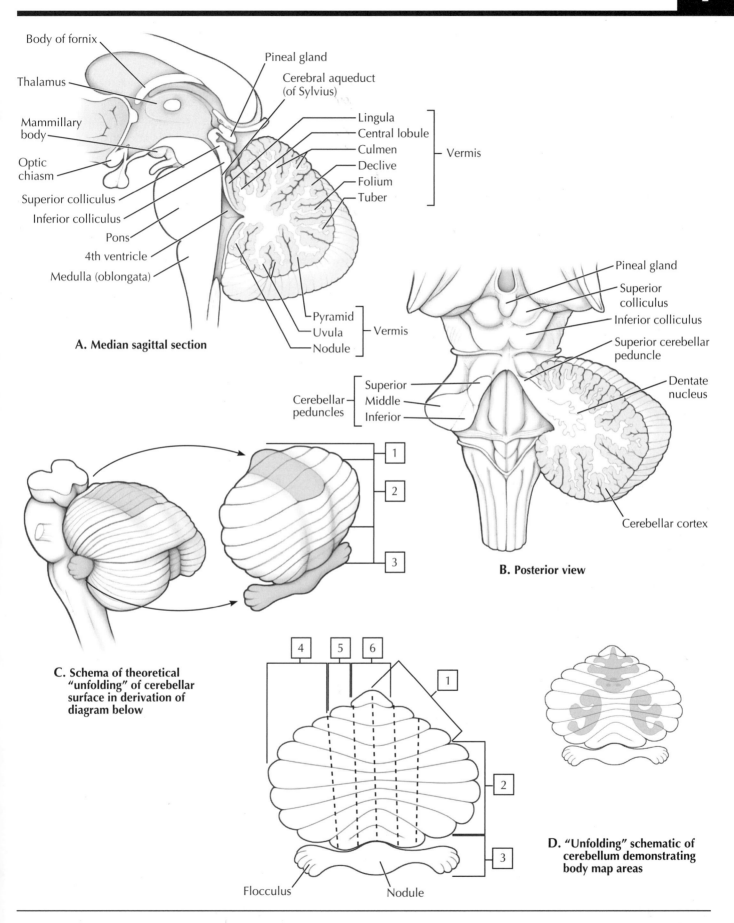

Body of fornix

Thalamus

Mammillary body

Optic chiasm

Superior colliculus

Inferior colliculus

Pons

4th ventricle

Medulla (oblongata)

Pineal gland

Cerebral aqueduct (of Sylvius)

Lingula
Central lobule
Culmen
Declive
Folium
Tuber
} Vermis

Pyramid
Uvula
Nodule
} Vermis

A. Median sagittal section

Superior
Middle
Inferior
} Cerebellar peduncles

Pineal gland

Superior colliculus

Inferior colliculus

Superior cerebellar peduncle

Dentate nucleus

Cerebellar cortex

B. Posterior view

C. Schema of theoretical "unfolding" of cerebellar surface in derivation of diagram below

Flocculus

Nodule

D. "Unfolding" schematic of cerebellum demonstrating body map areas

The spinal cord is a direct continuation of the medulla oblongata, extending below the foramen magnum at the base of the skull and passing through the vertebral (spinal) canal formed by the articulated vertebrae.

The spinal cord has a slightly larger diameter in the cervical and lumbar regions, due in large measure to the increased presence of neurons and axons in these regions related to the innervation of the large number of muscles in the upper and lower limbs. The spinal cord ends at a tapered region called the **conus medullaris**, which is situated at about the level of the L1-L2 vertebrae. From this point inferiorly, the nerve rootlets course to their respective levels and form a bundle called the **cauda equina**, because it resembles a horse's tail. The spinal cord is anchored inferiorly by the terminal filum, which is attached to the coccyx. Features of the spinal cord include:

- 31 pairs of spinal nerves (8 cervical pairs, 12 thoracic pairs, 5 lumbar pairs, 5 sacral pairs, and 1 coccygeal pair)
- Each spinal nerve is formed by dorsal and ventral roots
- Motor neurons reside in the spinal cord gray matter (anterior horn)
- Sensory neurons reside in the spinal nerve dorsal root ganglia
- Ventral rami of spinal nerves often converge to form plexuses (a mixed network of nerve axons)

The typical scheme for a somatic peripheral nerve (innervates skin and skeletal muscle) shows a motor neuron in the spinal cord anterior horn (gray matter) sending a myelinated axon through a ventral root and into a peripheral nerve that ends at a neuromuscular junction on a skeletal muscle. Likewise, a nerve ending in the skin sends a sensory axon toward the spinal cord in a peripheral nerve. Thus each peripheral nerve contains hundreds or thousands of somatic motor and sensory axons. The sensory neuron is a pseudounipolar neuron that resides in a dorsal root ganglion (a ganglion in the periphery is a collection of neurons, just as a nucleus is in the brain) and sends its central axon into the posterior horn (gray matter) of the spinal cord. At each level of the spinal cord, the gray matter is visible as a butterfly-shaped central collection of neurons, exhibiting a posterior and anterior horn.

COLOR the following features of the spinal cord, using a different color for each feature:

1. Spinal cord
2. Cauda equina: collection of nerve roots inferior to the spinal cord
3. White matter of spinal cord as seen in cross section: ascending and descending fiber tracts
4. **Sensory axon and its pseudounipolar neuron (in the dorsal root ganglion)**
5. **Central gray matter of the spinal cord (as seen in cross section)**
6. **Motor neuron and its axon to a skeletal muscle**

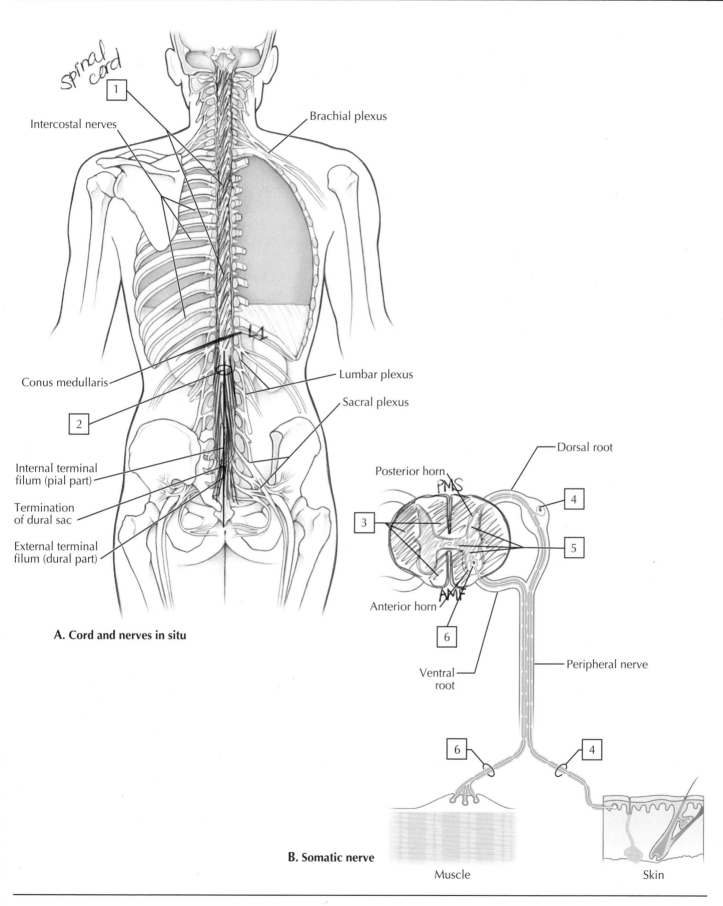

Spinal cord

1

Intercostal nerves

Brachial plexus

Conus medullaris

2

Lumbar plexus

Sacral plexus

Internal terminal filum (pial part)

Termination of dural sac

External terminal filum (dural part)

L1

A. Cord and nerves in situ

Dorsal root

Posterior horn

PMS

3

4

5

Anterior horn

AMF

6

Ventral root

Peripheral nerve

6

4

B. Somatic nerve

Muscle

Skin

The gray matter of the cerebral cortex lies on the surface of the brain, whereas in the spinal cord the gray matter and its associated neurons lie in the center of the cord, where they form a butterfly- or H-shaped region that can be discerned from the surrounding white matter. Spinal cord levels associated with the innervation of the limbs possess a larger amount of gray matter (C5-T1 and L1-S4 levels, corresponding to the brachial and lumbosacral plexuses, respectively). The gray matter is divided into a **posterior horn**, which receives sensory axons from the periphery, and an **anterior horn**, where efferent axons exit the cord to enter a spinal nerve. Between spinal cord levels T1 and L2, a lateral horn or cell column is present for sympathetic pre-ganglionic neurons of the ANS.

The white matter of the cord decreases as one continues inferiorly from rostral to caudal. The white matter is divided into dorsal, lateral, and anterior funiculi ("bundles") that contain multiple fiber tracts. In general, these tracts include:

• **Dorsal (posterior) funiculus**: ascending pathways that, generally speaking, convey proprioception (muscle and joint position), touch, and tactile discrimination (size and shape discrimination) from the leg (fasciculus gracilis) and arm (fasciculus cuneatus)
• **Lateral funiculus**: ascending pathways that convey proprioception, pain, temperature, and touch sensations to higher centers, and convey descending pathways concerned with skilled movements and autonomic information to preganglionic neurons
• **Anterior funiculus**: some ascending pathways that convey pain, temperature, and touch, and descending pathways that convey information that facilitates or inhibits flexor and extensor muscles; reflex movements that control tone, posture, and head movements; and some skilled movements

COLOR each of the following white matter tracts, using a different color for each tract:

☐ 1. **Dorsal funiculus (fasciculus cuneatus and fasciculus gracilis): ascending fibers conveying proprioception, touch, and tactile discrimination from limbs**

☐ 2. **Lateral corticospinal (pyramidal) tract: descending fibers conveying skilled movements**

☐ 3. **Rubrospinal tract: descending fibers that control movements of flexor muscle neurons**

☐ 4. **Lateral (medullary) reticulospinal tract: descending fibers that regulate autonomic preganglionic neurons**

☐ 5. **Anterior or medial (pontine) reticulospinal tract: descending fibers that control extensor muscle neurons**

☐ 6. **Anterior funiculus (vestibulospinal, tectospinal, and corticospinal) tracts: descending fibers conveying reflex movements that control tone, posture, and head movements, and some skilled movements**

☐ 7. **Anterior spinocerebellar tract: ascending fibers conveying proprioception**

☐ 8. **Spinothalamic and spinoreticular tracts: ascending fibers conveying pain, temperature, and touch**

☐ 9. **Posterior spinocerebellar tract: ascending fibers conveying proprioception**

Clinical Note:

Lower motor neurons are the neurons of the anterior horn that innervate skeletal muscle. Lesions of these neurons or their axons in the peripheral nerve result in the loss of voluntary and reflex responses of the muscles and cause muscle atrophy. The denervated muscles exhibit fibrillations (fine twitching) and fasciculations (brief contractions of muscle motor units).

Upper motor neurons are neurons at higher levels in the CNS that send axons either to the brainstem or spinal cord. In general, lesions of these neurons or their axons result in spastic paralysis, hyperactive muscle stretch reflexes, clonus (a series of rhythmic jerks), a "clasp-knife" response (muscle hypertonia) to passive movements, and lack of muscle atrophy (except by disuse).

Amyotrophic lateral sclerosis (ALS) is a progressive and fatal disease that results in the degeneration of motor neurons in cranial nerves and in the anterior horns of the spinal cord. Muscle weakness and atrophy occur in some muscles, whereas spasticity and hyperreflexia are present in other muscles.

Plate 4-14   **Nervous System**

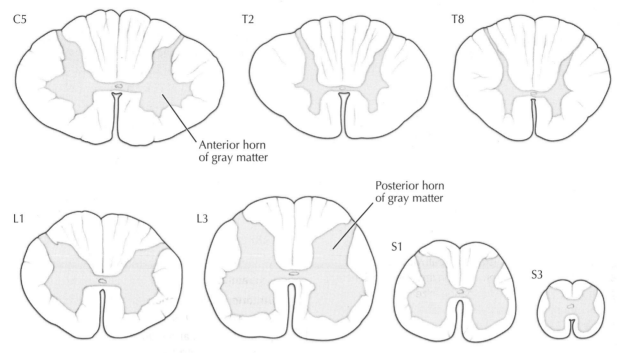

A. Sections through spinal cord at various levels

C5   T2   T8

Anterior horn
of gray matter

Posterior horn
of gray matter

L1   L3   S1   S3

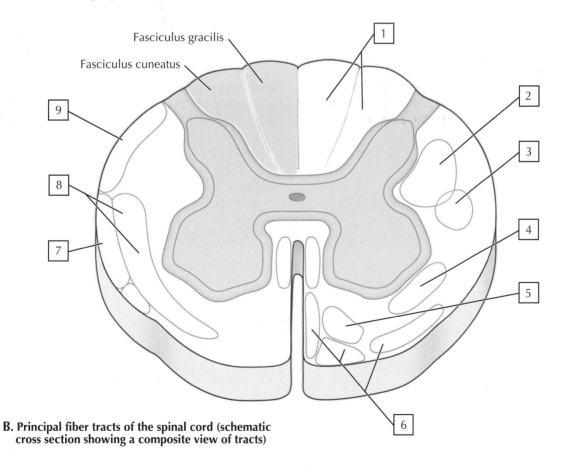

Fasciculus gracilis

Fasciculus cuneatus

1

2

3

4

5

6

7

8

9

**B. Principal fiber tracts of the spinal cord (schematic
cross section showing a composite view of tracts)**

The spinal cord gives rise to 31 pairs of spinal nerves, which then form two major branches (rami):

- Dorsal ramus: a small ramus that courses dorsally to the back conveys motor and sensory information to and from the skin and intrinsic back skeletal muscles (erector spinae and transversospinalis muscles) (see Plate 3-10)
- Ventral ramus: a much larger ramus that courses laterally and ventrally and innervates all the remaining skin and skeletal muscles of the neck, limbs, and trunk

Once nerve fibers (sensory or motor) are beyond, or peripheral to, the spinal cord proper, the fibers then reside in nerves of the peripheral nervous system (PNS). Components of the PNS include the:

- **Somatic nervous system**: sensory and motor fibers to skin, skeletal muscle, and joints (illustrated in part *B*, somatic components)
- **Autonomic nervous system (ANS)**: sensory and motor fibers to all smooth muscle (including viscera and vasculature), cardiac muscle (heart), and glands (illustrated in part *B*, efferent components)
- **Enteric nervous system**: plexuses and ganglia of the gastro-intestinal tract (GI) that regulate bowel secretion, absorption and motility (originally, considered part of the ANS); linked to the ANS for optimal regulation (see Plate 4-21).

Features of the somatic nervous system include:

- It is a one-neuron motor system
- The motor (efferent) neuron is in the CNS, and an axon projects to a peripheral target, such as a skeletal muscle
- The sensory (afferent) neuron (pseudounipolar) resides in a peripheral ganglion called the dorsal root ganglion (DRG) and conveys sensory information from the skin, muscle, or joint to the CNS (spinal cord)

Features of the ANS division of the PNS include:

- It is a two-neuron motor system; the first neuron resides in the CNS and the second neuron in a peripheral autonomic ganglion
- The axon of the first neuron is termed "preganglionic" and the axon of the second neuron is termed "postganglionic"
- The ANS has two divisions: sympathetic and parasympathetic
- The sensory neuron (pseudounipolar) resides in a dorsal root ganglion (DRG), just like the somatic system, and conveys sensory information from viscera to the CNS

COLOR the following features of the PNS, using a different color for each feature:

- [ ] 1. **Ventral root (contains efferent fibers)**
- [ ] 2. **Ventral ramus**
- [ ] 3. **Dorsal ramus (to intrinsic back muscles)**
- [ ] 4. **Dorsal root ganglion (contains sensory neurons)**
- [ ] 5. **Dorsal root (contains afferent fibers)**
- [ ] 6. **Sensory axon and nerve cell body in a DRG (in part *B*)**
- [ ] 7. **Somatic motor axon and nerve cell body (in part *B*, somatic) in anterior horn**
- [ ] 8. **Autonomic preganglionic fiber in ventral root passing to a sympathetic chain ganglion (ANS ganglion) (in part *B*, efferent autonomic components)**
- [ ] 9. **Autonomic postganglionic fiber in ventral root passing from a sympathetic chain ganglion to the skin (in part *B*, efferent autonomic components)**

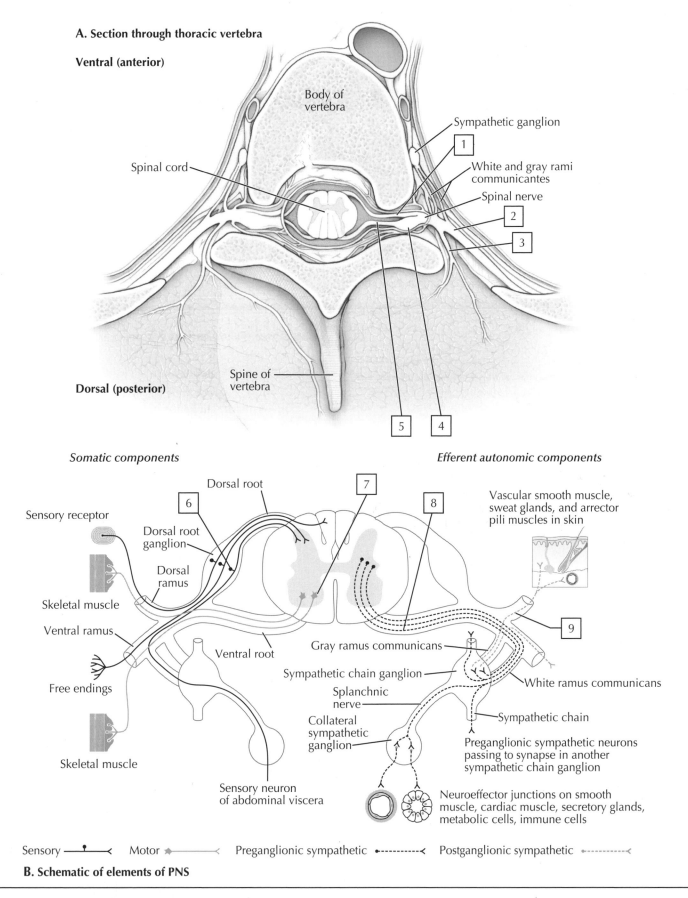

A. Section through thoracic vertebra

Ventral (anterior)

Body of vertebra

Spinal cord

Sympathetic ganglion

1

White and gray rami communicantes

Spinal nerve

2

3

Spine of vertebra

Dorsal (posterior)

5   4

Somatic components

Efferent autonomic components

Dorsal root

7

6

Sensory receptor

Dorsal root ganglion

8

Vascular smooth muscle, sweat glands, and arrector pili muscles in skin

Dorsal ramus

Skeletal muscle

Ventral ramus

Ventral root

9

Free endings

Gray ramus communicans

Skeletal muscle

Sympathetic chain ganglion

White ramus communicans

Splanchnic nerve

Sympathetic chain

Collateral sympathetic ganglion

Preganglionic sympathetic neurons passing to synapse in another sympathetic chain ganglion

Sensory neuron of abdominal viscera

Neuroeffector junctions on smooth muscle, cardiac muscle, secretory glands, metabolic cells, immune cells

Sensory ━━•━<   Motor ✹━━<   Preganglionic sympathetic •━━━━<   Postganglionic sympathetic ━━━━<

B. Schematic of elements of PNS

The region of skin innervated by the somatic sensory nerve fibers associated with a single dorsal root at a single spinal cord level is called a **dermatome**. (Likewise, over the anterolateral head, the skin is innervated by one of the three divisions of the trigeminal cranial nerve, which will be discussed later.) The neurons that give rise to these sensory fibers are pseudounipolar neurons that reside in the single dorsal root ganglion associated with the specific spinal cord level (realize that for each level we are speaking of a pair of nerves, roots, and ganglia, because there are 31 pairs of spinal nerves, one pair for each spinal cord level). C1, the first cervical spinal cord level, does possess sensory fibers but they provide little if any contribution to the skin, so at the top of the head the dermatome pattern begins with the C2 dermatome.

The dermatomes encircle the body segmentally, corresponding to the spinal cord level that receives sensory input from that segment of skin. The sensation conveyed by touching the skin is largely that of pressure and pain. Knowledge of the dermatome pattern is useful in localizing specific spinal cord segments and in assessing the integrity of the spinal cord at that level (intact or lesioned).

COLOR the dermatomes associated with the spinal cord segments of each region, using the color indicated for each region (the single coccygeal pair are not illustrated but encircle the anus):

- ☐ 1. Cervical dermatomes: C2-C8 (green)
- ☐ 2. Thoracic dermatomes: T1-T12 (blue)
- ☐ 3. Lumbar dermatomes: L1-L5 (purple)
- ☐ 4. Sacral dermatomes: S1-S5 (red)

The sensory nerve fibers that innervate a segment of skin and constitute the dermatome do exhibit some overlap of nerve fibers. Consequently, a segment of skin is innervated primarily by fibers from a single spinal cord level, but there will be some overlap with sensory fibers from the levels above and below the primary cord level. For example, dermatome T5 will have some overlap with sensory fibers associated with the T4 and T6 levels. Thus dermatomes give pretty good approximations of cord levels, but variation is common and overlap does exist.

Key dermatomes that are related to the body surface include the following:

C5	Clavicles	T10	Umbilicus (navel)
C5-C7	Lateral upper limb	T12-L1	Inguinal/groin region
C6	Thumb	L1-L4	Anterior & medial upper limb
C7	Middle finger	L4	Medial side of big toe
C8	Little finger	L4-S1	Foot
C8-T1	Medial upper limb	S1-S2	Posterior lower limb
T4	Nipple	S2-S4	Perineum

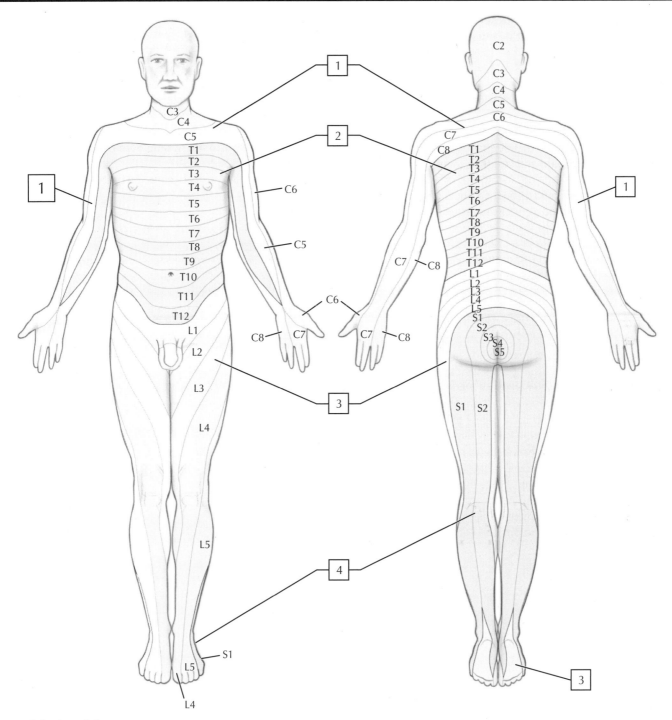

Spinal cord dermatomes

The small central canal of the spinal cord contains cerebrospinal fluid (CSF) and continues rostrally to expand into four brain ventricles, which include the:

- **4th ventricle**: situated above the pons and rostral portion of the medulla oblongata
- **3rd ventricle**: situated in the midline diencephalon between the thalamic nuclei
- **Lateral ventricles**: two lateral ventricles in the cerebral hemispheres that are C-shaped and extend forward, upward, and back, and then downward and forward into the temporal lobes

CSF fills these ventricles and is produced by the **choroid plexus** (a capillary network and its secretory epithelium), which is found in the floor of each lateral ventricle, with smaller accumulations in the roof of the 3rd and 4th ventricles. About 500 ml of CSF is produced in a 24-hour period, and it functions to:

- Support and cushion the brain and spinal cord
- Fulfill some of the functions normally provided by the lymphatic system
- Fill the 150-ml volume of the subarachnoid space and ventricular cavities
- Be reabsorbed largely by the arachnoid granulations that project into the superior sagittal dural venous sinus and by small pial veins of the brain and spinal cord

The flow of CSF is from the choroid plexus of the lateral ventricles to the 3rd ventricle via the interventricular foramen (of Monro), then to the 4th ventricle via the narrow cerebral aqueduct (of Sylvius) and then into the spinal canal, or through openings (lateral and median apertures) to access the subarachnoid space (between the pia and arachnoid mater) surrounding the brain and spinal cord. Secretion of CSF normally is matched by its absorption by the **arachnoid granulations** and small pial veins.

COLOR the following features of the ventricular system, using a different color for each feature:

☐ 1. 3rd ventricle
☐ 2. Lateral ventricles
☐ 3. 4th ventricle
☐ 4. Choroid plexus in the lateral ventricles (in part *B*)
☐ 5. Spinal canal in the middle of the spinal cord

Clinical Note:

The accumulation of excess CSF (overproduction or decreased absorption) within the brain's ventricular system is called **hydrocephalus**. Clinically, three types of hydrocephalus are recognized:

- Obstructive: usually a congenital stenosis (narrowing) of the cerebral aqueduct, interventricular foramina, or the lateral and median apertures; obstruction also may be caused by CNS tumors that block the normal flow of CSF through the ventricles
- Communicating: obstruction outside the ventricular system, perhaps because of pressure due to hemorrhage (bleeding) in the subarachnoid space or around the arachnoid granulations
- Normal pressure: an adult syndrome that results in progressive dementia, gait disorders, and urinary incontinence

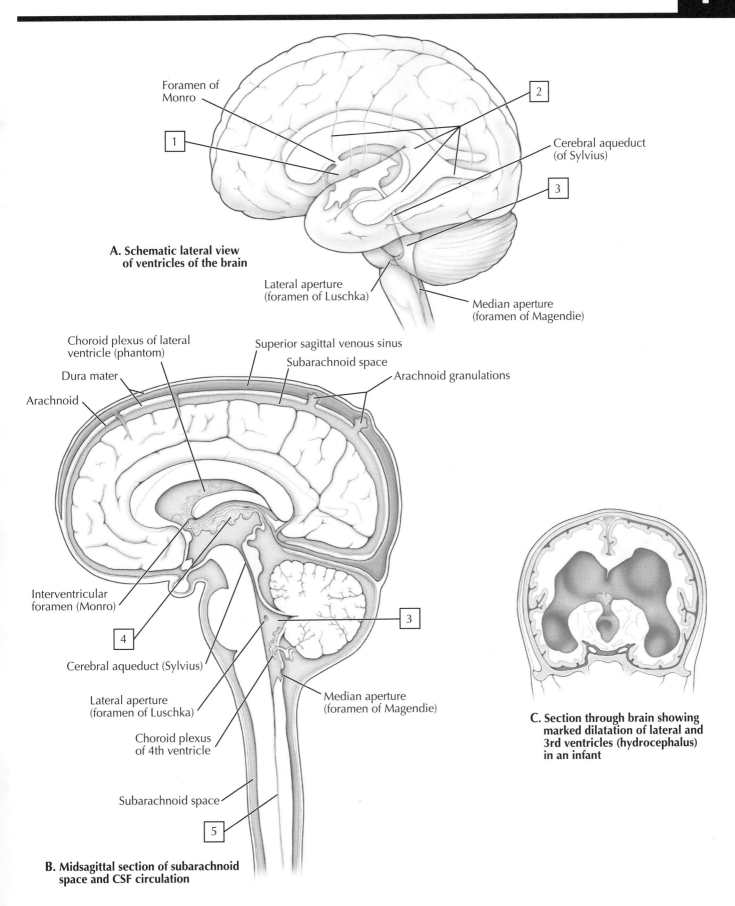

Foramen of
Monro

2

1

Cerebral aqueduct
(of Sylvius)

3

**A. Schematic lateral view
of ventricles of the brain**

Lateral aperture
(foramen of Luschka)

Median aperture
(foramen of Magendie)

Choroid plexus of lateral
ventricle (phantom)

Superior sagittal venous sinus

Subarachnoid space

Arachnoid granulations

Dura mater

Arachnoid

Interventricular
foramen (Monro)

4

Cerebral aqueduct (Sylvius)

Lateral aperture
(foramen of Luschka)

Median aperture
(foramen of Magendie)

3

Choroid plexus
of 4th ventricle

Subarachnoid space

5

**B. Midsagittal section of subarachnoid
space and CSF circulation**

**C. Section through brain showing
marked dilatation of lateral and
3rd ventricles (hydrocephalus)
in an infant**

The brain and spinal cord are covered by three membranes called the meninges and are bathed in cerebrospinal fluid (CSF).

COLOR the dura mater of the brain and spinal cord, and then color all three meningeal layers of the spinal cord as seen in section, using a different color for each layer:

☐ **1. Dura mater: a thick outer covering that is richly innervated by sensory nerve endings**

☐ **2. Arachnoid mater: a fine, weblike membrane that is avascular and lies directly beneath the dura mater**

☐ **3. Pia mater: a delicate, transparent inner layer that intimately covers the spinal cord**

The thick dura mater in the cranium is composed of two layers, a **periosteal layer** lining the inner aspect of the skull and a **meningeal layer** in close contact with the arachnoid mater. This layer also is continuous with the spinal dura. CSF fills a space, called the subarachnoid space, which lies between the arachnoid and pia meningeal layers. Thus CSF circulates through the brain ventricles and then gains access to the subarachnoid space via the lateral and median apertures, where it flows around and over the brain and spinal cord to the most caudal extent of the dural sac at the S2 vertebral level.

While CSF is secreted by the **choroid plexus**, it is absorbed largely by the **arachnoid granulations** associated with the superior sagittal dural venous sinus and, to a lesser degree, by small veins on the surface of the pia mater throughout the CNS. The arachnoid granulations are tufts of arachnoid mater that extend through a layer of split dura, which forms the dural venous sinus, and act as one-way valves that deliver CSF into the venous blood of the sinus.

COLOR the features of the arachnoid granulations, using the following color scheme:

☐ **4. Pia mater covering the cerebrum (green)**

☐ **5. Arachnoid mater and its granulations (villi) (red)**

☐ **6. Dura mater splitting to create the dural venous sinus (yellow)**

☐ **7. Venous blood in the superior sagittal dural venous sinus: note the connections with small emissary veins that pass from the scalp through the bony skull to join the sinus (also color blue)**

Clinical Note:

CSF may be sampled and examined clinically by performing a **lumbar puncture** (spinal tap). A needle is inserted into the subarachnoid space of the lumbar cistern, in the midline between the L3-L4 or L4-L5 vertebral spinal processes to avoid sticking the spinal cord proper (the cord ends at about the L1-L2 vertebrae; see part D).

Additionally, anesthetic agents may be administered into the epidural space (above the dura mater) to directly anesthetize the nerve fibers of the cauda equina. The **epidural anesthetic** infiltrates the dural sac to reach the nerve roots and is usually administered at the same levels as the lumbar puncture (see part E).

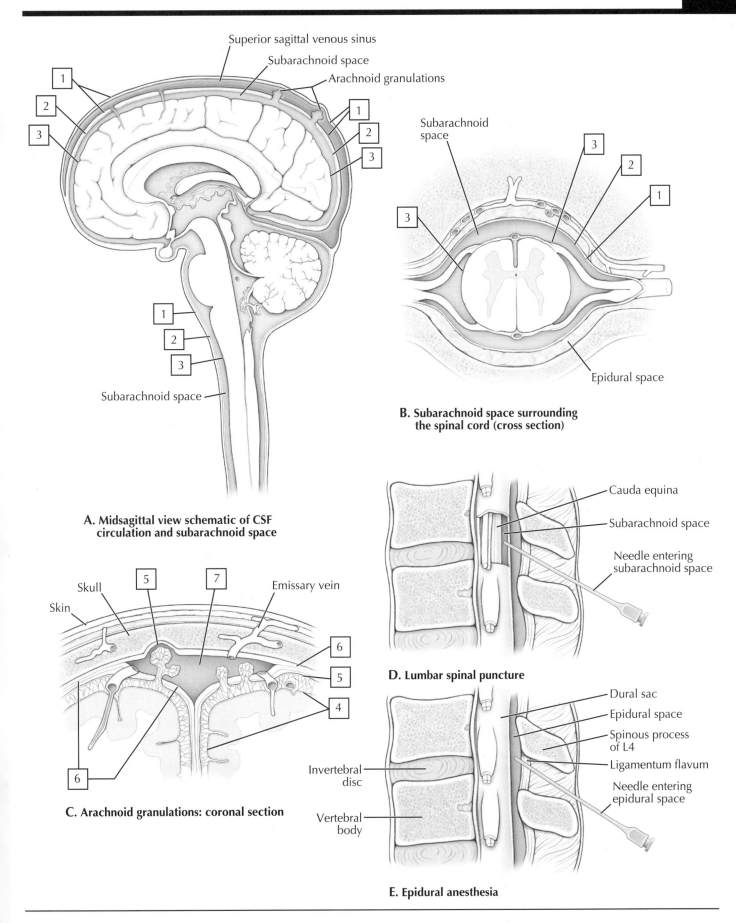

Superior sagittal venous sinus

Subarachnoid space

Arachnoid granulations

1
2
3

1
2
3

1
2
3

Subarachnoid space

A. Midsagittal view schematic of CSF circulation and subarachnoid space

Subarachnoid space

3

3
2
1

Epidural space

B. Subarachnoid space surrounding the spinal cord (cross section)

Skull

5   7   Emissary vein

Skin

6
5
4

6

C. Arachnoid granulations: coronal section

Cauda equina

Subarachnoid space

Needle entering subarachnoid space

D. Lumbar spinal puncture

Dural sac

Epidural space

Spinous process of L4

Ligamentum flavum

Needle entering epidural space

Invertebral disc

Vertebral body

E. Epidural anesthesia

The ANS is divided into the **sympathetic** and **parasympathetic divisions**. In contrast to the somatic division of the PNS, the ANS is a two-neuron system with a preganglionic neuron in the CNS that sends its axon into a peripheral nerve to synapse on a postganglionic neuron in a **peripheral autonomic ganglion**. The postganglionic neuron then sends its axon to the target (smooth muscle, cardiac muscle, and glands). The ANS is a visceral system because many of the body's organs are composed of smooth muscle walls and/or contain secretory glandular tissue.

The sympathetic division is also known as the **thoracolumbar division** because:
- Its preganglionic neurons are found only in the T1-L2 spinal cord levels
- Its preganglion neurons lie within the intermediolateral gray matter of the spinal cord in the 14 segments defined above

Preganglionic axons exit the T1-L2 spinal cord in a ventral root, and enter a spinal nerve and then a white ramus communicans to enter the **sympathetic chain**. The sympathetic chain is a bilateral chain of ganglia just lateral to the vertebral bodies that runs from the base of the skull to the coccyx. Once in the sympathetic chain, the preganglionic axon may do one of three things:
- Synapse on a sympathetic chain postganglionic neuron at the T1-L2 level or ascend or descend to synapse on a sympathetic chain neuron at any of the 31 spinal nerve levels
- Pass through the sympathetic chain, enter a **splanchnic (visceral) nerve**, and synapse in a **collateral ganglion** (celiac, superior mesenteric, inferior mesenteric) in the abdominopelvic cavity
- Pass through the sympathetic chain, enter a splanchnic nerve, pass through a collateral ganglion, and synapse on the cells of the **adrenal medulla**

Axons of the postganglionic sympathetic neurons may do one of four things:
- Those axons from sympathetic chain neurons re-enter the spinal nerve via a gray ramus communicans and join any one of the 31 spinal nerves as they distribute widely throughout the body
- Do the same as in the previous option but course along blood vessels in the head or join cardiopulmonary or hypogastric plexuses of nerves to distribute to head, thorax, and pelvic viscera
- Arise from postganglionic neurons in collateral ganglia and course with blood vessels to abdominopelvic viscera
- The postganglionic cells of the adrenal medulla are differentiated **endocrine cells (paraneurons)** that do not have axons but release their hormone (epinephrine and norepinephrine) directly into the bloodstream

COLOR the sympathetic preganglionic neuron and its axons red (solid lines), and color the postganglionic neuron and its axons green (dashed lines).

Preganglionic axons release **acetylcholine (ACh)** at their synapses, whereas **norepinephrine (NE)** is the transmitter released by postganglionic axons (except on sweat glands where it is ACh). The cells of the adrenal medulla (modified postganglionic sympathetic neurons) release **epinephrine** and some NE not as neurotransmitters but as hormones into the blood. The sympathetic system acts globally throughout the body to mobilize it in "fright-flight-fight" situations. The specific functions are summarized in the following table.

STRUCTURE	EFFECTS
Eyes	Dilates the pupil
Lacrimal glands	Reduces secretion slightly (vasoconstriction)
Skin	Causes goose bumps (arrector pili muscle contraction)
Sweat glands	Increases secretion
Peripheral vessels	Causes vasoconstriction
Heart	Increases heart rate and force of contraction
Coronary arteries	Assists in vasodilation
Lungs	Assists in bronchodilation and reduced secretion
Digestive tract	Decreases peristalsis, contracts internal anal sphincter muscle, causes vasoconstriction to shunt blood elsewhere
Liver	Causes glycogen breakdown, glucose synthesis and release
Salivary glands	Reduces and thickens secretion via vasoconstriction
Genital system	Causes ejaculation and orgasm, and remission of erection
	Constricts male internal urethral sphincter muscle
Urinary system	Decreases urine production via vasoconstriction
	Constricts male internal urethral sphincter muscle
Adrenal medulla	Increases secretion of epinephrine or norepinephrine

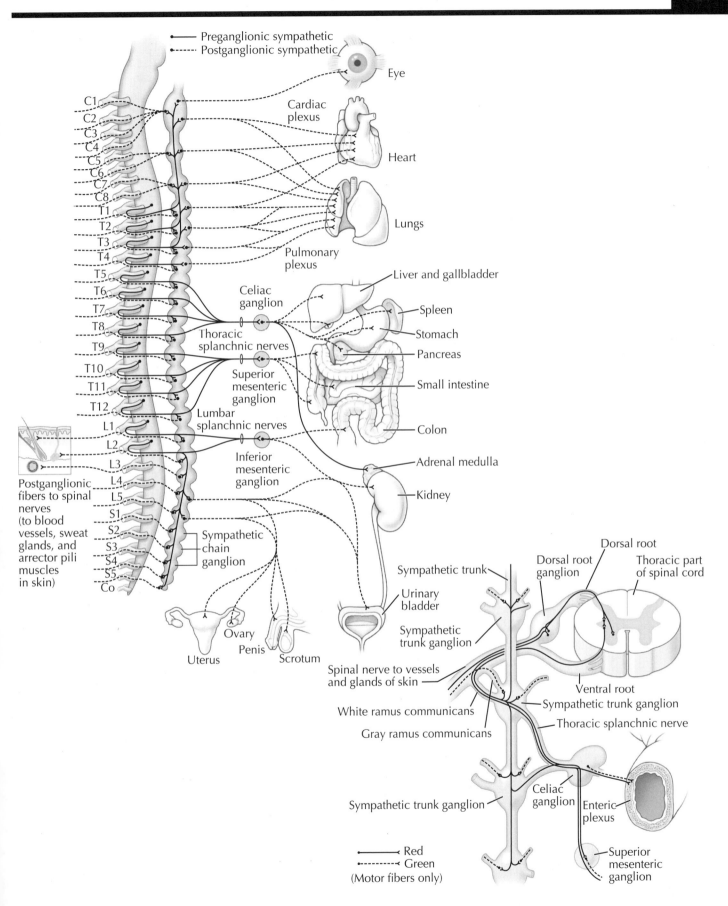

Preganglionic sympathetic
Postganglionic sympathetic

Eye

Cardiac plexus

Heart

Lungs

Pulmonary plexus

C1
C2
C3
C4
C5
C6
C7
C8
T1
T2
T3
T4
T5
T6
T7
T8
T9
T10
T11
T12
L1
L2
L3
L4
L5
S1
S2
S3
S4
S5
Co

Celiac ganglion

Thoracic splanchnic nerves

Superior mesenteric ganglion

Lumbar splanchnic nerves

Inferior mesenteric ganglion

Liver and gallbladder
Spleen
Stomach
Pancreas
Small intestine
Colon
Adrenal medulla
Kidney

Postganglionic fibers to spinal nerves (to blood vessels, sweat glands, and arrector pili muscles in skin)

Sympathetic chain ganglion

Ovary
Uterus
Penis
Scrotum

Urinary bladder

Sympathetic trunk

Sympathetic trunk ganglion

Spinal nerve to vessels and glands of skin

White ramus communicans

Gray ramus communicans

Sympathetic trunk ganglion

Dorsal root
Dorsal root ganglion
Thoracic part of spinal cord

Ventral root
Sympathetic trunk ganglion

Thoracic splanchnic nerve

Celiac ganglion
Enteric plexus

Superior mesenteric ganglion

Red
Green
(Motor fibers only)

The parasympathetic division of the ANS also is a two-neuron system with its preganglionic neuron in the CNS and postganglionic neuron in a peripheral ganglion. The parasympathetic division also is known as the **craniosacral division** because:

- Its preganglionic neurons are found in cranial nerves III, VII, IX and X, and in the sacral spinal cord at levels S2-S4
- Its preganglionic neurons reside in the four cranial nuclei associated with the four cranial nerves listed previously, or in the lateral gray matter of the sacral spinal cord at levels S2-S4

Preganglionic parasympathetic axons may do one of two things:

- Exit the brainstem in the cranial nerve (except CN X, see below) and pass to a peripheral ganglion in the head (ciliary, pterygopalatine, submandibular, and otic ganglia) to synapse on the parasympathetic postganglionic neurons residing in these ganglia
- Exit the sacral spinal cord via a ventral root and then enter the **pelvic splanchnic nerves** to synapse on postganglionic neurons in **terminal ganglia** located in or near the viscera to be innervated

Axons of the postganglionic parasympathetic neurons may do one of two things:

- Pass from the **parasympathetic ganglion in the head** on existing nerves or blood vessels to innervate smooth muscle and glands of the head
- Pass from **terminal ganglia** in or near the viscera innervated and synapse on smooth muscle, cardiac muscle, or glands in the neck, thorax, and abdominopelvic cavity

CN X (vagus nerve) is unique. Its preganglionic axons exit the brainstem and synapse on terminal ganglia in or near the targets in the neck, thorax (heart, lungs, glands, smooth muscle), and abdominal cavity (proximal two thirds of the GI tract and its accessory organs). Axons of the terminal ganglia neurons then synapse on their targets.

COLOR the preganglionic parasympathetic neurons and their axons (solid lines) arising from a cranial nerve or S2-S4 red, and color the postganglionic neuron and axon (dashed lines) in the peripheral or terminal ganglion green.

The sympathetic axons pass into the limbs, but the parasympathetic axons do not. Therefore the vascular smooth muscle, arrector pili muscles of the skin (attached to hair follicles), and sweat glands are all innervated only by the sympathetic system. ACh is the neurotransmitter at all parasympathetic synapses. The parasympathetic system is concerned with feeding and sexual arousal and acts more slowly and focally than the sympathetic system. For example, CN X can slow the heart rate without affecting input to the stomach. In general, the sympathetic and parasympathetic systems maintain **homeostasis**, although as a protective measure, the body does maintain a low level of "sympathetic tone" and can activate this division on a moment's notice. ANS function is regulated ultimately by the **hypothalamus**. The specific functions of the parasympathetic division of the ANS are summarized in the table below.

STRUCTURE	EFFECTS
Eyes	Constricts pupil
Ciliary body	Constricts muscle for accommodation (near vision)
Lacrimal glands	Increases secretion
Heart	Decreases heart rate and force of contraction
Coronary arteries	Causes vasoconstriction with reduced metabolic demand
Lungs	Causes bronchoconstriction and increased secretion
Digestive tract	Increases peristalsis, increases secretion, inhibits internal anal sphincter for defecation
Liver	Aids glycogen synthesis and storage
Salivary glands	Increases secretion
Genital system	Promotes engorgement of erectile tissues
Urinary system	Contracts bladder (detrusor muscle) for urination, inhibits contraction of internal urethral sphincter, increases urine production

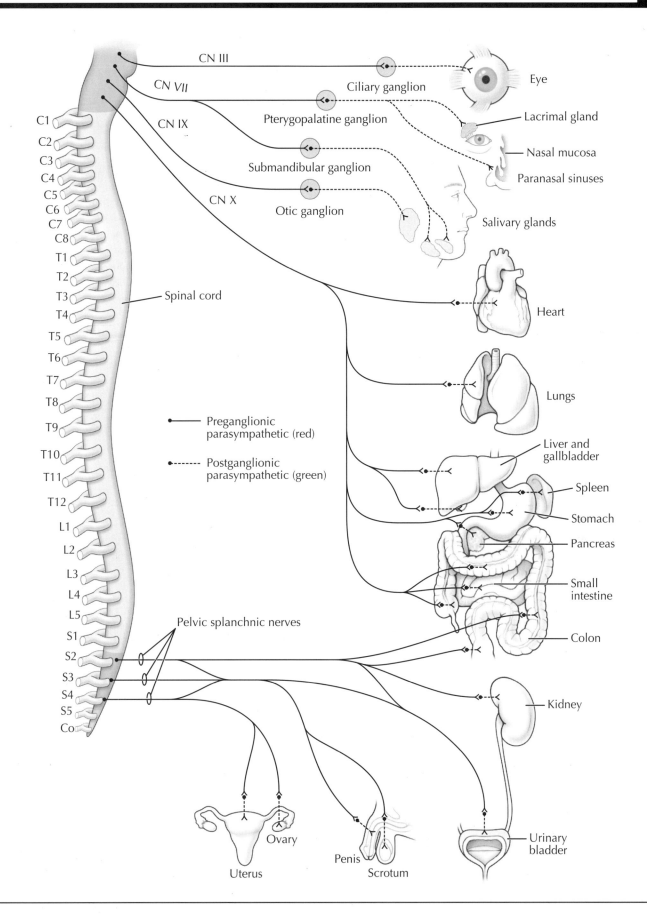

CN III

CN VII

CN IX

CN X

C1
C2
C3
C4
C5
C6
C7
C8
T1
T2
T3
T4
T5
T6
T7
T8
T9
T10
T11
T12
L1
L2
L3
L4
L5
S1
S2
S3
S4
S5
Co

Spinal cord

Ciliary ganglion

Pterygopalatine ganglion

Submandibular ganglion

Otic ganglion

Eye

Lacrimal gland

Nasal mucosa

Paranasal sinuses

Salivary glands

Heart

Lungs

Liver and gallbladder

Spleen

Stomach

Pancreas

Small intestine

Colon

Kidney

Urinary bladder

Preganglionic parasympathetic (red)

Postganglionic parasympathetic (green)

Pelvic splanchnic nerves

Ovary

Uterus

Penis

Scrotum

Historically, the third division of the ANS was the enteric nervous system (the intrinsic neurons and nerve plexus found in the myenteric and submucosal layers of the bowel). Because the enteric neurons can function somewhat independently, it was simplistically viewed as having a "brain of its own." However, the enteric nervous system is linked to the sympathetic and parasympathetic divisions of the ANS, and these are required for optimal regulation of bowel secretion, absorption, and motility. Some have characterized the enteric system as a "computer terminal" that has connections with the ANS and to the hypothalamus, which functions as the "master computer."

The neurons and nerve plexuses of the enteric nervous system use a variety of neurotransmitters and neuromodulators to communicate with one another and coordinate bowel function. More than 20 such substances have been identified, and it is estimated that the number of neurons in the gut are at least equivalent to the number found in the spinal cord!

ANS connections to the enteric nervous system include:
- Vagal parasympathetic input to the esophagus, stomach, small intestine, and proximal half of the colon
- S2-S4 parasympathetic input via pelvic splanchnic nerves to the distal half of the colon and to the rectum
- Sympathetic input from thoracic splanchnic nerves (T5-T12) to the stomach, small intestine, and proximal half of the colon
- Sympathetic input from lumbar splanchnic nerves (L1-L2) to the distal half of the colon and to the rectum

COLOR the following pathways from the ANS to the enteric nerve plexuses, using a different color for each pathway:

- [ ] 1. **Vagus nerves**
- [ ] 2. **Pelvic splanchnic nerves**
- [ ] 3. **Thoracic splanchnic nerves**
- [ ] 4. **Lumbar splanchnic nerves**

Clinical Note:

Congenital megacolon (distended large bowel) (also known as **Hirschsprung's disease**) results from a developmental defect that leads to an aganglionic segment of bowel that lacks both a submucosal and myenteric plexus. Distention of the bowel proximal to the aganglionic region may occur shortly after birth or may cause symptoms only later, in early childhood.

Plate 4-21

Nervous System

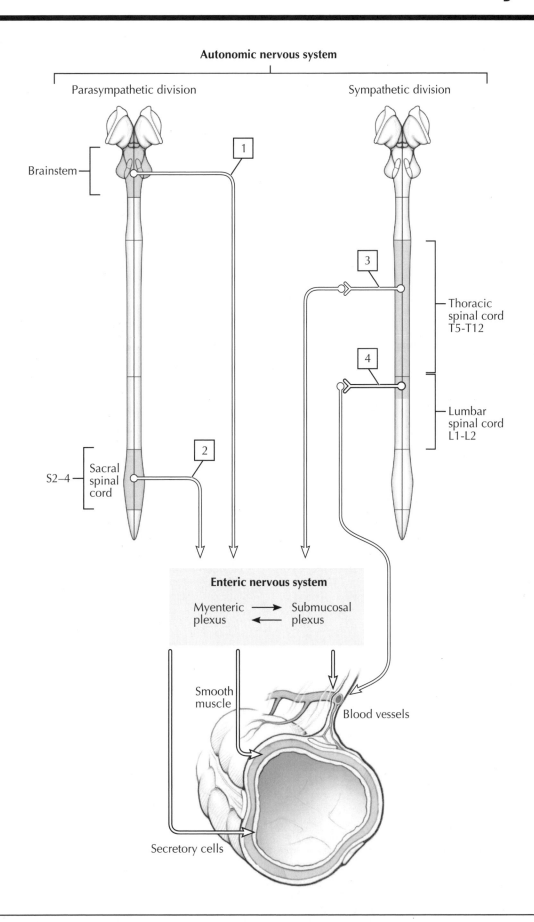

Autonomic nervous system

Parasympathetic division

Sympathetic division

Brainstem

1

3

Thoracic
spinal cord
T5-T12

4

Lumbar
spinal cord
L1-L2

2

S2–4 | Sacral
spinal
cord

Enteric nervous system

Myenteric → Submucosal
plexus ← plexus

Smooth
muscle

Blood vessels

Secretory cells

In addition to the 31 pairs of spinal nerves, 12 pairs of cranial nerves arise from the brain, and they are identified both by their names and by **Roman numerals I through XII**. The cranial nerves are somewhat unique and can contain multiple functional components:

- **General**: same general functions as spinal nerves
- **Special**: functions found only in cranial nerves
- **Afferent and efferent**: sensory or motor functions, respectively
- **Somatic and visceral**: related to skin and skeletal muscle (somatic), or to smooth muscle and glands (visceral)

Hence, each cranial nerve may possess multiple functional components, such as GSA (general somatic afferents), meaning it contains nerve fibers that are sensory from the skin, not unlike those of the spinal nerve; GVE (general visceral efferents), meaning it contains motor fibers to visceral structures (smooth muscle and/or glands) like a parasympathetic fiber from the sacral spinal cord (S2-S4 gives rise to parasympathetics); or SSA (special somatic afferents), meaning it contains special sensory fibers, such as those for vision or hearing.

In general, CN I and II arise from the forebrain and are really tracts of the brain for the special senses of smell and sight. CN III, IV, and VI move the extra-ocular skeletal muscles of the eyeball. CN V has three divisions: V_1 and V_2 are sensory, and V_3 is both motor to skeletal muscle and sensory. CN VII, IX and X are both motor and sensory. CN VIII is the special sense of hearing and balance. CN XI and XII are motor to skeletal muscle. CN III, VII, IX and X also contain parasympathetic fibers of origin (visceral), although many of the ANS fibers will "jump" onto the branches of CN V to reach their targets. The following table summarizes the types of fibers in each cranial nerve.

COLOR each cranial nerve as it arises from the brain or brainstem:

- ☐ 1. **I, olfactory nerve**
- ☐ 2. **II, optic nerve**
- ☐ 3. **III, oculomotor nerve**
- ☐ 4. **IV, trochlear nerve**
- ☐ 5. **V, trigeminal nerve**
- ☐ 6. **VI, abducent nerve**
- ☐ 7. **VII, facial nerve**
- ☐ 8. **VIII, vestibulocochlear nerve**
- ☐ 9. **IX, glossopharyngeal nerve**
- ☐ 10. **X, vagus nerve**
- ☐ 11. **XI, accessory nerve**
- ☐ 12. **XII, hypoglossal nerve**

CRANIAL NERVE	FUNCTIONAL COMPONENT
I Olfactory nerve	SSA (special sense of smell)
II Optic nerve	SSA (special sense of sight)
III Oculomotor nerve	GSE (motor to extra-ocular muscles)
	GVE (parasympathetic to smooth muscle in eye)
IV Trochlear nerve	GSE (motor to 1 extra-ocular muscle)
V Trigeminal nerve	GSA (sensory to face, orbit, nose, anterior tongue)
	SVE (motor to skeletal muscles)
VI Abducent nerve	GSE (motor to 1 extra-ocular muscle)
VII Facial nerve	GSA (sensory to skin of ear)
	SVA (special sense of taste to anterior tongue)
	GVE (motor to glands—salivary, nasal, lacrimal)
	SVE (motor to facial muscles)
VIII Vestibulocochlear nerve	SSA (special sense of hearing and balance)
IX Glossopharyngeal nerve	GSA (sensory to posterior tongue)
	SVA (special sense of taste—posterior tongue)
	GVA (sensory from middle ear, pharynx, carotid body, and sinus)
	GVE (motor to parotid gland)
	SVE (motor to 1 muscle of pharynx)
X Vagus nerve	GSA (sensory external ear)
	SVA (special sense of taste—epiglottis)
	GVA (sensory from pharynx, larynx, and thoracic and abdominal organs)
	GVE (motor to thoracic and abdominal organs)
	SVE (motor to muscles of pharynx/larynx)
XI Accessory nerve	GSE (motor to 2 muscles)
XII Hypoglossal nerve	GSE (motor to tongue muscles)

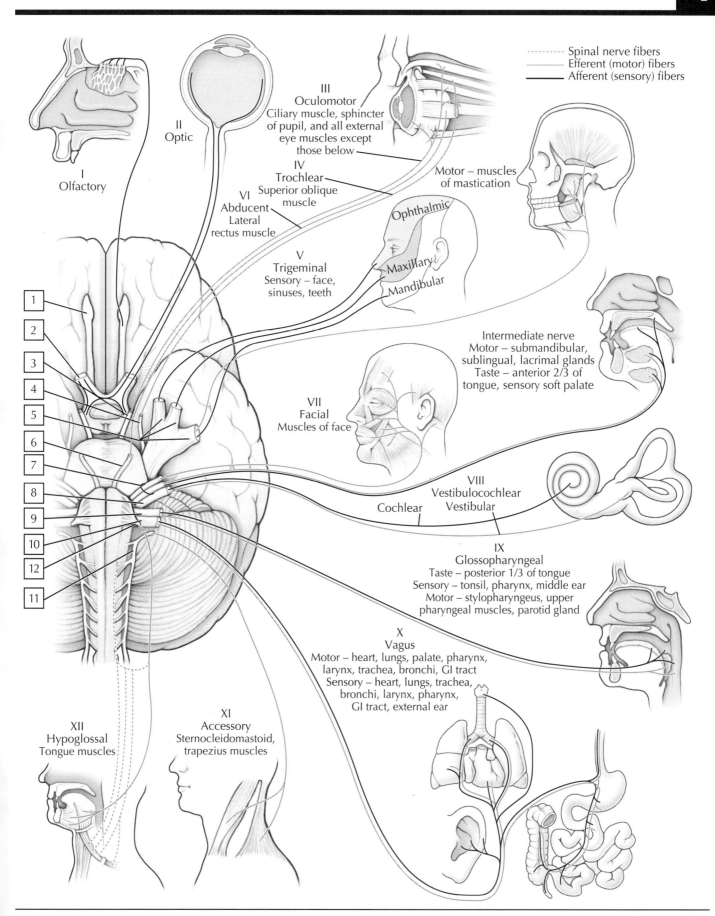

Spinal nerve fibers
Efferent (motor) fibers
Afferent (sensory) fibers

III
Oculomotor
Ciliary muscle, sphincter
of pupil, and all external
eye muscles except
those below

IV
Trochlear
Superior oblique
muscle

VI
Abducent
Lateral
rectus muscle

II
Optic

I
Olfactory

Motor – muscles
of mastication

Ophthalmic

Maxillary

Mandibular

V
Trigeminal
Sensory – face,
sinuses, teeth

Intermediate nerve
Motor – submandibular,
sublingual, lacrimal glands
Taste – anterior 2/3 of
tongue, sensory soft palate

VII
Facial
Muscles of face

VIII
Vestibulocochlear
Vestibular

Cochlear

IX
Glossopharyngeal
Taste – posterior 1/3 of tongue
Sensory – tonsil, pharynx, middle ear
Motor – stylopharyngeus, upper
pharyngeal muscles, parotid gland

X
Vagus
Motor – heart, lungs, palate, pharynx,
larynx, trachea, bronchi, GI tract
Sensory – heart, lungs, trachea,
bronchi, larynx, pharynx,
GI tract, external ear

XII
Hypoglossal
Tongue muscles

XI
Accessory
Sternocleidomastoid,
trapezius muscles

1
2
3
4
5
6
7
8
9
10
12
11

The eyeball (globe) is protected by the eyelid, which, in combination with the lacrimal apparatus, keeps the cornea moist by laying down a thin layer of tear film that coats the exposed surface of the eyeball (conjunctiva and cornea).

COLOR the following features of the lacrimal apparatus, using a different color for each feature:

☐ **1. Lacrimal gland: secretes tears under control of the parasympathetic fibers that originate in the facial nerve (CN VII)**

☐ **2. Lacrimal ducts: excretory ducts of the lacrimal gland**

☐ **3. Lacrimal sac: receives tears that are collected by the lacrimal canaliculi associated with the superior and inferior lacrimal punctum**

☐ **4. Nasolacrimal duct: conveys tears from the lacrimal sac into the nasal cavity**

Excessive irritation, pain, or emotional triggers can increase tear production (crying). Excess tears overwhelm the collecting system of the lacrimal ducts such that the tears will spill over the lower eyelid and run down the cheek. Likewise, copious tears collected in the lacrimal sacs will flow into the nasal cavity and cause a "runny" nose. Tears contain albumins, lactoferrin, lysozyme, lipids, metabolites, and electrolytes.

The human eyeball measures about 25 mm in diameter, is tethered in the bony orbit by six **extra-ocular muscles** that move the globe (see Plate 3-3), and is cushioned by fat that surrounds the posterior two thirds of the globe. The eyeball is composed of three concentric layers:
- **Fibrous**: an outer layer that includes the cornea and sclera
- **Vascular**: the middle (uveal) layer that includes the choroid, and the stroma of the ciliary body and iris
- **Retina**: an outer, pigmented epithelium upon which the neural retina (photosensitive) lies

COLOR the following layers of the eyeball, using a different color for each layer:

☐ **5. Cornea**

☐ **6. Iris**

☐ **7. Ciliary body**

☐ **8. Retina**

☐ **9. Choroid**

☐ **10. Sclera**

The large chamber behind the lens is the **vitreous chamber** (body) and is filled with a gel-like substance called the **vitreous humor**, which helps cushion and protect the fragile retina during rapid movements of the eye. The chamber between the cornea and the iris is the **anterior chamber**, and the space between the iris and lens is the **posterior chamber**. Both of these chambers are filled with **aqueous humor**, which is produced by the **ciliary body** and circulates from the posterior chamber through the pupil (central opening in the iris) and into the anterior chamber where it is absorbed by the trabecular meshwork into the **scleral venous sinus** at the angle of the cornea and iris.

The **ciliary body** contains smooth muscle that is arranged in a circular fashion like a sphincter muscle. When this muscle is relaxed, it pulls a set of zonular fibers attached to the elastic lens taut and flattens the lens for viewing objects at some distance from the eye. When focusing on near objects, the sphincter-like ciliary muscle contracts and constricts in closer to the lens, relaxing the zonular fibers and allowing the elastic lens to round up for accommodation. This **accommodation reflex** is controlled by parasympathetic fibers that originate in the oculomotor (CN III) nerve.

The iris also contains smooth muscle. Contraction of the circular **sphincter pupillae muscle**, under the control of CN III parasympathetic fibers, makes the pupil smaller, whereas contraction of the radially oriented **dilator pupillae muscle** under sympathetic control makes the pupil larger.

COLOR the following features of the anterior portion of the eyeball, using a different color for each feature:

☐ **11. Sphincter pupillae muscle of the iris**

☐ **12. Lens**

☐ **13. Dilator pupillae muscle of the iris**

☐ **14. Zonular fibers**

FEATURE	DEFINITION
Sclera	Outer fibrous layer of eyeball
Cornea	Transparent part of outer layer; very sensitive to pain
Choroid	Vascular middle layer of eyeball
Ciliary body	Vascular and muscular extension of choroid anteriorly
Ciliary process	Radiating pigmented folds on ciliary body; secrete aqueous humor that fills posterior and anterior chambers
Iris	Contractile diaphragm with central aperture (pupil)
Lens	Transparent lens supported in capsule by zonular fibers
Retina	Optically receptive part of optic nerve (optic retina)
Macula lutea	Retinal area of most acute vision
Optic disc	Nonreceptive area where optic nerve axons leave retina for brain

Clinical Note:

A **cataract** is an opacity, or cloudy area, in the crystalline lens. Treatment is often surgical, involving lens removal with vision correction with glasses, or an implanted plastic lens (intraocular lens).

Glaucoma is an optic neuropathy; the cause of glaucoma usually is an increase to resistance to outflow of aqueous humor in the anterior chamber, which leads to an increase in the intraocular pressure.

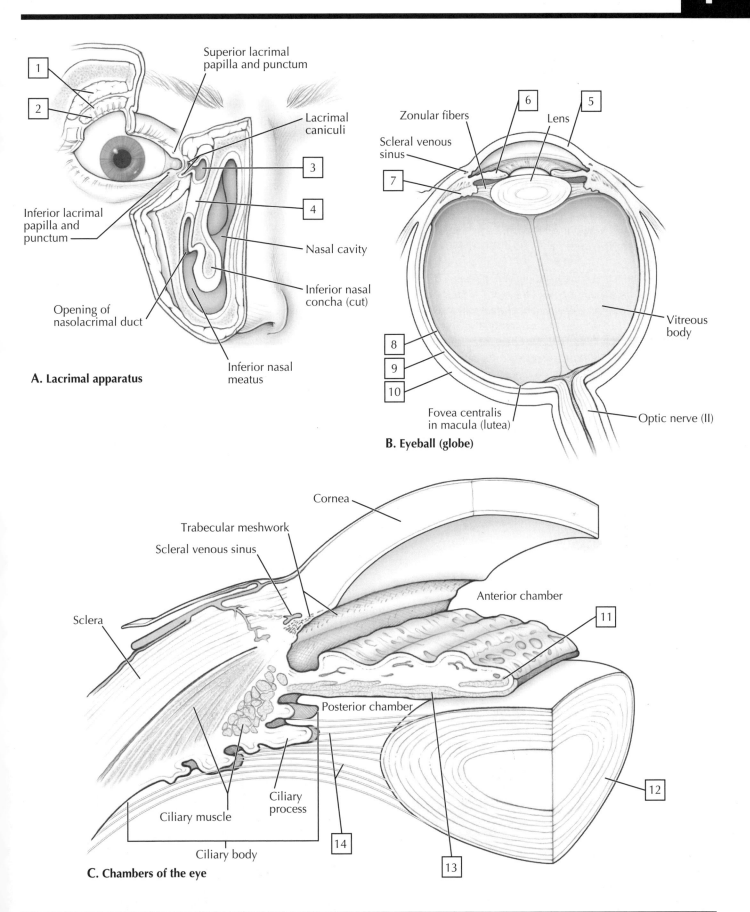

1

2

Superior lacrimal
papilla and punctum

Lacrimal
caniculi

3

4

Inferior lacrimal
papilla and
punctum

Nasal cavity

Inferior nasal
concha (cut)

Opening of
nasolacrimal duct

Inferior nasal
meatus

A. Lacrimal apparatus

Zonular fibers

6

5

Lens

Scleral venous
sinus

7

Vitreous
body

8

9

10

Fovea centralis
in macula (lutea)

Optic nerve (II)

B. Eyeball (globe)

Cornea

Trabecular meshwork

Scleral venous sinus

Anterior chamber

Sclera

11

Posterior chamber

12

Ciliary
process

Ciliary muscle

14

Ciliary body

13

C. Chambers of the eye

The **retina** is a very thin layer of tissue that is a direct extension of the brain, with most of its ganglion cell axons coursing back through the optic nerve to reach their first synapse in the lateral geniculate bodies of the thalamus. Light passes through the refractile media of the eye (cornea, aqueous humor, lens, and vitreous humor) to impinge on the neural retina, where it passes through the thickness of the retina to finally encounter the **photoreceptor cells** resting on a layer of **pigmented epithelium** (this epithelium prevents backscatter). The photoreceptors (rods and cones) synapse with bipolar cells, which synapse with the ganglion cells, whereas amacrine and horizontal cells provide interconnections. **Cones** are specialized for bright-light (color) vision and rods for low-light (night) vision. Each human retina contains about 7 million cones and about 120 million rods.

The portion of the retina directly in line with the focus of the lens and situated at the posterior pole of the globe is specialized. Here there is an area called the **macula lutea** with a very small pit, about the size of the head of a pin, called the **fovea centralis** in the middle of the lutea. In the fovea, the retina is very thin and consists only of cones and ganglion cells, and it represents our area of greatest visual acuity. The macula lutea contains mostly cones and some rods, and outside of the macula, the rods predominate over cones.

COLOR the cells of the neural retina, using the suggested colors for each cell:

- ☐ 1. **Pigmented epithelium (brown)**
- ☐ 2. **Ganglion cells and their axons (yellow)**
- ☐ 3. **Bipolar cells (red)**
- ☐ 4. **Rods (gray) (the thinner cells)**
- ☐ 5. **Cones (blue) (the thicker cells)**

The visual pathway is organized topographically throughout its course to the occipital lobe. **Nasal** (medial side of the retina) ganglion cells send axons that cross the midline at the **optic chiasm** whereas **temporal** (lateral side of the retina) ganglion cell axons remain ipsilateral (on the same side). Ganglion cell axons in the optic tracts:

- Largely terminate in the lateral geniculate body, which is organized in six layers
- Optic radiations from the geniculate body pass to the calcarine cortex of the occipital lobe, where conscious visual perception occurs
- From this region of the primary visual cortex, axons pass to the association visual cortex for processing of form, color, and movement
- Connections to the temporal lobe provide high-resolution object recognition (faces, and classification of objects)
- Connections to the parietal cortex provide analysis of motion of positional relationships of objects in the visual scene

Clinical Note:

Ametropias are the aberrant focusing of light rays on a site other than the optimal retinal site, the macula lutea. Optically, the cornea, lens, and axial length of the eyeball must be in precise balance to achieve sharp focus. Common disorders include:

- Myopia (nearsightedness): 80% of ametropias, where the point of focus is in front of the retina
- Hyperopia (farsightedness): age-related occurrence, where the point of focus is behind the retina
- Astigmatism: a nonspheroidal cornea causes focusing at multiple locations instead of at a single point; affects about 25% to 40% of the population
- Presbyopia: age-related progressive loss of the ability to accommodate the lens because of a loss of elasticity in the lens, requiring correction for seeing near objects or reading

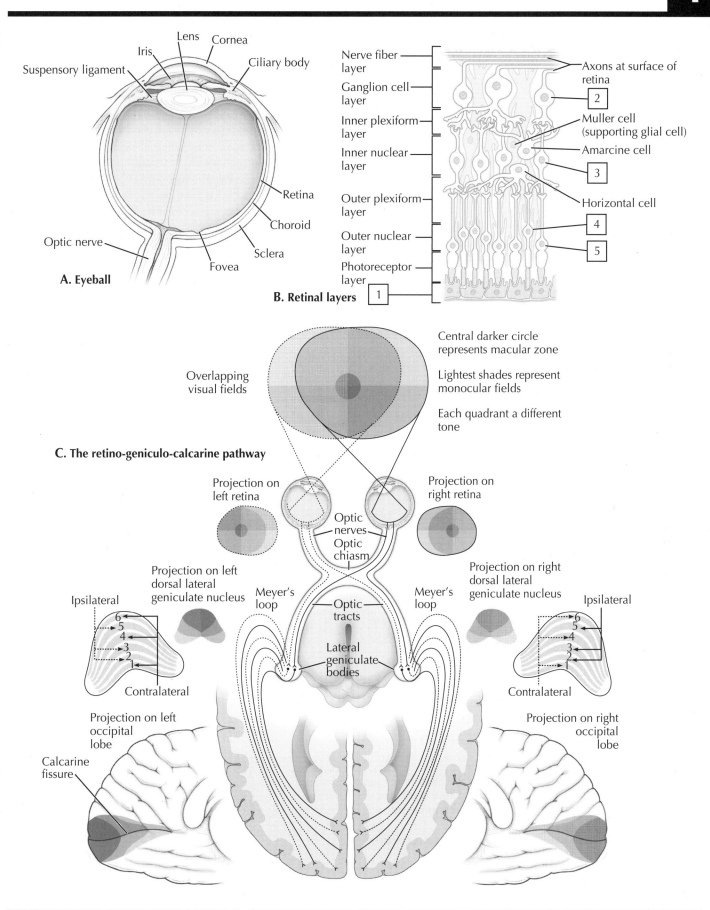

A. Eyeball

Suspensory ligament · Iris · Lens · Cornea · Ciliary body · Retina · Choroid · Sclera · Fovea · Optic nerve

B. Retinal layers

Nerve fiber layer · Ganglion cell layer · Inner plexiform layer · Inner nuclear layer · Outer plexiform layer · Outer nuclear layer · Photoreceptor layer · 1

Axons at surface of retina · 2 · Muller cell (supporting glial cell) · Amarcine cell · 3 · Horizontal cell · 4 · 5

C. The retino-geniculo-calcarine pathway

Overlapping visual fields

Central darker circle represents macular zone

Lightest shades represent monocular fields

Each quadrant a different tone

Projection on left retina · Projection on right retina

Optic nerves · Optic chiasm

Projection on left dorsal lateral geniculate nucleus · Meyer's loop · Optic tracts · Meyer's loop · Projection on right dorsal lateral geniculate nucleus

Ipsilateral · 6 5 4 3 2 1 · Contralateral

Lateral geniculate bodies

Ipsilateral · 6 5 4 3 2 1 · Contralateral

Projection on left occipital lobe · Projection on right occipital lobe

Calcarine fissure

The transduction mechanism of the ear (hearing) and vestibular system (equilibrium) are closely aligned anatomically. The ear consists of three parts:
- **External**: the auricle (pinna), external acoustic meatus (canal), and the tympanic membrane (eardrum)
- **Middle**: the tympanic cavity that contains the ear ossicles (malleus, incus, and stapes); communicates with the mastoid antrum posteriorly and with the auditory (eustachian) tube anteriorly
- **Inner (internal)**: the acoustic apparatus (cochlea) and vestibular apparatus (vestibule with the utricle and saccule, and semicircular canals)

COLOR the following features of the ear, using a different color for each feature:

☐ 1. **Middle ear ossicles (malleus, incus, and stapes) (also known as the hammer, anvil, and stirrup, respectively)**

☐ 2. **Cochlea**

☐ 3. **Tympanic membrane**

☐ 4. **External acoustic meatus**

Sound waves travel through the external ear and set up vibrations of the tympanic membrane. These vibrations, in turn, cause the middle ear ossicles to vibrate, causing the stapes to vibrate against the **oval (vestibular) window**, initiating a wave action within the fluid-filled (perilymph) **scala vestibuli** and **scala tympani of the cochlea** that causes deflection and depolarization of tiny hair cells within the **organ of Corti**. This stimulates action potentials in the afferent axons of the spiral ganglion cells, which are then conveyed centrally to the cochlear nuclei of the medulla oblongata. From this point, impulses are conveyed to higher brain centers for auditory processing, ending in the auditory cortex in the temporal lobe.

COLOR the following features of the bony and membranous labyrinths of the cochlea and vestibular apparatus, using a different color for each feature:

☐ 5. **Semicircular canals (anterior, lateral, and posterior): which are arranged at 90 degrees to each other and represent the x-, y-, and z-axes**

☐ 6. **Utricle**

☐ 7. **Saccule**

☐ 8. **Round (cochlear) window: closed by a secondary tympanic membrane, which dissipates the fluid wave initiated at the oval window by the vibratory action of the stapes**

The final step in the auditory transduction pathway from mechanical vibrations to neuronal action potentials, which then are conveyed to the brain, occurs at the level of the organ of Corti within the cochlea. Cochlear hair cells (inner and outer rows) rest on a basilar membrane and are arranged functionally. Traveling pressure waves in the scala vestibuli are transmitted through the **vestibular membrane** to the endolymph-filled cochlear duct. These traveling pressure waves displace the **basilar membrane** (louder sounds cause more displacement), and **tectorial membrane**. The hair cells on the basilar membrane have their tufts attached to the tectorial membrane, and the different displacements of these two membranes cause a shearing effect of the hair cells. This shearing effect deflects the hairs, depolarizes the hair cells, causes the release of neurotransmitters, and initiates an action potential in the afferent axons of the spiral ganglion cells.

COLOR the following features of the organ of Corti, using a different color for each feature:

☐ 9. **Cochlear nerve, spiral ganglion and axons**

☐ 10. **Inner hair cells**

☐ 11. **Outer hair cells**

☐ 12. **Basilar membrane**

☐ 13. **Tectorial membrane**

Clinical Note:
Several kinds of **hearing loss** can occur:
- **Conductive loss:** usually due to a disorder or damage to the tympanic membrane and/or the middle ear ossicles
- **Sensorineural loss:** disorder of the inner ear or cochlear division of the vestibulocochlear nerve (CN VIII), which may include such causes as infection, exposure to loud noises, tumors, or adverse reactions to certain administered drugs

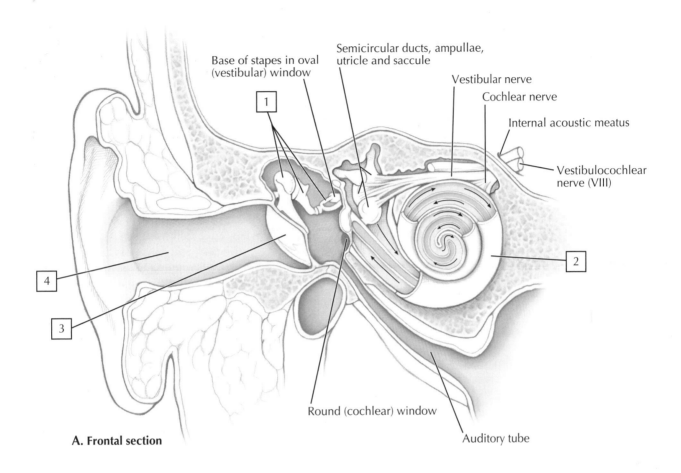

Base of stapes in oval (vestibular) window

Semicircular ducts, ampullae, utricle and saccule

Vestibular nerve

Cochlear nerve

Internal acoustic meatus

Vestibulocochlear nerve (VIII)

1

2

4

3

Round (cochlear) window

Auditory tube

A. Frontal section

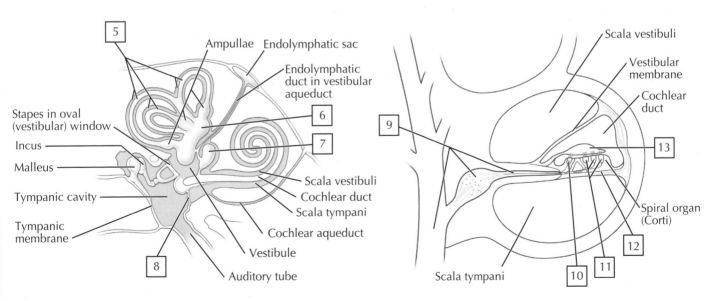

5

Ampullae Endolymphatic sac

Endolymphatic duct in vestibular aqueduct

Stapes in oval (vestibular) window

Incus

Malleus

Tympanic cavity

Tympanic membrane

6

7

Scala vestibuli
Cochlear duct
Scala tympani

Cochlear aqueduct

Vestibule

Auditory tube

8

B. Bony and membranous labryinths: schema

Scala vestibuli

Vestibular membrane

Cochlear duct

9

13

Spiral organ (Corti)

12

Scala tympani

10   11

C. Section through turn of cochlea

While half of the vestibulocochlear nerve (CN VIII) is concerned with hearing, the other half conveys sensory information that is important in maintaining the special sense of equilibrium. Receptors for equilibrium involve two functional components:

• **Static**: a special receptor called the macula resides in each utricle and saccule and is concerned with the position of the head and linear acceleration, as well as gravity and low-frequency vibrations (saccule only)

• **Dynamic**: special receptors called the crista ampullaris reside in the ampulla of each semicircular canal and are concerned with angular (rotational) movements of the head

The maculae also have hair cells (like the organ of Corti), but a single kinocilium also exists at the edge of each bundle of hairlike stereocilia (really long microvilli). The "hair" tufts are embedded in a gelatinous polysaccharide mass called the **otolithic membrane**, which is capped by very small **otoliths** (calcium carbonate crystals), giving the mass a rigidity that resists a change in motion. During linear acceleration, the hairs are displaced and will increase their release of neurotransmitters onto the primary sensory axons of the vestibular ganglion cells. This occurs as the hairs are bent toward the kinocilium, thus depolarizing the hair cells. Movement of the hairs away from the kinocilium hyperpolarizes the hair cells, decreasing their release of neurotransmitters. Finally, the utricle's macula senses acceleration on a horizontal plane, whereas the saccule's macula is better at sensing vertical acceleration, the sensation one feels when one starts to ascend in an elevator.

COLOR the following features of the vestibular system (part A) and maculae (part B), using a different color for each feature:

☐ **1. Maculae of the saccule and utricle**

☐ **2. Vestibular ganglion and its afferent axons**

☐ **3. Cristae within the ampulla of the semicircular canals**

☐ **4. Otoliths (on the surface of the otolithic membrane)**

☐ **5. Gelatinous otolithic membrane**

☐ **6. Hair cells and "hair" tufts extending into the otolithic membrane**

The **crista** in the ampullae of the semicircular canals also have hair cells and a kinocilium just like the maculae. However, the gelatinous protein-polysaccharide mass is called a **cupula** (pointed cap) and it projects into the endolymph of the semicircular canal. During rotational movements, the cupula is swayed by the movement of the endolymph and the deflection of the hair cells causes depolarization and release of neurotransmitter on the sensory nerve endings.

COLOR the following features of the crista, using a different color for each feature:

☐ **7. Gelatinous cupula**

☐ **8. Hair cells and "hair" tufts extending into the cupula**

Vestibular afferent axons terminate in the vestibular nuclei in the brainstem or directly in the cerebellum, to modulate and coordinate muscle movement, tone, and posture. Descending axons from the vestibular nuclei course to the spinal cord to regulate head and neck movements, while other projections coordinate eye movements (CN III, IV, and VI). Finally, some axons ascend to the thalamus and then to the insular, temporal, and parietal cortex.

Clinical Note:

Vertigo is the sensation of movement or rotation with a loss of equilibrium (dizziness). It can be produced by excessive stimulation of the vestibular system, as occurs in seasickness, carsickness, or carnival rides. Viral infections, certain medications, and tumors also can lead to vertigo.

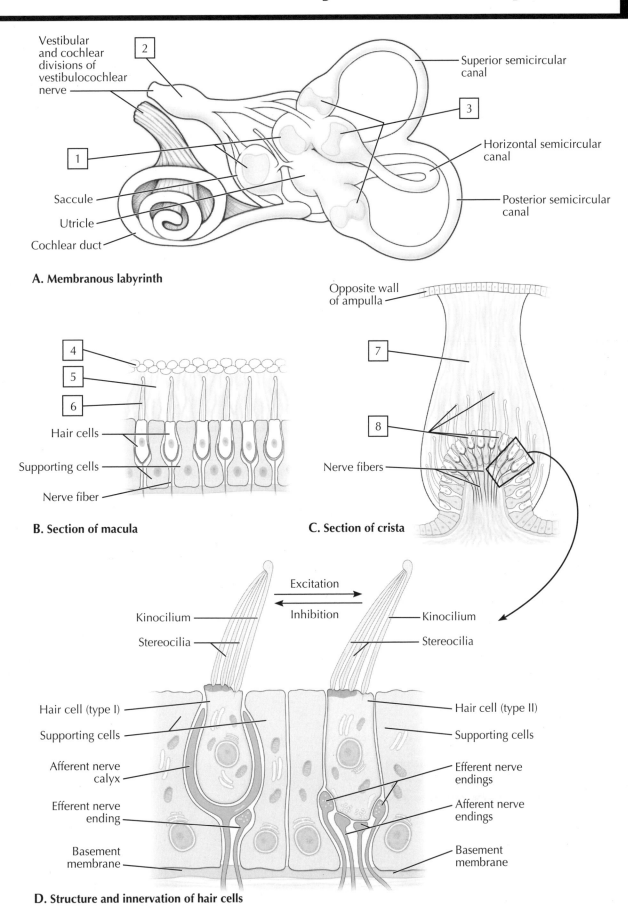

Vestibular and cochlear divisions of vestibulocochlear nerve

2

Superior semicircular canal

3

Horizontal semicircular canal

1

Posterior semicircular canal

Saccule

Utricle

Cochlear duct

A. Membranous labyrinth

4

5

6

Hair cells

Supporting cells

Nerve fiber

B. Section of macula

Opposite wall of ampulla

7

8

Nerve fibers

C. Section of crista

Excitation

Inhibition

Kinocilium

Stereocilia

Kinocilium

Stereocilia

Hair cell (type I)

Supporting cells

Afferent nerve calyx

Efferent nerve ending

Basement membrane

Hair cell (type II)

Supporting cells

Efferent nerve endings

Afferent nerve endings

Basement membrane

D. Structure and innervation of hair cells

Taste buds are chemoreceptors that transduce chemical "tastes" into electrical signals that are conveyed to the CNS for higher processing. We have about 2,000 to 5,000 taste buds (each with 50-150 taste receptor cells) mostly located on the dorsal tongue (also present on the epiglottis and palate), which can distinguish the following taste sensations:

- **Salty**: inorganic salts
- **Sweet**: organic molecules, such as sugar, alcohol, saccharin, and some amino acids
- **Sour**: acids and protons (hydrogen ions)
- **Bitter**: alkaloids and poisons
- **Umami**: glutamate (the taste of MSG)

On the tongue, various mucosal specializations called **lingual papillae** are evident and include four types, three of which possess taste buds:

- **Filiform**: small and the most numerous papillae, they serve only a mechanical function and do not possess taste buds
- **Fungiform**: mushroom-shaped papillae that are more numerous near the tip of the tongue and possess taste buds
- **Foliate**: parallel rows of papillae concentrated near the lateral edge of the tongue that contain many taste buds
- **Circumvallate**: large papillae (about 8-12) close to the back of the body of the tongue that possess taste buds

Most taste buds respond to multiple "tastes," and our gustatory and olfactory receptors function in parallel; most flavors are enhanced by both taste and smell. Pinching your nose shut while eating will significantly diminish your sensation of the taste! Molecules, dissolved in saliva, contact the gustatory microvilli in the taste pore and depolarize the taste cells, causing the release of neurotransmitter onto afferent nerve endings. Nerve impulses are conveyed to the CNS via the facial (from the anterior two thirds of the tongue), glossopharyngeal (posterior one third of the tongue), and vagus (epiglottis and palate) nerves to the pontine taste area (parabrachial nucleus in the pons). Axons then project to the thalamus, hypothalamus, and amygdala, and to the gustatory cortex.

COLOR the following features of the tongue and taste bud, using a different color for each feature:

- [ ] 1. Circumvallate papillae
- [ ] 2. Foliate papillae
- [ ] 3. Filiform papillae
- [ ] 4. Microvilli of the taste cells in the taste pore
- [ ] 5. Taste cells

Olfactory chemoreceptors lie in the olfactory epithelium at the roof of the nasal cavity. The receptors are bipolar neurons whose dendritic end projects into the nasal cavity and ends in a tuft of microvilli in a mucous film. Odors, dissolved in the mucous film, bind to specific odorant-binding proteins and interact with the microvilli, depolarizing the olfactory neuron. Impulses then are conveyed along the neuron's central process through the cribriform plate to neurons in the olfactory bulb. The olfactory tract (CN I) projects centrally, bypassing the thalamus and distributing to various cortical areas, the amygdala, and the entorhinal cortex.

It is estimated that we can sense thousands of substances, but most can be reduced to the following six categories: floral, ethereal (pears), musky, camphor (eucalyptus), putrid, and pungent (vinegar, peppermint).

COLOR the following features of the olfactory receptors, using a different color for each feature:

- [ ] 6. **Region of olfactory epithelium distribution in the nose**
- [ ] 7. **Olfactory receptor cells: their dendrites and microvilli projecting into the nasal cavity, and their axons coursing through the cribriform plate**

Clinical Note:
The olfactory axons are very fragile and can be easily injured by trauma. If they are permanently damaged one can lose their sense of smell, which is termed **anosmia**. The olfactory receptor cells survive for about one month and then are replaced (bipolar neurons), representing one of a few nerve cells that can be replaced throughout life.

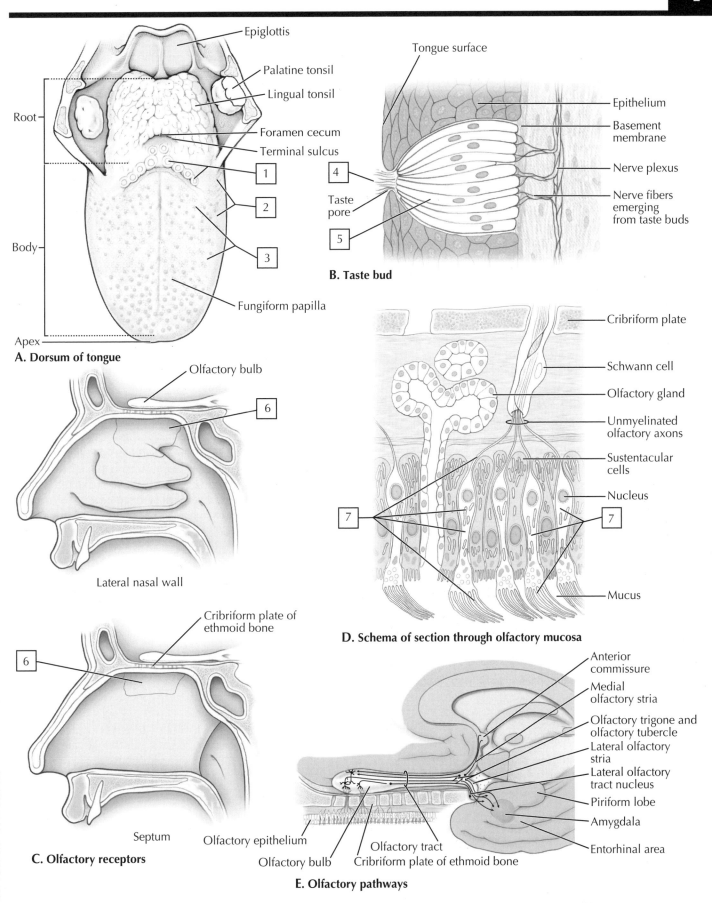

A. Dorsum of tongue

Epiglottis
Palatine tonsil
Lingual tonsil
Foramen cecum
Terminal sulcus
1
2
3
Fungiform papilla

Root
Body
Apex

B. Taste bud

Tongue surface
Epithelium
Basement membrane
Nerve plexus
Nerve fibers emerging from taste buds
4
Taste pore
5

Olfactory bulb
6
Lateral nasal wall

C. Olfactory receptors

Cribriform plate of ethmoid bone
6
Septum

D. Schema of section through olfactory mucosa

Cribriform plate
Schwann cell
Olfactory gland
Unmyelinated olfactory axons
Sustentacular cells
Nucleus
7
7
Mucus

E. Olfactory pathways

Anterior commissure
Medial olfactory stria
Olfactory trigone and olfactory tubercle
Lateral olfactory stria
Lateral olfactory tract nucleus
Piriform lobe
Amygdala
Entorhinal area
Olfactory epithelium
Olfactory bulb
Olfactory tract
Cribriform plate of ethmoid bone

The ventral rami of the 31 pairs of spinal nerves often join one another shortly after they branch from the spinal nerve and form a network or **plexus of nerves**. A plexus is not unlike a vast network of different railway tracks that interconnect in a major rail terminal or switching yard. The nerve plexus is a mixing of nerve fibers from several adjacent spinal cord levels that ultimately gives rise to several "terminal" nerve branches, which then pass into the periphery and innervate skeletal muscle, joints, and the skin. Although a muscle may be innervated by a single nerve, that nerve usually has fibers from several spinal cord levels in it.

The first and most rostral of the nerve plexuses is the **cervical (neck) plexus**, composed of the ventral rami of the first four cervical nerves. The motor branches of the plexus, as is typical of all spinal nerves, contain hundreds or thousands of three types of nerve fibers (**somatic motor** to skeletal muscle; **postganglionic sympathetics** to innervate smooth muscle of the hair follicles, vasculature, and sweat glands; and **sensory** fibers).

The major motor branches include the:
- **Ansa cervicalis**: innervates the infrahyoid or "strap" muscles of the anterior neck
- **Phrenic nerve**: from C3, C4, and C5, this nerve "keeps the diaphragm alive"; it innervates the abdominal diaphragm, which is critical to our breathing
- **Minor branches**: several smaller motor branches innervate individual neck muscles

The remaining branches of the cervical plexus are largely sensory, and innervate the skin of the neck and even send sensory branches superiorly to the skin around the ear and back of the scalp. The table summarizes the branches of the cervical plexus.

NERVE	INNERVATION
C1	Travels with CN XII to innervate geniohyoid and thyrohyoid muscles
Ansa cervicalis	Is C1-C3 loop that sends motor branches to infrahyoid muscles
Lesser occipital	From C2, is sensory to neck and scalp posterior to ear
Great auricular	From C2 to C3, is sensory over parotid gland and posterior ear
Transverse cervical	From C2 to C3, is sensory to anterior triangle of neck
Supraclavicular	From C3 to C4, are anterior, middle, and posterior sensory branches to skin over clavicle and shoulder region
Phrenic	From C3 to C5, is motor and sensory nerve to diaphragm
Motor branches	Are small twigs that supply scalene muscles, levator scapulae, and prevertebral muscles

Clinical Note:

The phrenic nerve (C3-C5) receives two of its three nerve segment contributions from the cervical plexus and is an important nerve, because it innervates the abdominal diaphragm. This nerve passes through the thorax in close association with the heart and its pericardial sac, so any surgeon operating in the thorax must identify this nerve and be certain to preserve it. Likewise, a person with cervical spine injuries above the level of C3 that severely damage the spinal cord will need mechanical ventilation, because the nerve fibers to the phrenic nerve will degenerate. In fact, all motor function below the level of the spinal cord injury will be lost.

COLOR the following branches of the cervical plexus. Color the motor branches one color and the sensory branches a different color:

- ☐ 1. **Nerves to the geniohyoid and thyrohyoid muscles**
- ☐ 2. **Transverse cervical: sensory**
- ☐ 3. **Ansa cervicalis (*ansa* means "loop"): motor branch**
- ☐ 4. **Supraclavicular nerves: sensory**
- ☐ 5. **Phrenic nerve: motor branch**
- ☐ 6. **Lesser occipital: sensory**
- ☐ 7. **Great auricular: sensory**

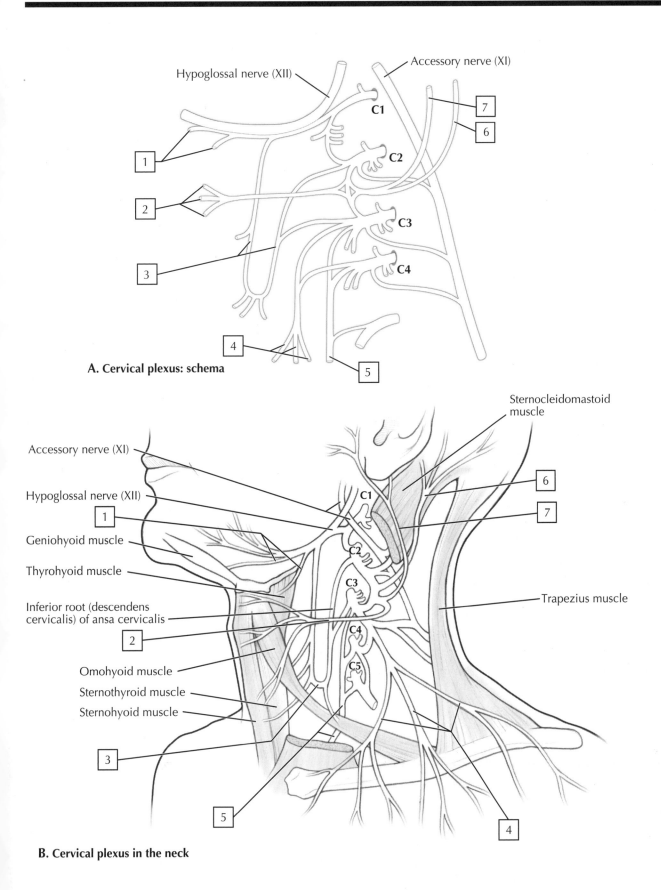

Hypoglossal nerve (XII)

Accessory nerve (XI)

C1

7

6

1

2

3

C2

C3

C4

4

5

A. Cervical plexus: schema

Sternocleidomastoid muscle

Accessory nerve (XI)

Hypoglossal nerve (XII)

1

Geniohyoid muscle

Thyrohyoid muscle

Inferior root (descendens cervicalis) of ansa cervicalis

2

Omohyoid muscle

Sternothyroid muscle

Sternohyoid muscle

3

C1

C2

C3

C4

C5

6

7

Trapezius muscle

5

4

B. Cervical plexus in the neck

The brachial plexus is formed by the ventral rami of spinal nerves C5-T1. This plexus consists of the following descriptive components:

- **Roots**: five ventral rami of C5-T1 form the "roots" of the plexus
- **Trunks**: the five roots sort into three trunks, called superior, middle, and inferior, all lying beneath the clavicle and above the 1st rib
- **Divisions**: each trunk divides into an anterior and posterior division, forming six divisions
- **Cords**: all the posterior divisions combine to form the posterior cord; the lateral and medial cords are formed by combinations of the anterior divisions
- **Terminal branches**: the plexus gives rise to five large terminal branches that innervate the muscles of the shoulder, arm, forearm, and hand

The three cords of the plexus are named for their relationship to the axillary artery, because they wrap around this artery in the axilla (armpit) and its accompanying vein(s), with the entire neurovascular bundle being wrapped in a fascial sheath called the axillary sheath. A number of other, smaller nerves also arise from components of the brachial plexus to innervate some muscles of the back, and lateral and anterior chest wall. The following table summarizes some of the more important nerves of the brachial plexus and the muscles they innervate (see individual muscle tables for more detail).

COLOR the five roots, three trunks, six divisions, three cords, and five terminal branches of the brachial plexus (part *A*), using a different color for each component, for example, red for roots, blue for trunks, and so on. Also, **color** the five terminal branches of the cord as they pass into the upper limb (part *B*), using a different color for each nerve:

- ☐ **1. Axillary**
- ☐ **2. Musculocutaneous**
- ☐ **3. Median**
- ☐ **4. Radial**
- ☐ **5. Ulnar**

Clinical Note:

Various injuries to the upper limb can result in damage to one or more of the terminal branches of the brachial plexus.

Musculocutaneous nerve: because this nerve runs through the arm and is protected by overlying muscles, it is not frequently injured.

Axillary nerve: damage results in weakened ability to abduct the limb at the shoulder. A dislocated shoulder injury could stretch this nerve and damage its axons.

Radial nerve: because this nerve innervates all extensors, a proximal injury would result in a weakened ability to extend at the elbow, wrist, and fingers. A somewhat lower injury might only result in "wrist drop" (inability to extend the wrist and fingers).

Median nerve: damage results in weakness in flexing the wrist and weakened flexion of the thumb, index, and middle finger when asked to make a fist. Compression of the nerve at the wrist (carpal tunnel syndrome) would not affect wrist movement but would weaken the function of the thenar muscles of the hand.

Ulnar nerve: damage results in weakness in flexing the wrist, little, and ring fingers, and, with hyperextended metacarpophalangeal (MP) joints of these same fingers, results in a "claw hand," indicative of an ulnar nerve injury. Atrophy of the hypothenar eminence may also occur. The ulnar nerve is the most frequently injured nerve of the upper limb.

ARISE FROM	NERVE	MUSCLES INNERVATED
Roots	Dorsal scapular	Levator scapulae and rhomboids
	Long thoracic	Serratus anterior
Upper trunk	Suprascapular	Supraspinatus and infraspinatus
	Subclavius	Subclavius
Lateral cord	Lateral pectoral	Pectoralis major
	Musculocutaneous	Anterior compartment muscles of arm
Medial cord	Medial pectoral	Pectoralis minor and major
	Ulnar	Some forearm and most hand muscles
Medial and lateral cords	Median	Most forearm and some hand muscles
Posterior cord	Upper subscapular	Subscapularis
	Thoracodorsal	Latissimus dorsi
	Lower subscapular	Subscapularis and teres major
	Axillary	Deltoid and teres minor
	Radial	Posterior compartment muscles of the arm and forearm

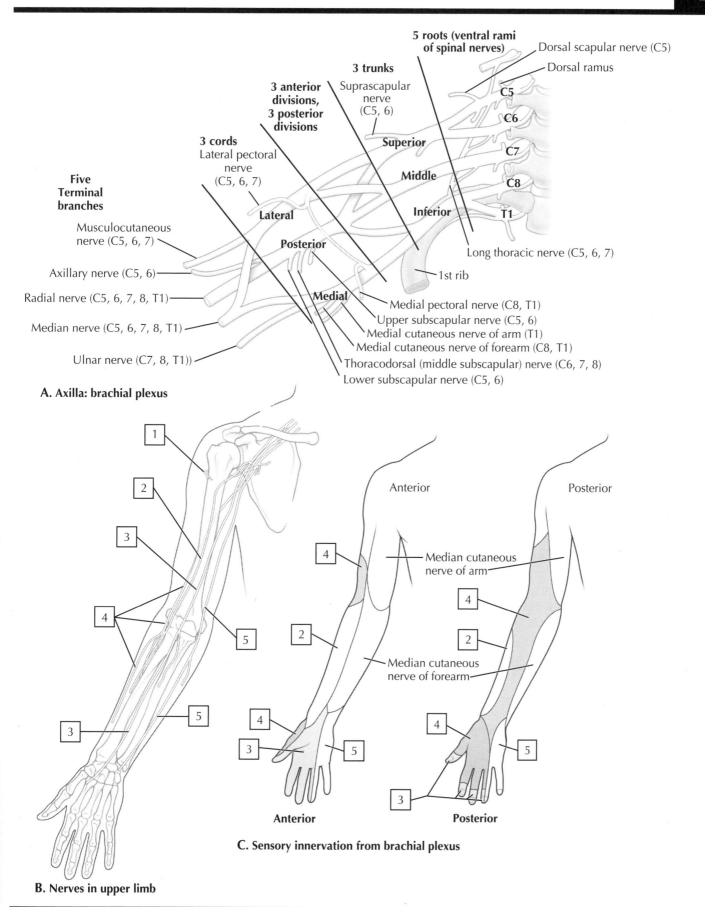

5 roots (ventral rami of spinal nerves)

Dorsal scapular nerve (C5)

Dorsal ramus

3 trunks

Suprascapular nerve (C5, 6)

C5

C6

C7

C8

T1

3 anterior divisions, 3 posterior divisions

Superior

Middle

Inferior

3 cords

Lateral pectoral nerve (C5, 6, 7)

Lateral

Posterior

Long thoracic nerve (C5, 6, 7)

1st rib

Five Terminal branches

Musculocutaneous nerve (C5, 6, 7)

Axillary nerve (C5, 6)

Radial nerve (C5, 6, 7, 8, T1)

Median nerve (C5, 6, 7, 8, T1)

Ulnar nerve (C7, 8, T1))

Medial

Medial pectoral nerve (C8, T1)

Upper subscapular nerve (C5, 6)

Medial cutaneous nerve of arm (T1)

Medial cutaneous nerve of forearm (C8, T1)

Thoracodorsal (middle subscapular) nerve (C6, 7, 8)

Lower subscapular nerve (C5, 6)

A. Axilla: brachial plexus

Anterior

Posterior

Median cutaneous nerve of arm

Median cutaneous nerve of forearm

Anterior

Posterior

C. Sensory innervation from brachial plexus

B. Nerves in upper limb

The lumbar plexus is formed by the ventral rami of spinal nerves L1-L4. The major motor components of this plexus are included in the following nerves:

- **Femoral nerve**: from L2-L4, this nerve innervates the anterior thigh muscles (largely extensors of the knee)
- **Obturator nerve**: from L2-L4, this nerve innervates the medial thigh muscles (largely adductors of the hip)
- **Genitofemoral nerve**: motor to the cremaster muscle (a covering of the spermatic cord) in males, and sensory to the anteromedial thigh in both sexes

A large nerve trunk from the inferior portion of the lumbar plexus, called the **lumbosacral trunk**, will continue into the pelvis and join ventral rami of sacral nerves to form the **sacral plexus** (L4-S4). Nerves from these two plexuses innervate muscles of the pelvis, perineum, and all the muscles of the lower limb.

The sensory components of the lumbar plexus innervate the inguinal region, groin, and the medial, anterior, and lateral aspects of the thigh, and anteromedial leg and ankle (see individual muscle tables for more detail).

COLOR the following nerves of the lumbar plexus, using a different color for each nerve:

- ☐ 1. **Iliohypogastric: largely sensory to the inguinal region but does provide some motor fibers to several abdominal wall muscles (internal oblique and transversus abdominis) (L1)**

- ☐ 2. **Ilio-inguinal: largely sensory to the inguinal region and external genitalia but does supply some motor fibers to the same abdominal muscles listed above (L1)**

- ☐ 3. **Genitofemoral: motor to the cremaster muscle in males and sensory to the anteromedial thigh in both sexes (L1-L2)**

- ☐ 4. **Lateral cutaneous nerve of the thigh: largely sensory to the lateral thigh (L2-L3)**

- ☐ 5. **Femoral: motor to anterior compartment thigh muscles and sensory over the anterior thigh, and anteromedial leg and ankle; passes deep to the inguinal ligament (L2-L4)**

- ☐ 6. **Obturator: motor to medial compartment thigh muscles and sensory to the medial thigh; passes through the obturator foramen to enter the medial thigh (L2-L4)**

Clinical Note:

Various injuries to the lower limb can result in damage to one or more of the large nerves innervating the muscles of the thigh. (The resulting conditions will make more sense if you also review the muscle compartments of the lower limb.) Some examples include:

Femoral nerve: damage results in a weakened ability to extend the knee. A patient may have to push on their anterior thigh when placing their affected limb on the ground during walking to "force" the knee into an extended position.

Obturator nerve: damage results in a weakened ability to adduct the hip. The obturator nerve lies beneath several layers of muscle and is well protected in the thigh, except if cut by a deep laceration. Most injuries of the nerve occur as it passes through the pelvis (e.g., pelvic trauma from automobile accidents).

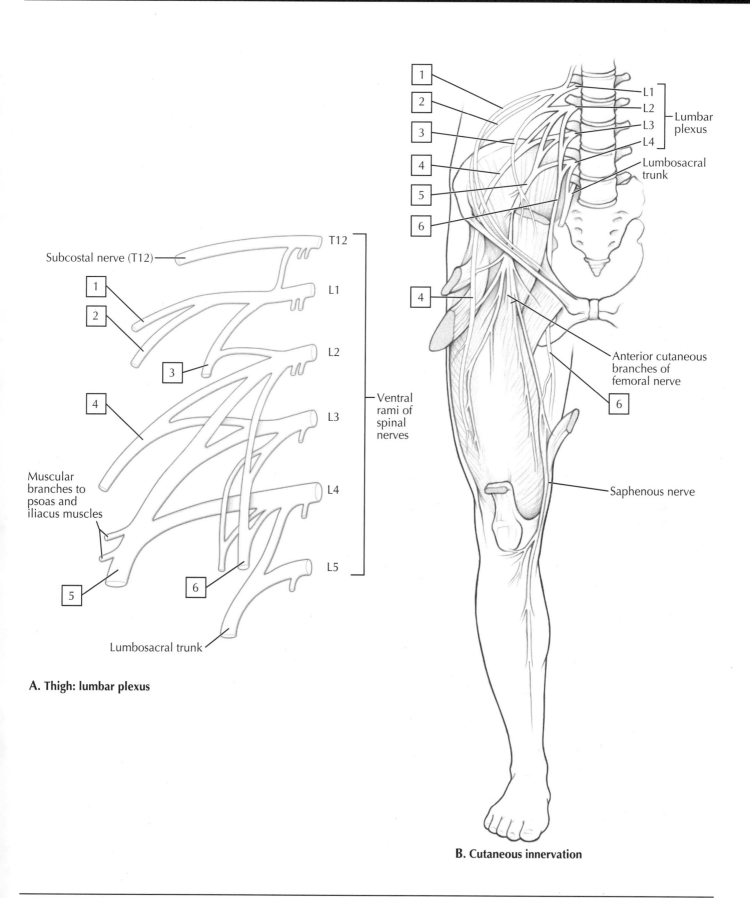

Subcostal nerve (T12)

T12

L1

2

3

L2

4

L3

L4

Muscular
branches to
psoas and
iliacus muscles

L5

5

6

Lumbosacral trunk

Ventral
rami of
spinal
nerves

1

L1

2

L2

3

L3

4

L4

Lumbar
plexus

Lumbosacral
trunk

4

6

Anterior cutaneous
branches of
femoral nerve

Saphenous nerve

A. Thigh: lumbar plexus

B. Cutaneous innervation

The sacral plexus is formed by the ventral primary rami of spinal nerves L4-S4. The major motor components of the sacral plexus are summarized in the table. In general, the sacral plexus innervates:
• Muscles forming the walls and floor of the pelvic cavity
• Muscles of the gluteal (buttocks) region
• Muscles of the perineum
• Muscles of the posterior thigh (hamstrings)
• All the muscles of the leg and foot

The largest nerve in the body, the **sciatic nerve**, arises from the sacral (sometimes referred to as the lumbosacral) plexus, with nerve fiber contributions from L4-S3. The lumbar contribution comes from the union of the lumbosacral trunk (L4-L5), which joins the first four sacral nerves to form the plexus. The sciatic nerve is really two nerves combined to form one:
• **Tibial nerve**: innervates the three hamstring muscles of the posterior thigh, the posterior compartment of the leg and all the muscles of the foot (via plantar branches)
• **Common fibular**: innervates the short head of the biceps femoris in the posterior thigh, and the lateral and anterior compartments of the leg (see individual muscle tables for more detail)

Sensory distribution of the sacral plexus includes the perineum, gluteal region, posterior thigh, posterolateral leg and ankle, and all of the foot.

DIVISION AND NERVE	INNERVATION
Anterior	
Pudendal (S2-S4)	Supplies motor and sensory innervation to perineum
Tibial (L4-S3)	Innervates posterior thigh muscles, posterior leg muscles, and foot; with common fibular nerve, it forms sciatic nerve (largest nerve in body)
Posterior	
Superior gluteal (L4-S1)	Innervates several gluteal muscles
Inferior gluteal (L5-S2)	Innervates gluteus maximus muscle
Common fibular (L4-S2)	Portion of sciatic nerve (with tibial) that innervates lateral and anterior muscle compartments of leg

COLOR the following nerves of the sacral plexus, using a different color for each nerve:

☐ 1. **Superior gluteal**: motor and sensory to two of the three gluteal muscles and tensor fasciae latae muscle

☐ 2. **Inferior gluteal**: motor and sensory to the gluteus maximus muscle

☐ 3. **Sciatic**: motor to the posterior thigh and all muscles below the knee; sensory to the posterior thigh, posterolateral leg and ankle, and all of the foot

☐ 4. **Pudendal (means "shameful")**: motor and sensory to the perineum and external genitalia

Clinical Note:
Athletically active individuals may report pain when an injury is actually related to the lumbar spine (**herniated disc** impinging on L4, L5, or S1 nerve roots), buttocks (**bursitis** or **hamstring muscle pulls**), or pelvic region (intrapelvic disorders). **Sciatica** is the pain associated with the large sciatic nerve and is often felt in the buttocks and/or radiating down the posterior thigh and into the posterolateral leg. As noted above, it can be due to multiple problems (disc herniation, direct trauma, inflammation, compression).

The common fibular nerve is the nerve most often injured in the lower limb. It is most vulnerable to trauma where it passes around the fibular head. Weakness of the muscles of the anterior and lateral compartments of the leg leads to "**foot drop**" (an inability to adequately dorsiflex the foot) and weakened eversion of the foot.

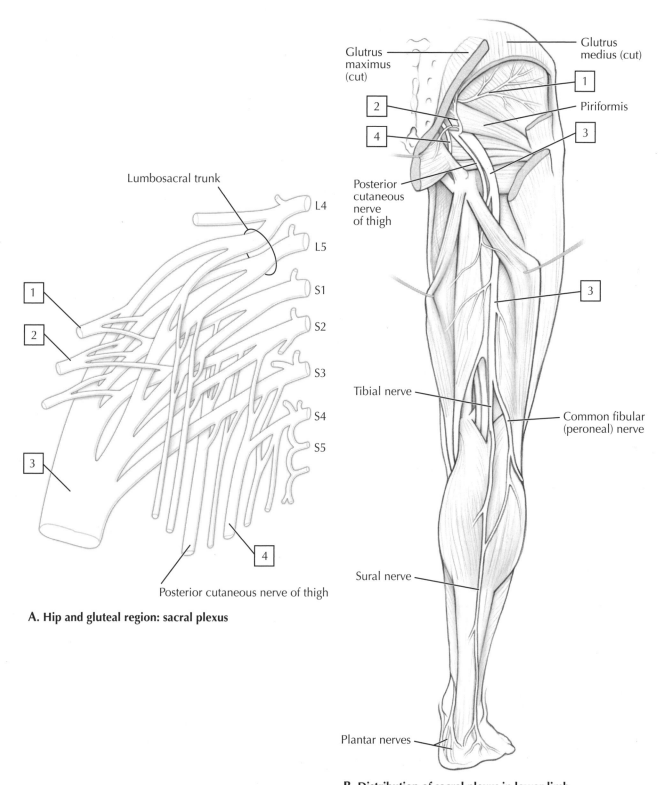

Glutrus medius (cut)

Glutrus maximus (cut)

1

2

Piriformis

4

3

Posterior cutaneous nerve of thigh

Lumbosacral trunk

L4

L5

S1

S2

S3

S4

S5

1

2

3

3

Tibial nerve

Common fibular (peroneal) nerve

4

Posterior cutaneous nerve of thigh

Sural nerve

A. Hip and gluteal region: sacral plexus

Plantar nerves

B. Distribution of sacral plexus in lower limb

For each description below (1-3), color the relevant structure in the image.

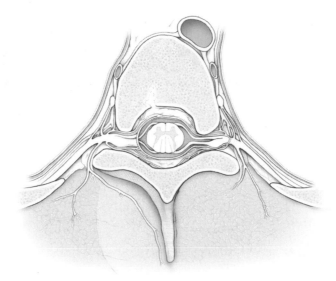

1. The nerve cell bodies (soma) of afferent (sensory) nerves are found in this structure (color it red).

2. This structure innervates the intrinsic back muscles (color it blue).

3. This structure contains somatic efferent and preganglionic sympathetic fibers (color it green).

4. In multiple sclerosis, the CNS myelin is progressively destroyed. Which of the following cells myelinates CNS axons?
   A. Astrocytes
   B. Microglia
   C. Oligodendrocytes
   D. Schwann cells
   E. Tanycytes

5. The primary motor cortex is located in which of the following structures?
   A. Cingulate gyrus
   B. Corpus callosum
   C. Insula
   D. Precentral gyrus
   E. Thalamus

6. Bradykinesia (slow movements) and resting tremor suggest that a patient has Parkinson's disease and a reduction of dopamine release from the substantia nigra. Which of the following brain regions is the target area for these dopamine-secreting neurons?
   A. Amygdaloid body
   B. Cingulate gyrus
   C. Hippocampus
   D. Globus pallidus
   E. Thalamus

7. A patient presents with a fractured humerus and wrist drop. Which of the following nerves is most likely injured?
   A. Axillary
   B. Median
   C. Musculocutaneous
   D. Radial
   E. Ulnar

8. Which is the largest nerve in the human body (hint: innervates most of the muscles of the lower limb)? _____ _____

9. Which cranial nerve has three large divisions? _____

10. Which cranial nerve innervates the submandibular salivary glands?_____

ANSWER KEY

1. Dorsal root ganglion

2. Dorsal ramus (of a spinal nerve)

3. Ventral root

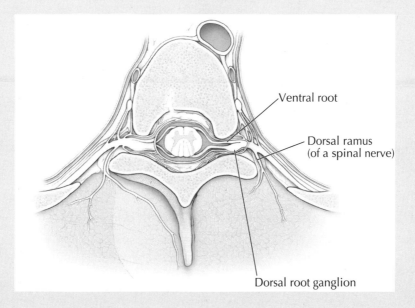

4. C

5. D

6. D

7. D

8. Sciatic nerve (combined tibial and common fibular nerves)

9. Trigeminal nerve (CN V)

10. Facial nerve (CN VII) via its parasympathetic fibers

Chapter 5 **Cardiovascular System**

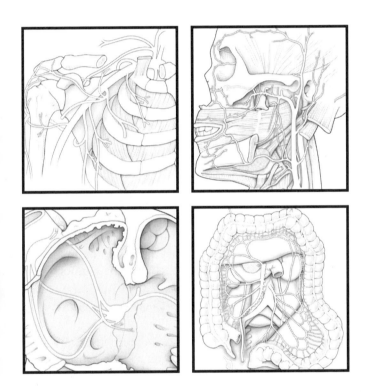

The blood consists of the following formed elements:
- Platelets
- White blood cells (WBCs)
- Red blood cells (RBCs)
- Plasma

Blood is a **fluid connective tissue** that circulates through the arteries to reach the body's tissues and returns to the heart through the veins. The functions of blood include:
- Transport of dissolved gases, nutrients, metabolic waste products, and hormones to and from tissues
- Prevention of fluid loss via clotting mechanisms
- Immune defense activities
- Regulation of pH and electrolyte balance
- Thermoregulation via blood vessel constriction and dilation

When blood is "spun down" in a centrifuge, the RBCs precipitate to the bottom of the tube where they comprise about 45% of the blood volume. The next layer is a "buffy coat" that comprises slightly less than 1% of the blood volume and includes the WBCs (leukocytes) and platelets. The remaining 55% of the blood volume is the **plasma** (**serum** is plasma with the clotting factors removed), which includes:
- Water
- Plasma proteins
- Other solutes (electrolytes, organic nutrients, organic wastes)

The volume of the packed RBCs represents the **hematocrit**, which normally ranges from about 40% to 50% in males to 35% to 45% in females. The "buffy coat" includes platelets and the WBCs. The WBCs include the following types of leukocytes (see Plate 6-2):
- **Neutrophils**: the most numerous of the granular WBCs (and all WBCs, granular and agranular), they possess a multilobed nucleus, function as phagocytes at sites of inflammation, live 8 to 12 hours in the blood and about 1 to 2 days in the extravascular compartment
- **Eosinophils**: are granular WBCs that respond to allergic reactions, participate in immune responses, phagocytose antigen-antibody complexes, live about 8 to 12 hours in the blood and for an unknown period of time in the connective tissues

- **Lymphocytes**: the most common type of agranular WBCs, they are one of three types (B cells that are derived from the bone marrow and produce circulating antibodies; T cells that are derived from the bone marrow but complete their differentiation in the thymus, they are either cytotoxic, helper, or suppressor cell-mediated immune cells; and natural killer (NK) cells that kill virus-infected cells)
- **Basophils**: least numerous WBCs, they are granular, function in immune, allergic, and inflammatory reactions, release vasoactive substances that can lead to hypersensitivity or allergic reactions, live in the blood for about 8 hours and for an unknown period of time in connective tissues
- **Monocytes**: the largest of the WBCs, they are agranular, travel from the bone marrow into the connective tissue where they differentiate into macrophages, live as monocytes in the blood about 16 hours and for an unknown period of time in connective tissues as macrophages

COLOR the following blood cells, using the colors suggested:

☐ 1. **Red blood cells: do not possess a nucleus as mature cells (red)**

☐ 2. **Platelets (yellow)**

☐ 3. **Neutrophil (color the multilobed nucleus purple or dark blue and the cytoplasm light blue)**

☐ 4. **Monocyte (color the crescent-shaped nucleus purple or dark blue and the cytoplasm light blue)**

☐ 5. **Eosinophil (color the nucleus dark blue or purple, the small cytoplasmic granules red, and the surrounding cytoplasm light blue)**

☐ 6. **Lymphocyte (color the nucleus blue or purple and the cytoplasm light blue)**

☐ 7. **Basophil (color the nucleus dark blue or purple, the cytoplasmic granules dark blue, and the surrounding cytoplasm light blue)**

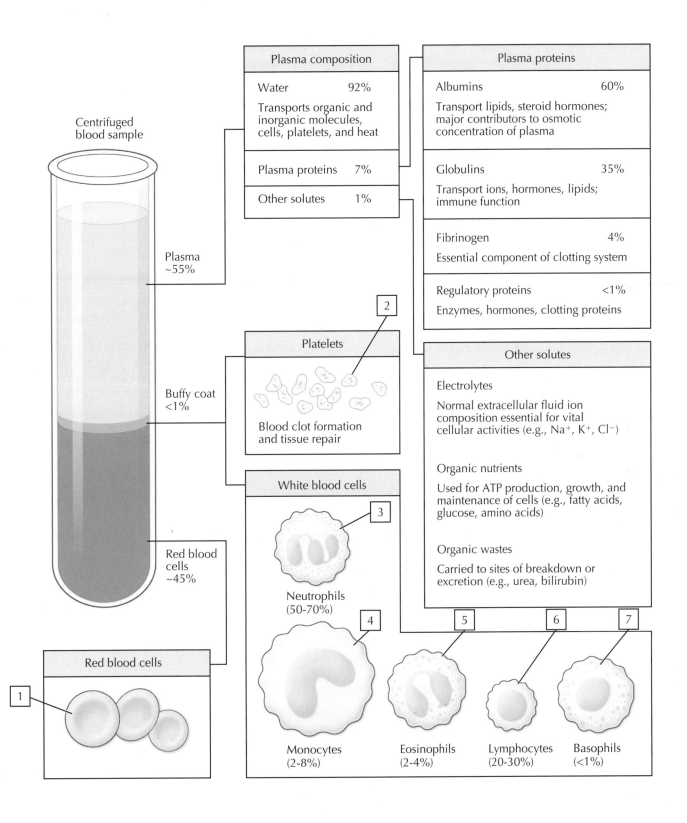

Centrifuged
blood sample

Plasma
~55%

Buffy coat
<1%

Red blood
cells
~45%

Plasma composition

Water	92%
Transports organic and inorganic molecules, cells, platelets, and heat	
Plasma proteins	7%
Other solutes	1%

Plasma proteins

Albumins	60%
Transport lipids, steroid hormones; major contributors to osmotic concentration of plasma	
Globulins	35%
Transport ions, hormones, lipids; immune function	
Fibrinogen	4%
Essential component of clotting system	
Regulatory proteins	<1%
Enzymes, hormones, clotting proteins	

2

Platelets

Blood clot formation
and tissue repair

Other solutes

Electrolytes

Normal extracellular fluid ion
composition essential for vital
cellular activities (e.g., Na^+, K^+, Cl^-)

Organic nutrients

Used for ATP production, growth, and
maintenance of cells (e.g., fatty acids,
glucose, amino acids)

Organic wastes

Carried to sites of breakdown or
excretion (e.g., urea, bilirubin)

White blood cells

3

Neutrophils
(50-70%)

4

Monocytes
(2-8%)

5

Eosinophils
(2-4%)

6

Lymphocytes
(20-30%)

7

Basophils
(<1%)

Red blood cells

1

The cardiovascular system consists of the following components:
- **Heart**: pumps the blood throughout the circulation
- **Pulmonary circulation**: a closed loop circulation between the heart and lungs for gas exchange
- **Systemic circulation**: a closed loop circulation between the heart and all the tissues of the body

The circulatory system's vessels include the following:
- **Arteries**: any vessel that carries blood away from the heart
- **Veins**: any vessel that returns blood to the heart

At rest, the cardiac output is about 5 L/min in both the pulmonary and systemic circulations. The amount of blood flow per minute ($\dot{Q}$), as a percent of cardiac output, and relative to the percent oxygen used per minute ($\dot{V}O_2$) in various organ systems are shown for the resting state in the illustration. Note that the brain uses over 20% of the available oxygen. At any point, most of the blood (64%) resides in the veins (a low pressure system) and is returned to the right side of the heart. The arterial side of the systemic circulation (a high pressure system) possesses significant amounts of smooth muscle in the vessel walls, and the small arteries and arterioles are largely responsible for most of the vascular resistance in the circulatory system.

COLOR

☐ 1. **The arterial side (right side) of the central schematic figure red**

☐ 2. **The venous side (left side) blue. Note that the vessels passing from the right ventricle (RV) to the lungs are the pulmonary arteries (even though the blood is less saturated with oxygen) and that the vessels from the lungs to the left atrium (LA) are called pulmonary veins (fully saturated with oxygen).**

Clinical Note:

Hypertension (high blood pressure) is a major risk factor for atherogenesis, atherosclerotic cardiovascular disease, stroke, coronary artery disease, and renal failure. Hypertension can result from an unknown cause (idiopathic, or essential hypertension) or secondary causes (e.g., medications, hormone imbalance, tumors). Hypertension is defined as two or more blood pressure readings of systolic pressure higher than 140 mm Hg or a diastolic pressure higher than 90 mm Hg. One reading of over 210 mm Hg systolic or over 120 mm Hg diastolic also indicates hypertension.

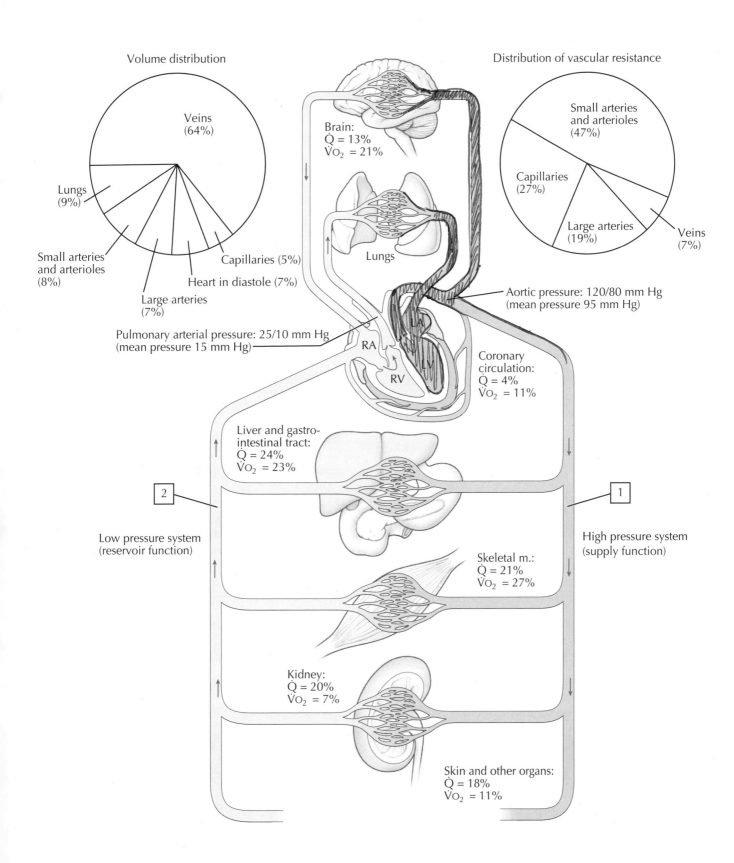

Volume distribution

Veins (64%)

Lungs (9%)

Small arteries and arterioles (8%)

Large arteries (7%)

Capillaries (5%)

Heart in diastole (7%)

Distribution of vascular resistance

Small arteries and arterioles (47%)

Capillaries (27%)

Large arteries (19%)

Veins (7%)

Brain:
$\dot{Q}$ = 13%
$\dot{V}O_2$ = 21%

Lungs

Aortic pressure: 120/80 mm Hg (mean pressure 95 mm Hg)

Pulmonary arterial pressure: 25/10 mm Hg (mean pressure 15 mm Hg)

RA

RV

LA

LV

Coronary circulation:
$\dot{Q}$ = 4%
$\dot{V}O_2$ = 11%

Liver and gastro-intestinal tract:
$\dot{Q}$ = 24%
$\dot{V}O_2$ = 23%

2

Low pressure system (reservoir function)

1

High pressure system (supply function)

Skeletal m.:
$\dot{Q}$ = 21%
$\dot{V}O_2$ = 27%

Kidney:
$\dot{Q}$ = 20%
$\dot{V}O_2$ = 7%

Skin and other organs:
$\dot{Q}$ = 18%
$\dot{V}O_2$ = 11%

The thoracic cavity is divided into a left and right pleural sac, which contains the lungs, and a "middle space" called the **mediastinum**. The mediastinum is further subdivided into the following regions:
- **Superior**: lies deep to the manubrium of the sternum and contains the great vessels (superior vena cava and aorta)
- **Inferior**: has 3 subdivisions of its own:
  - **Anterior**: lies deep to the body of the sternum and contains some fat and connective tissue
  - **Middle**: lies deep to the anterior mediastinum and contains the heart encased in its pericardial sac
  - **Posterior**: lies deep to the heart and contains the descending thoracic aorta, thoracic lymphatic duct, and esophagus

COLOR the following subdivisions of the mediastinum, using a different color for each subdivision:
- ☐ 1. Middle mediastinum
- ☐ 2. Anterior mediastinum
- ☐ 3. Superior mediastinum
- ☐ 4. Posterior mediastinum

The heart lies in the middle mediastinum and is encased within a tough fibrous sac called the **pericardium**. The pericardium has a tough outer layer called the **fibrous pericardium**, which reflects onto the great vessels in the superior mediastinum. A parietal layer of the serous pericardium lines the inner aspect of the fibrous pericardium and then reflects onto the heart itself as the visceral serous pericardium (**epicardium**). The serous layers secrete a thin film of serous fluid that lubricates the walls of the pericardium and reduces the friction created by the beating of the heart. The features of the pericardium are summarized in the table below.

FEATURE	DEFINITION
Fibrous pericardium	Tough, outer layer that reflects onto great vessels
Serous pericardium	Layer that lines inner aspect of fibrous pericardium (parietal layer); reflects onto heart as epicardium (visceral layer)
Innervation	Phrenic nerve (C3-5) for conveying pain; vasomotor innervation via sympathetics
Transverse sinus	Space posterior to aorta and pulmonary trunk; can clamp vessels with fingers in this sinus and above
Oblique sinus	Pericardial space posterior to heart

COLOR the components of the pericardium, using a different color for each component:
- ☐ 5. Fibrous pericardium
- ☐ 6. Parietal layer of the serous pericardium
- ☐ 7. Visceral layer of the serous pericardium (epicardium)

Note that when viewed in situ, the heart cannot be seen because it is encased within the pericardial sac. The great vessels in the superior mediastinum are visible superior to the pericardium and the fatty thymus gland can be seen overlying the upper portion of the pericardium. The base of the pericardium and heart lies upon the abdominal diaphragm, with the lungs bordering the pericardium on each side.

COLOR the following features of the pericardium in situ, using the colors suggested:
- ☐ 8. Arch of the aorta (red)
- ☐ 9. Thymus gland (yellow)
- ☐ 10. Superior vena cava (blue)
- ☐ 11. Pericardium (gray or tan)

Clinical Note:
Diseases of the pericardium involve inflammatory conditions (**pericarditis**) and effusions (fluid accumulation in the pericardial sac). Additionally, bleeding into the pericardial cavity can cause **cardiac tamponade**. The bleeding may be from a ruptured aortic aneurysm, ruptured myocardial infarct, or a penetrating injury (stab wound). The collection of blood in the pericardial cavity is called **hemopericardium** and it compromises the beating of the heart, decreases venous return to the heart, and affects cardiac output. The accumulating blood needs to be drawn out of the pericardial cavity and the appropriate repair initiated, because this is often a life-threatening condition.

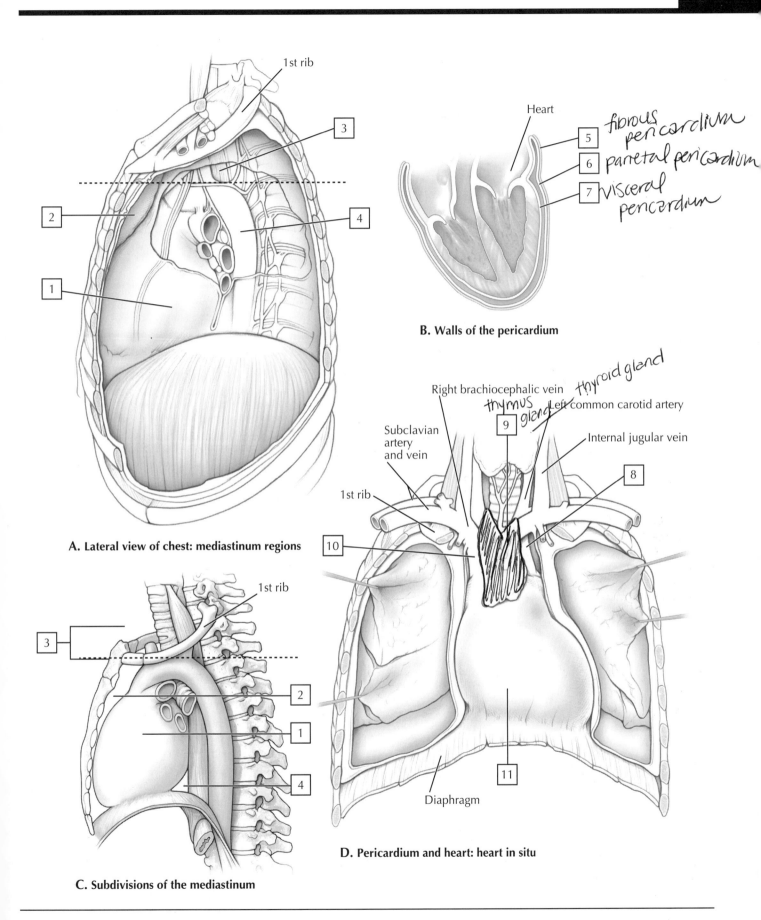

1st rib

3

2

4

1

A. Lateral view of chest: mediastinum regions

Heart

5 fibrous pericardium

6 parietal pericardium

7 visceral pericardium

B. Walls of the pericardium

1st rib

3

2

1

4

C. Subdivisions of the mediastinum

thyroid gland

Right brachiocephalic vein

thymus gland · Left common carotid artery

9

Subclavian artery and vein

Internal jugular vein

8

1st rib

10

11

Diaphragm

D. Pericardium and heart: heart in situ

The human heart has four chambers: two atria and two ventricles. Blood returning from the **systemic circulation** enters the right atrium and right ventricle and is pumped into the **pulmonary circulation** for gas exchange. Blood returning from the pulmonary circulation enters the left atrium and ventricle and then is pumped into the systemic circulation.

The atria and ventricles are separated by atrioventricular valves (tricuspid on the right and mitral on the left side), which prevent blood from refluxing into the atria when the ventricles contract. Likewise, the two major outflow vessels, the pulmonary trunk from the right ventricle and the ascending aorta from the left ventricle also possess valves called semilunar valves (pulmonic and aortic valves). Each semilunar valve has three valve leaflets that look like the crescent moon, hence "semilunar." Details of the features of each heart chamber are summarized in the table below.

FEATURE	DEFINITION
Right Atrium	
Auricle	Pouchlike appendage of atrium; embryonic heart tube derivative
Pectinate muscles	Ridges of myocardium inside auricle
Crista terminalis	Ridge that runs from the inferior (IVC) to superior (SVC) vena cava openings; its superior extent marks the site of the SA node
Fossa ovalis	Depression in interatrial septum; former site of foramen ovale
Atrial openings	One each for SVC, IVC, and coronary sinus (venous return from cardiac veins)
Right Ventricle	
Trabeculae carneae	Irregular ridges of ventricular myocardium
Papillary muscles	Anterior, posterior, and septal projections of myocardium extending into ventricular cavity; prevent valve leaflet prolapse
Chordae tendineae	Fibrous cords that connect papillary muscles to valve leaflets
Moderator band	Muscular band that conveys AV bundle from septum to base of ventricle at site of anterior papillary muscle
Ventricular openings	One to pulmonary trunk through pulmonary valve; one to receive blood from right atrium through tricuspid valve
Left Atrium	
Auricle	Small appendage representing primitive embryonic atrium whose wall has pectinate muscle
Atrial wall	Wall slightly thicker than thin-walled right atrium
Atrial openings	Usually four openings for four pulmonary veins

FEATURE	DEFINITION
Left Ventricle	
Papillary muscles	Anterior and posterior muscles, larger than those of right ventricle
Chordae tendineae	Fibrous cords that connect papillary muscles to valve leaflets
Ventricular wall	Wall much thicker than that of right ventricle
Membranous septum	Very thin superior portion of IVS and site of most ventricular septal defects (VSDs)
Ventricular openings	One to aorta through aortic valve; one to receive blood from left atrium through mitral valve

COLOR the following features of the heart chambers, using a different color for each feature, except where a color is suggested:

- [ ] 1. **Outflow to the pulmonary trunk (blue)**
- [ ] 2. **Left atrium**
- [ ] 3. **Pulmonary veins (usually two from each side) (light red)**
- [ ] 4. **Mitral valve**
- [ ] 5. **Ascending aorta and aortic arch (red)**
- [ ] 6. **Superior vena cava (blue)**
- [ ] 7. **Aortic semilunar valve**
- [ ] 8. **Right atrium**
- [ ] 9. **Tricuspid valve**
- [ ] 10. **Right ventricle**
- [ ] 11. **Inferior vena cava (blue)**
- [ ] 12. **Papillary muscles**
- [ ] 13. **Left ventricle**
- [ ] 14. **Pulmonic semilunar valve**

Clinical Note:

Typically, the **heart sounds** are described as "lub-dub," signifying the sounds made by the closing of the atrioventricular valves followed rapidly by the closing of the semilunar valves. Two additional sounds occur with the filling of the ventricles but are more difficult to discern. Using a stethoscope, one can listen to the four valves to determine if they are functioning properly. To do so, it is best to place the stethoscope over the chest wall and heart at a point where the blood has passed through the valve, to the heart chamber or vessel downstream, because the sound is better carried in the fluid medium. The gray dots in part *C* show the proper placement of a stethoscope to auscultate each valve.

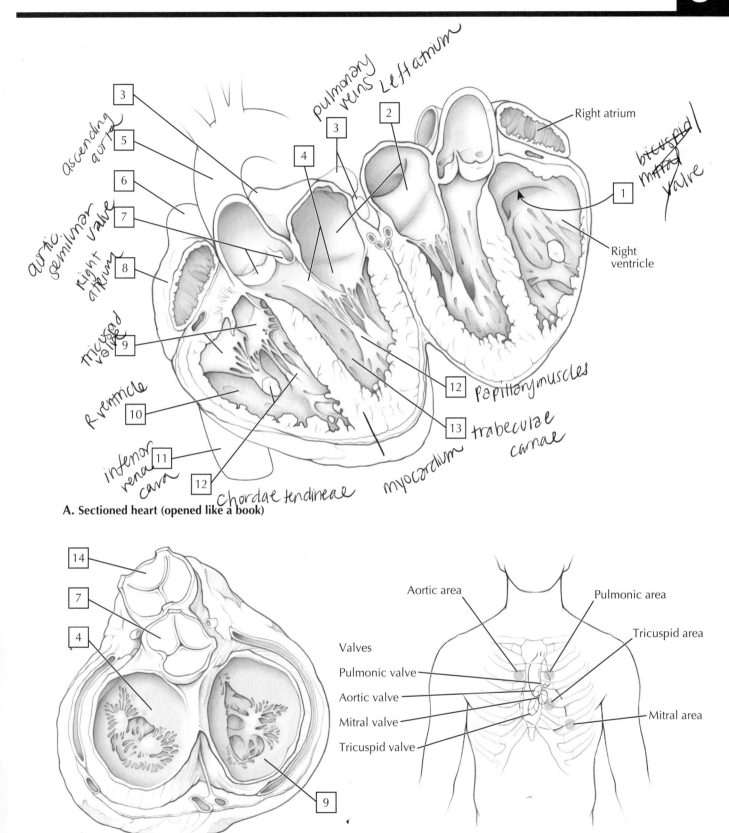

A. Sectioned heart (opened like a book)

ascending aorta

aortic semilunar valve

right atrium

tricuspid valve

R. ventricle

inferior vena cava

chordae tendineae

pulmonary veins

Left atrium

Right atrium

bicuspid mitral valve

Right ventricle

papillary muscles

trabeculae carnae

myocardium

B. Heart in diastole: viewed from base with atria removed

C. Precordial areas of auscultation

Aortic area

Pulmonic area

Tricuspid area

Valves

Pulmonic valve

Aortic valve

Mitral valve

Tricuspid valve

Mitral area

The pericardium is innervated by somatic pain fibers that course in the phrenic nerves (C3-C5), whereas the heart itself is innervated by the autonomic nervous system. The chief components of this innervation pattern include:

- **Parasympathetics**: derived from the vagus nerve (CN X), which courses to the cardiac plexus; parasympathetic stimulation slows the heart rate and decreases the force of contraction
- **Sympathetics**: derived from cervical and thoracic cardiac nerves originating in the T1-T4 intermediolateral cell column, these fibers course to the cardiac plexus; sympathetic stimulation increases heart rate and the force of contraction
- **Afferents**: sensory nerve fibers course from the heart in the sympathetic nerves to dorsal root ganglia associated with T1-T4 spinal cord levels; these fibers convey pain associated with myocardial ischemia

The heart maintains an intrinsic spontaneous rhythm of about 100 beats/min, but the normal parasympathetic tone overrides this intrinsic rate and maintains the resting heart rate at about 72 beats/min. The cardiac muscle of the heart exists in two forms:
- Contractile myocardium
- Specialized conducting myocardium

The specialized conducting myocardium does not contract but does spread the wave of depolarization rapidly throughout the chambers of the heart. Impulses are initiated in the sinu-atrial (SA) node and are conveyed to the atrioventricular (AV) node. From here, the impulses pass through the common AV bundle (of His) and then spread through the ventricles via the right and left bundle branches and Purkinje fiber system. Components of this intrinsic conduction system are summarized in the table below.

FEATURE	DEFINITION
SA node	Pacemaker of heart; site where action potential is initiated
AV node	Node that receives impulses from SA node and conveys them to the common AV bundle (of His)
Bundle branches	Right and left bundles that convey impulses down either side of IVS to subendocardial Purkinje system

The wave of depolarization, beginning at the SA node, and the repolarization of the myocardium generates the familiar electrocardiographic (ECG) pattern (P, QRS, and T waves) used clinically to assess the heart's conduction system.

COLOR the features of the heart's intrinsic conduction pathway and the elements (action potential wave forms) of the ECG listed below using the colors suggested:

- [ ] 1. **SA node (blue)**
- [ ] 2. **AV node (yellow)**
- [ ] 3. **Common AV bundle (of His)**
- [ ] 4. **Ventricular bundle branches (Purkinje system)**

Clinical Note:

Atrial fibrillation is the most common arrhythmia (although uncommon in children) and affects about 4% of people older than 60 years. **Ventricular tachycardia** is a dysrhythmia originating from a ventricular focus with a heart rate typically greater than 120 beats/min. It is usually associated with coronary artery disease, because myocardial ischemia often affects the ventricular endocardium where the Purkinje conduction system is localized.

Plate 5-5   See Netter: *Atlas of Human Anatomy*, 6th Edition, Plate 222; also see *Netter's Clinical Anatomy*, 3rd Edition, Figure 3-20

Cardiovascular System

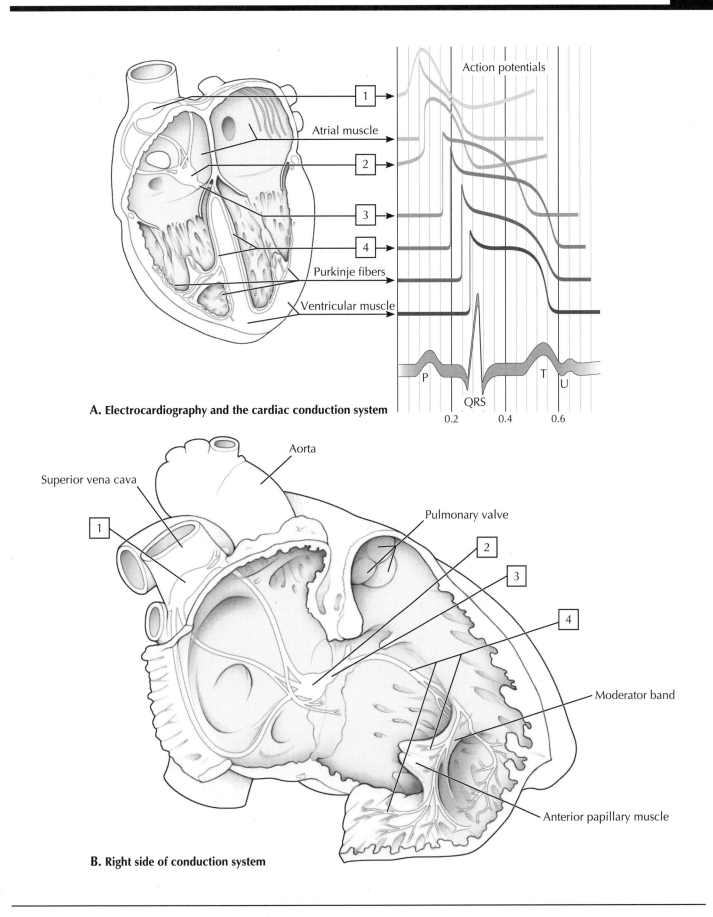

A. Electrocardiography and the cardiac conduction system

Action potentials

Atrial muscle

Purkinje fibers

Ventricular muscle

P

QRS

T

U

0.2   0.4   0.6

Aorta

Superior vena cava

Pulmonary valve

Moderator band

Anterior papillary muscle

B. Right side of conduction system

The first set of arteries to arise from the ascending aorta as it leaves the heart are the **coronary arteries**, which literally "crown" the heart, hence the reference to coronary (coronation). Thus the heart gets the first and most oxygen-saturated blood to meet its high metabolic needs. There are two coronary arteries, left and right, and three major **cardiac veins**, great, middle, and small. These veins return most of the blood to the **coronary sinus** and the right atrium, although several other small veins also return coronary blood flow to the heart chambers. The vascular supply to the heart is summarized in the following table.

VESSEL	COURSE
Right coronary artery	Consists of major branches: sinu-atrial (SA) nodal, right marginal, posterior interventricular (posterior descending), atrioventricular (AV) nodal
Left coronary artery	Consists of major branches: circumflex, anterior interventricular (left anterior descending) (LAD), left marginal
Great cardiac vein	Parallels LAD artery and drains into coronary sinus
Middle cardiac vein	Parallels posterior descending artery and drains into coronary sinus
Small cardiac vein	Parallels right marginal artery and drains into coronary sinus
Anterior cardiac veins	Are several small veins that drain directly into right atrium
Smallest cardiac veins	Drain through the cardiac wall directly into all four heart chambers

Coronary blood flow varies with the aortic pressure but also is influenced by physical factors such as compression of the vessels during contraction of the heart chambers (coronary flow is significantly decreased as the contracting ventricular myocardium compresses the coronary arteries) and by metabolic factors released from the myocytes. A number of metabolic factors have been implicated in the regulation of coronary blood flow:

- H^+
- CO_2
- Decreased O_2
- K^+
- Lactic acid
- Nitric oxide
- Adenosine (probably the most important factor)

When cardiac work demand increases, adenosine is released by the myocytes and this leads to vasodilation and increased blood flow in the coronary arteries.

COLOR each of the coronary arteries and cardiac veins listed below, using the colors suggested:

- [ ] 1. **Left coronary artery and its major branches (anterior interventricular [anterior descending] branch, circumflex branch, left marginal branch) (orange)**
- [ ] 2. **Great cardiac vein (blue)**
- [ ] 3. **Small cardiac vein (brown)**
- [ ] 4. **Right coronary artery and its major branches (SA nodal branch, right marginal branch, and posterior interventricular [posterior descending] branch) (red)**
- [ ] 5. **Coronary sinus (purple)**
- [ ] 6. **Middle cardiac vein (green)**

Clinical Note:

Angina pectoris is the sensation caused by myocardial ischemia and is usually described as pressure, discomfort, or a feeling of choking in the left chest or substernal region that radiates to the left shoulder and arm as well as the neck, jaw and teeth, abdomen, and back. This radiating pattern is an example of "referred pain," in which visceral afferents from the heart enter the upper thoracic spinal cord along with somatic afferents, both converging in the spinal cord's dorsal horn. Interpretation of the visceral pain may initially be confused with somatic sensations from the same cord levels. Myocardial ischemia due to atherosclerosis and coronary artery thrombosis is the major cause of **myocardial infarction** (MI), which affects more than 1 million Americans each year. If the ischemia is severe enough, necrosis (tissue death) of the myocardium can occur and usually begins in the subendocardium, because this region is the most poorly perfused region of the ventricular wall.

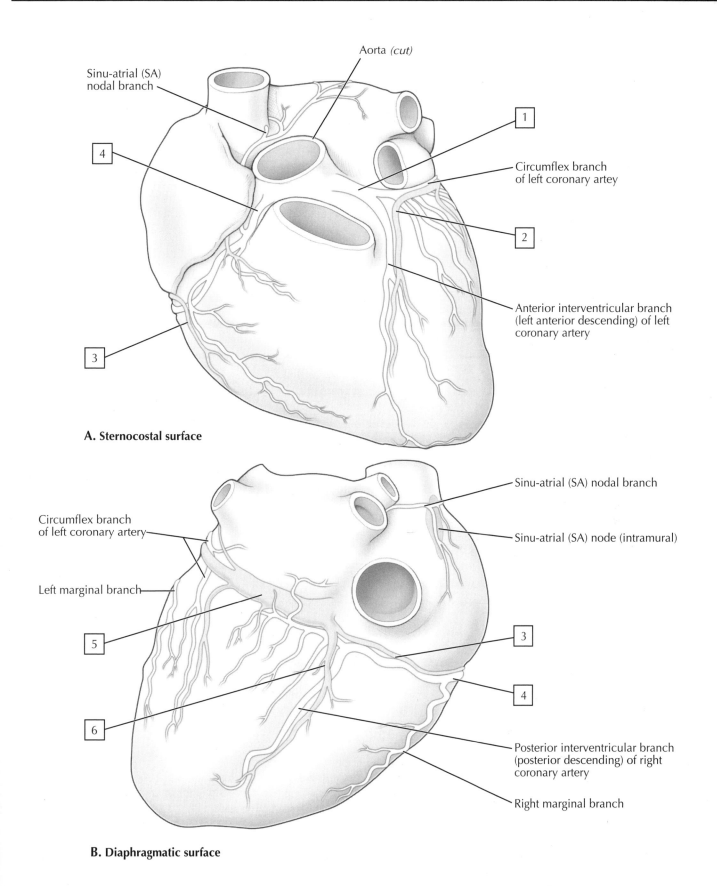

Sinu-atrial (SA)
nodal branch

Aorta *(cut)*

[1]

Circumflex branch
of left coronary artey

[4]

[2]

Anterior interventricular branch
(left anterior descending) of left
coronary artery

[3]

A. Sternocostal surface

Circumflex branch
of left coronary artery

Sinu-atrial (SA) nodal branch

Sinu-atrial (SA) node (intramural)

Left marginal branch

[5]

[3]

[4]

[6]

Posterior interventricular branch
(posterior descending) of right
coronary artery

Right marginal branch

B. Diaphragmatic surface

Arteries and veins are composed of three essential layers (tunics) (except capillaries and postcapillary venules), which include the:

- **Tunica intima**: an inner layer of simple squamous epithelium, called the endothelium, that lines all arteries, veins, and capillaries
- **Tunica media**: a middle layer of concentrically oriented layers of smooth muscle; in large arteries (aorta), elastic lamellae are interspersed between the smooth muscle layers
- **Tunica adventitia**: an outer layer of connective tissue, composed primarily of collagen and a few elastic fibers

Arteries can be classified into four different types based upon their size and the relative thickness or presence of the tunics:

- **Large (elastic) arteries**: aorta and proximal portions of the subclavian and common carotid arteries
- **Medium (muscular) arteries**: most of the commonly "named" arteries in the body
- **Small arteries and arterioles**: responsible for most of the vascular resistance; arterioles regulate the blood flow into the capillary beds

- **Capillaries**: consist of only an endothelium and are functionally responsible for the exchange of gases and metabolites between the tissues and the blood

Veins can be classified into three different types based on their size and the relative thickness of the tunica media:

- **Venules and small veins**: venules include postcapillary venules (endothelium and pericytes only) and muscular venules (1-2 layers of smooth muscle in the tunica media); small veins have two to three smooth muscle layers
- **Medium veins**: most of the commonly "named" veins in the body; these veins in the extremities contain valves that assist in the venous return against gravity
- **Large veins**: a much thicker tunica adventitia compared with the tunica media, and include the subclavian veins and venae cavae

The human body contains over 50,000 miles of blood vessels and the key distinguishing features of these vessels are summarized in the table below.

VESSEL	DIAMETER	INNER LAYER (TUNICA INTIMA)	MIDDLE LAYER (TUNICA MEDIA)	OUTER LAYER (TUNICA ADVENTITIA)
Arteries				
Large artery (elastic artery)	>1 cm	Endothelium; connective tissue; smooth muscle	Smooth muscle; elastic lamellae	Connective tissue; elastic fibers; thinner than media
Medium artery (muscular artery)	2-10 mm	Endothelium; connective tissue; smooth muscle	Smooth muscle; collagen fibers; little elastic tissue	Connective tissue; some elastic fibers; thinner than media
Small artery	0.1-2 cm	Endothelium; connective tissue; smooth muscle	Smooth muscle (8-10 cell layers); collagen fibers	Connective tissue; some elastic fibers; thinner than media
Arteriole	10-100 μm	Endothelium; connective tissue; smooth muscle	Smooth muscle (1-2 cell layers)	Thin, ill-defined
Capillary	4-10 μm	Endothelium	None	None
Veins				
Postcapillary venule	10-50 μm	Endothelium; pericytes	None	None
Muscular venule	50-100 μm	Endothelium; pericytes	Smooth muscle (1-2 cell layers)	Connective tissue; some elastic fibers; thicker than media
Small vein	0.1-1 mm	Endothelium; connective tissue; smooth muscle (2-3 layers)	Smooth muscle (2-3 layers continuous with intima)	Connective tissue; some elastic fibers; thicker than media
Medium vein	1-10 mm	Endothelium; connective tissue; smooth muscle; some have valves	Smooth muscle; collagen fibers	Connective tissue; some elastic fibers; thicker than tunica media
Large vein	>1 cm	Endothelium; connective tissue; smooth muscle	Smooth muscle (2-15 layers); collagen fibers	Connective tissue; some elastic fibers, longitudinal smooth muscles; much thicker than media

COLOR the following features of the blood vessels, using a different color for each feature:

- [ ] 1. Tunica intima (endothelium)
- [ ] 2. Tunica media
- [ ] 3. Tunica adventitia

Clinical Note:

A thickening and narrowing of the arterial wall and eventual deposition of lipid into the wall can lead to one form of **atherosclerosis**. The narrowed artery may not be able to meet the metabolic needs of the adjacent tissues, with the danger that they may become ischemic (lack of oxygen). Multiple factors, including focal inflammation of the arterial wall, may result in this condition.

Plate 5-7   **Cardiovascular System**

Features of Blood Vessels

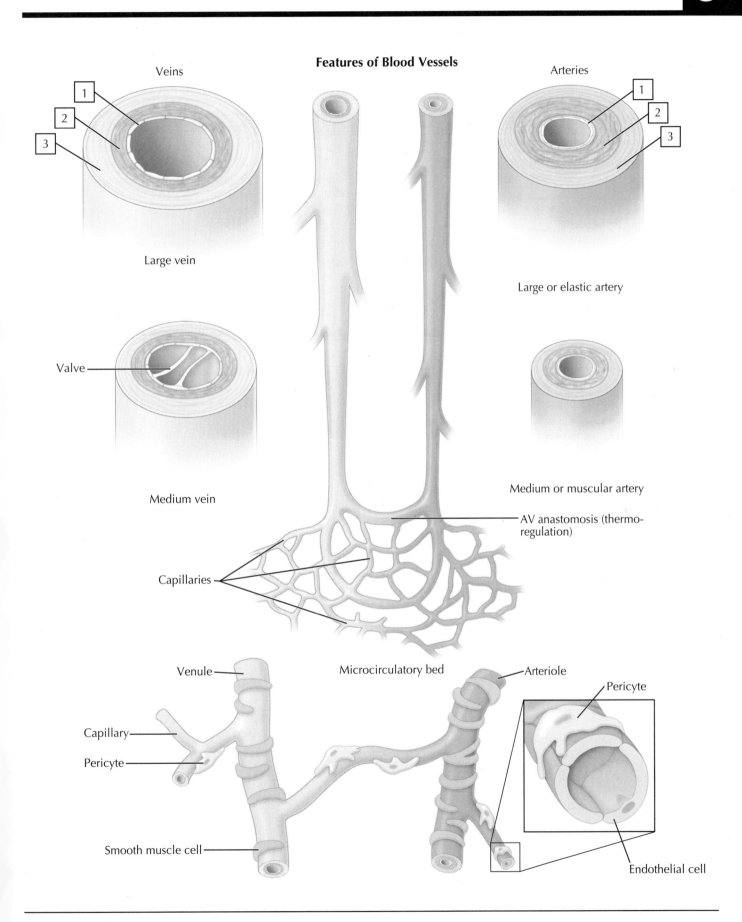

Veins

1
2
3

Large vein

Valve

Medium vein

Capillaries

Venule

Capillary

Pericyte

Smooth muscle cell

Microcirculatory bed

Arteries

1
2
3

Large or elastic artery

Medium or muscular artery

AV anastomosis (thermo-regulation)

Arteriole

Pericyte

Endothelial cell

Arteries supplying the head and neck region arise principally from the **subclavian** and **common carotid arteries**. The subclavian artery is divided into three parts by the anterior scalene muscle. Part 1 lies medial, part 2 posterior, and part 3 lateral to the anterior scalene muscle. Branches of the subclavian are summarized in the following table.

BRANCH	COURSE
Part 1	
Vertebral	Ascends through C6-C1 foramen transversarium and enters foramen magnum
Internal thoracic	Descends parasternally to anastomose with superior epigastric artery
Thyrocervical trunk	Gives rise to inferior thyroid, transverse cervical, and suprascapular arteries
Part 2	
Costocervical trunk	Gives rise to deep cervical and superior intercostal arteries
Part 3	
Dorsal scapular	Is inconstant; may also arise from transverse cervical artery

COLOR the following branches of the subclavian artery, using a different color for each branch:

☐ 1. **Vertebral: provides blood to the posterior portion of the brain**

☐ 2. **Costocervical trunk: its deep cervical branch supplies the deep lateral neck**

☐ 3. **Thyrocervical trunk: its transverse cervical and inferior thyroid branches supply portions of the neck and the thyroid and parathyroid glands**

The **common carotid artery** ascends in the carotid sheath, which also contains the internal jugular vein and vagus nerve, and divides into the internal and external carotid branches. The **internal carotid artery** essentially does not give off any branches in the neck (it does, but they are very small and seldom mentioned), but does pass into the carotid canal to supply the middle and anterior portions of the brain, and orbit. The **external carotid artery** gives rise to eight branches that supply the neck, face, scalp, dura, nasal and paranasal regions, and the oral cavity. Its branches are summarized in the following table.

BRANCH	COURSE AND STRUCTURES SUPPLIED
Superior thyroid	Supplies thyroid gland, larynx, and infrahyoid muscles
Ascending pharyngeal	Supplies pharyngeal region, middle ear, meninges, and prevertebral muscles
Lingual	Passes deep to hyoglossus muscle to supply the tongue
Facial	Courses over the mandible and supplies the face
Occipital	Supplies sternocleidomastoid muscle and anastomoses with costocervical trunk
Posterior auricular	Supplies region posterior to ear
Maxillary	Passes into infratemporal fossa (described later)
Superficial temporal	Supplies face, temporalis muscle, and lateral scalp

COLOR the following branches of the external carotid artery, using a different color for each branch:

☐ 4. **Maxillary**

☐ 5. **Facial**

☐ 6. **Lingual**

☐ 7. **Superior thyroid**

☐ 8. **Superficial temporal**

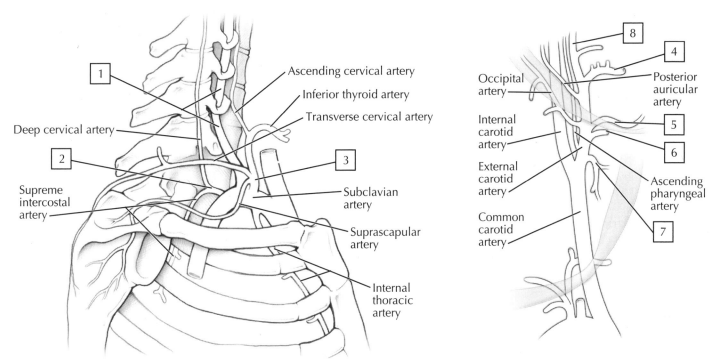

Ascending cervical artery

Inferior thyroid artery

Transverse cervical artery

1

Deep cervical artery

2

Supreme intercostal artery

3

Subclavian artery

Suprascapular artery

Internal thoracic artery

A. Neck: subclavian artery

Occipital artery

8

4

Posterior auricular artery

Internal carotid artery

External carotid artery

Common carotid artery

5

6

Ascending pharyngeal artery

7

B. Right external carotid branches: schema

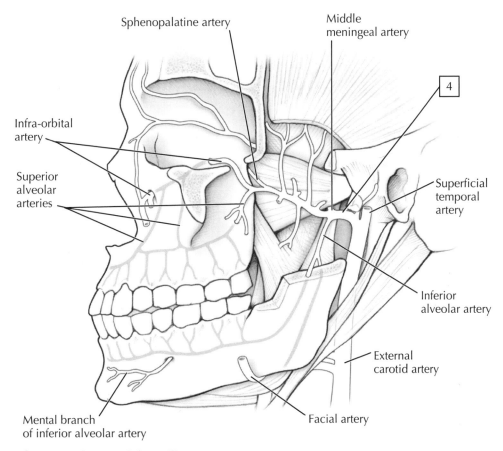

Sphenopalatine artery

Middle meningeal artery

4

Infra-orbital artery

Superior alveolar arteries

Superficial temporal artery

Inferior alveolar artery

External carotid artery

Facial artery

Mental branch of inferior alveolar artery

C. Temporal region: left maxillary artery

The **maxillary artery** supplies the infratemporal region, dura mater, nasal region, and a portion of the oral cavity. It is the largest and has the most extensive distribution of the branches of the external carotid artery. It gives rise to 15 or more branches of its own but, for descriptive purposes, is divided into three parts:

- **Retromandibular**: arteries enter foramina of the skull or jaw and supply the dura, mandibular teeth and gums, ear, and chin
- **Pterygoid**: branches supply the muscles of mastication and buccinator muscle
- **Pterygopalatine**: branches enter foramina of the skull and supply maxillary teeth and gums, orbital floor, nose, paranasal sinuses, palate, auditory tube, and superior pharynx

COLOR the following major branches of the maxillary artery using the color red:

☐ 1. **Maxillary artery and only these major branches arising from it:**
☐ 2. **Inferior alveolar (to mandibular teeth and gums)**
☐ 3. **Middle meningeal (to dura mater covering the brain)**
☐ 4. **Superior alveolar (its branches to maxillary teeth and gums)**
☐ 5. **Infra-orbital (to floor of orbit)**
☐ 6. **Sphenopalatine (to nose, paranasal sinuses, palate, and superior pharynx)**

The maxillary artery passes through the infratemporal fossa, enmeshed within the medial and lateral pterygoid muscles and a large venous plexus called the pterygoid plexus of veins (see Plate 5-11).

Clinical Note:

Because of the extensive arterial supply and venous drainage in the infratemporal fossa region, trauma to this area of the face and head can cause significant bleeding. Numerous nerves, muscles, and other structures lie within this region, and hemostasis and infection control must be a priority for the healthcare team.

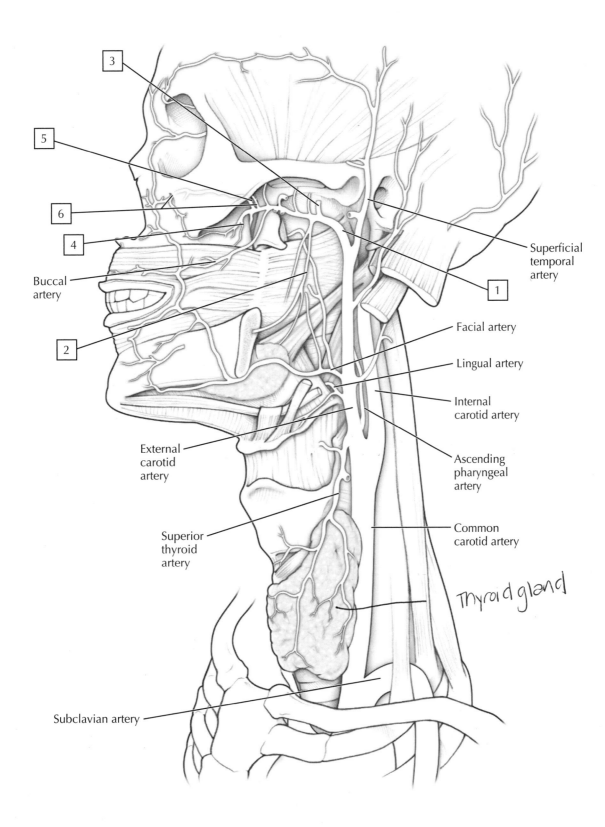

3

5

6

4

Buccal
artery

2

Superficial
temporal
artery

1

Facial artery

Lingual artery

Internal
carotid artery

Ascending
pharyngeal
artery

External
carotid
artery

Common
carotid artery

Superior
thyroid
artery

Thyroid gland

Subclavian artery

The arteries supplying the brain arise largely from two pairs of arteries:
- **Vertebrals**: arise from the subclavian in the neck, ascend through the foramen transversarium of the cervical vertebrae, and enter the foramen magnum of the skull to supply the posterior portion of the brain
- **Internal carotids**: arise from the common carotid in the neck, ascend in the neck to enter the carotid canal, and traverse the foramen lacerum to terminate as the middle and anterior cerebral arteries, which anastomose with the circle of Willis around the optic chiasm, hypophysis, and basal hypothalamus

COLOR the following arteries that supply the brain, using a different color for each artery:
- [ ] 1. **Anterior communicating**
- [ ] 2. **Anterior cerebral**
- [ ] 3. **Middle cerebral**
- [ ] 4. **Posterior communicating**
- [ ] 5. **Posterior cerebral**
- [ ] 6. **Basilar**
- [ ] 7. **Anterior inferior cerebellar**
- [ ] 8. **Vertebral**

ARTERY	COURSE AND STRUCTURES SUPPLIED
Vertebral	From subclavian artery, supplies cerebellum
Posterior inferior cerebellar	From vertebral artery, goes to posteroinferior cerebellum
Basilar	From both vertebrals, goes to brainstem, cerebellum, cerebrum
Anterior inferior cerebellar	From basilar, supplies inferior cerebellum
Superior cerebellar	From basilar, supplies superior cerebellum
Posterior cerebral	From basilar, supplies inferior cerebrum, occipital lobe
Posterior communicating	Cerebral arterial circle (of Willis)
Internal carotid (IC)	From common carotid, supplies cerebral lobes and eye
Middle cerebral	From IC, goes to lateral aspect of cerebral hemispheres
Anterior communicating	Cerebral arterial circle (of Willis)
Anterior cerebral	From IC, goes to cerebral hemispheres (except occipital lobe)

Clinical Note:

Bleeding from an artery supplying the dura mater results in arterial blood collecting in the space between the dura and the skull and is called an **epidural hematoma**. This often occurs from blunt trauma to the head and involves bleeding from the middle meningeal artery (from the maxillary artery) or one of its branches.

A **subarachnoid hemorrhage** usually occurs from the rupture of a saccular, or berry, aneurysm (a ballooning of an artery) involving one of the branches of the vertebral, internal carotid, or circle of Willis arteries.

Occlusion (by an atherosclerotic plaque or thrombus) of the:
- Anterior cerebral artery can disrupt sensory and motor functions on the contralateral lower extremity
- Middle cerebral artery can disrupt sensory and motor functions on the contralateral upper extremity or, if the internal capsule is affected, the entire contralateral body
- Posterior cerebral artery can disrupt visual functions from the contralateral visual field

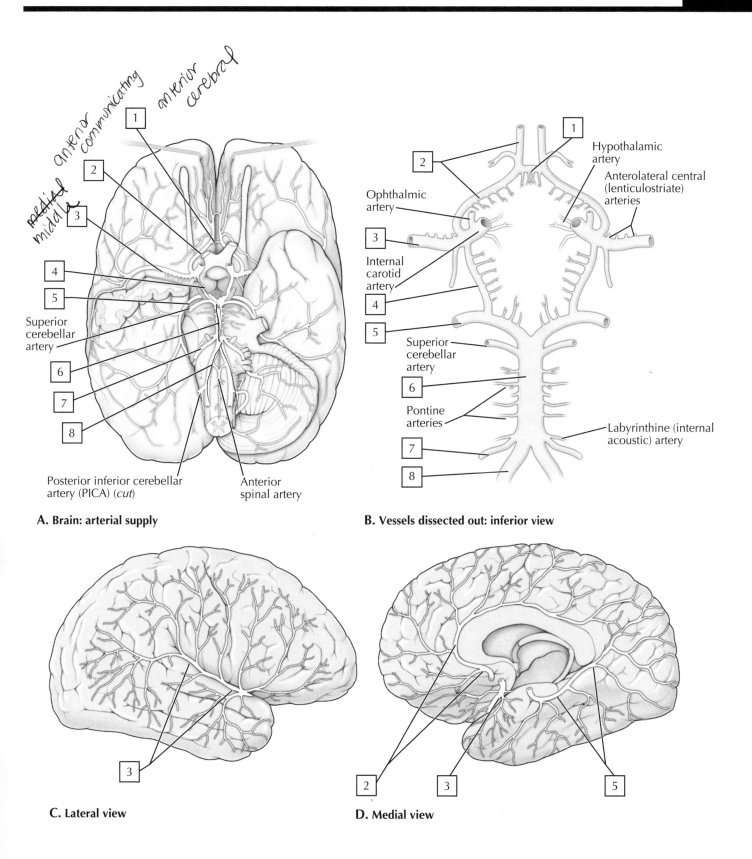

anterior communicating
anterior cerebral
medial
anterior
middle

1
2
3
4
5

Superior
cerebellar
artery

6
7
8

Posterior inferior cerebellar
artery (PICA) (*cut*)

Anterior
spinal artery

A. Brain: arterial supply

1
2

Ophthalmic
artery

3

Internal
carotid
artery

4

5

Superior
cerebellar
artery

6

Pontine
arteries

7

8

Hypothalamic
artery

Anterolateral central
(lenticulostriate)
arteries

Labyrinthine (internal
acoustic) artery

B. Vessels dissected out: inferior view

3

C. Lateral view

2
3
5

D. Medial view

Much of the blood drained from the brain collects into various **dural venous sinuses** (the dural layers separate to form a large vein or sinus) (see Plates 4-17 and 4-18), which tend to direct the flow of venous blood posteriorly along the superior and inferior sagittal sinuses to the confluence of sinuses. From here, blood flows in the right and left transverse and sigmoid sinuses to collect into the origin of the **internal jugular veins**.

COLOR the following venous sinuses, using a different color for each sinus:

☐ 1. Cavernous
☐ 2. Sigmoid
☐ 3. Transverse
☐ 4. Superior sagittal
☐ 5. Straight sinus
☐ 6. Superior petrosal

The venous drainage of the head and neck ultimately collects blood into the following major veins (numerous anastomoses exist between these veins):

• **Retromandibular**: receives tributaries from the temporal and infratemporal regions (pterygoid plexus), nasal cavity, pharynx, and oral cavity
• **Internal jugular**: drains the brain, face, thyroid gland, and neck
• **External jugular**: drains the superficial neck, lower neck and shoulder, and upper back (often communicates with the retro-mandibular vein)

COLOR the following veins, using a different color for each vein:

☐ 7. Facial
☐ 8. Superior, middle, and inferior thyroid
☐ 9. Retromandibular
☐ 10. Internal jugular

Clinical Note:
The cavernous sinus surrounds the pituitary gland and has connections to ophthalmic veins, the pterygoid plexus of veins, the basilar plexus, and superior and inferior petrosal sinuses. Venous blood flow through this sinus is stagnant because the interior of the sinus is filled with a trabecular web of connective tissue fibers that impede blood flow. Consequently, blood-borne infections can "seed" themselves in this sinus and cause a **cavernous sinus thrombosis**. Additionally, pituitary tumors can expand laterally into this sinus and stretch its dural wall, potentially placing pressure on a number of cranial nerves (CN III, IV, V_1, V_2, and VI) related to the sinus.

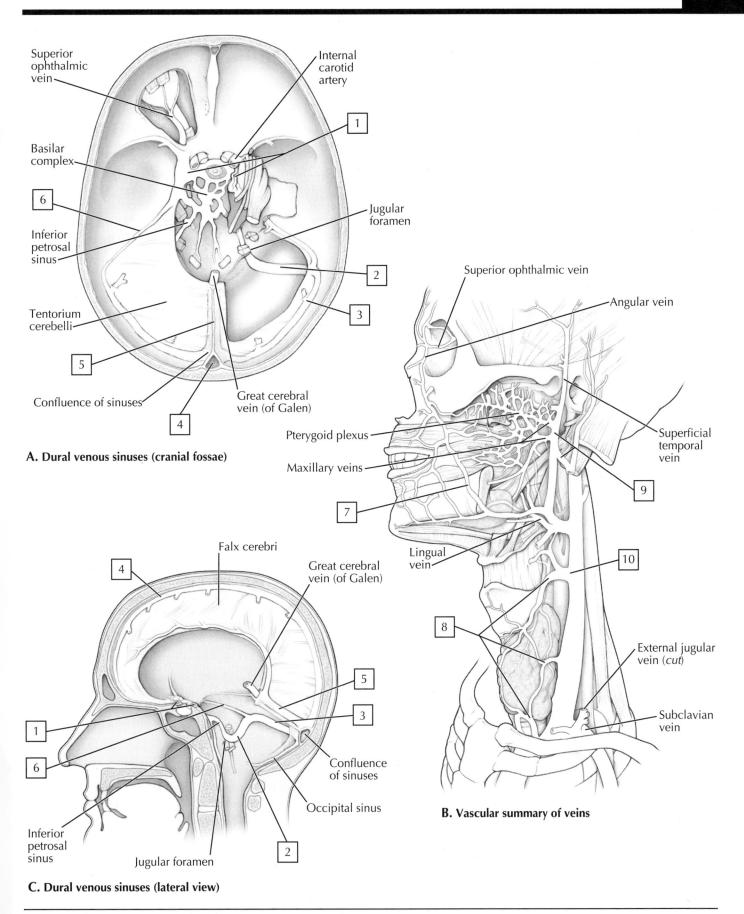

A. Dural venous sinuses (cranial fossae)

Superior ophthalmic vein

Internal carotid artery

Basilar complex

Inferior petrosal sinus

Jugular foramen

Tentorium cerebelli

Confluence of sinuses

Great cerebral vein (of Galen)

1, 6, 2, 3, 5, 4

B. Vascular summary of veins

Superior ophthalmic vein

Angular vein

Superficial temporal vein

Pterygoid plexus

Maxillary veins

Lingual vein

External jugular vein (*cut*)

Subclavian vein

7, 9, 10, 8

C. Dural venous sinuses (lateral view)

Falx cerebri

Great cerebral vein (of Galen)

Confluence of sinuses

Occipital sinus

Inferior petrosal sinus

Jugular foramen

4, 5, 3, 1, 6, 2

Arteries of the upper limb arise from a continuation of the **subclavian arteries**. Once the subclavian artery emerges from beneath the clavicle and crosses the first rib, its name changes to the **axillary artery** as it courses through the axillary region (armpit). Once the axillary artery reaches the inferior border of the teres major muscle, it becomes the **brachial artery**, which it-self divides into the **ulnar** and **radial arteries** in the cubital fossa (region anterior to the elbow).

The **axillary artery** begins at the 1st rib and descriptively is divided into three parts by the presence of the overlying pectoralis minor muscle. Branches of the subclavian and axillary artery form a rich anastomosis around the scapula, supplying the muscles acting on the shoulder joint.

PART OF AXILLARY ARTERY	BRANCH	COURSE AND STRUCTURES SUPPLIED
1	Superior thoracic	Supplies first two intercostal spaces
2	Thoraco-acromial	Has clavicular, pectoral, deltoid, and acromial branches
	Lateral thoracic	Runs with long thoracic nerve and supplies muscles that it traverses
3	Subscapular	Divides into thoracodorsal and circumflex scapular branches
	Anterior humeral circumflex	Passes around surgical neck of humerus circumflex
	Posterior humeral circumflex	Runs with axillary nerve through the quadrangular space to anastomose with anterior circumflex branch

The **brachial artery** is a direct continuation of the axillary artery inferior to the teres major muscle.

ARTERY	COURSE
Brachial	Begins at inferior border of teres major and ends at its bifurcation in cubital fossa
Deep artery of arm	Runs with radial nerve around humeral shaft
Superior ulnar collateral	Runs with ulnar nerve
Inferior ulnar collateral	Passes anterior to medial epicondyle of humerus
Radial	Is smaller lateral branch of brachial artery
Ulnar	Is larger medial branch of brachial artery

The brachial artery divides into the ulnar and radial arteries in the cubital fossa.

ARTERY	COURSE
Radial	Arises from brachial artery in cubital fossa
Radial recurrent branch	Anastomoses with radial collateral artery in arm
Palmar carpal branch	Anastomoses with carpal branch of ulnar artery
Ulnar	Arises from brachial artery in cubital fossa
Anterior ulnar recurrent	Anastomoses with inferior ulnar collateral in arm

ARTERY	COURSE
Posterior ulnar recurrent	Anastomoses with superior ulnar collateral in arm
Common interosseous	Gives rise to anterior and posterior interosseous arteries
Palmar carpal branch	Anastomoses with carpal branch of radial artery

The **ulnar** and **radial arteries** anastomose in the palm of the hand by forming **two palmar arches**. Common digital and proper digital branches arise from the superficial palmar arch to supply the fingers. The ulnar and radial arteries are summarized in the following table.

ARTERY	COURSE
Radial	
Superficial palmar branch	Forms superficial palmar arch with ulnar artery
Princeps pollicis	Passes under flexor pollicis longus tendon and divides into two proper digital arteries to thumb
Radialis indicis	Passes to index finger on its lateral side
Deep palmar arch	Is formed by terminal part of radial artery
Ulnar	
Deep palmar branch	Forms deep palmar arch with radial artery
Superficial palmar arch	Is formed by termination of ulnar artery; gives rise to three common digital arteries, each of which gives rise to two proper digital arteries

COLOR the following arteries, using a different color for each artery:

- [ ] 1. **Subclavian**
- [ ] 2. **Axillary**
- [ ] 3. **Brachial**
- [ ] 4. **Deep brachial**
- [ ] 5. **Radial**
- [ ] 6. **Ulnar**
- [ ] 7. **Deep palmar arch**
- [ ] 8. **Superficial palmar arch**

Clinical Note:
Pulse points of the upper limb include:
- Brachial: in the proximal third of the medial arm, where the brachial artery can be pressed against the humerus
- Cubital: brachial artery in the cubital fossa, medial to the biceps tendon and just before it divides into the ulnar and radial branches
- Radial: common site for taking a pulse, felt just lateral to the flexor carpi radialis tendon in the distal forearm (at the wrist)
- Ulnar: in the distal forearm (wrist), just lateral to the flexor carpi ulnaris tendon

A. Arteries of upper limb

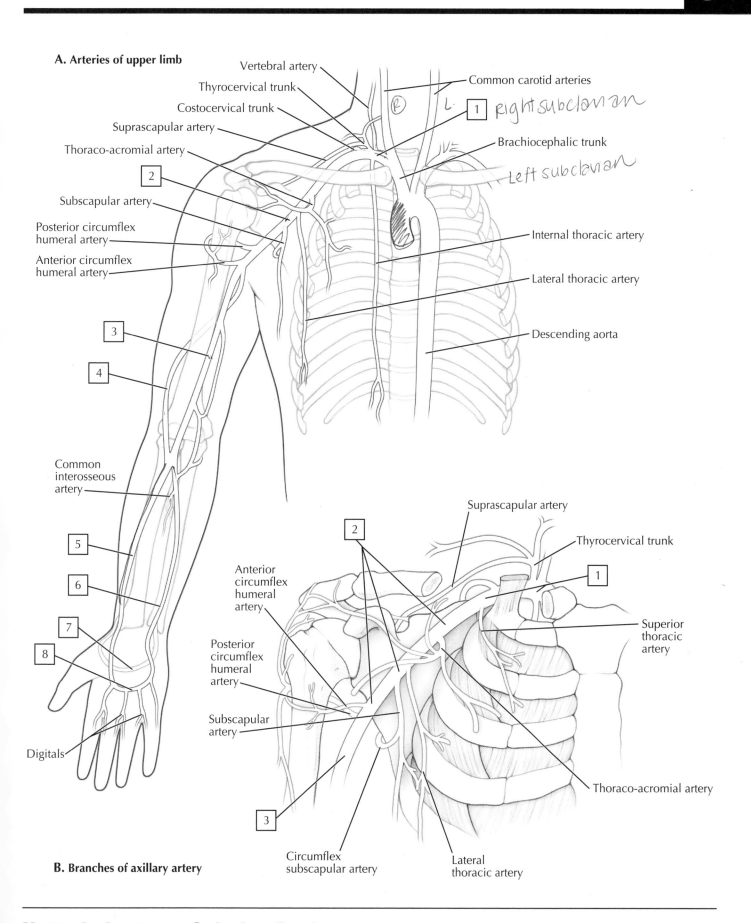

Vertebral artery

Thyrocervical trunk

Costocervical trunk

Suprascapular artery

Thoraco-acromial artery

[2]

Subscapular artery

Posterior circumflex humeral artery

Anterior circumflex humeral artery

Common carotid arteries

[1] Right subclavian

Brachiocephalic trunk

Left subclavian

Internal thoracic artery

Lateral thoracic artery

Descending aorta

[3]

[4]

Common interosseous artery

[5]

[6]

[7]

[8]

Digitals

Suprascapular artery

[2]

Anterior circumflex humeral artery

Posterior circumflex humeral artery

Subscapular artery

Thyrocervical trunk

[1]

Superior thoracic artery

Thoraco-acromial artery

[3]

Circumflex subscapular artery

Lateral thoracic artery

B. Branches of axillary artery

Arteries of the lower limb arise from the pelvis. The **obturator artery** arises from the internal iliac artery and supplies the medial compartment of the thigh. The much larger **femoral artery** arises as a direct continuation of the external iliac artery as it passes beneath the inguinal ligament. These two arteries are summarized in the following table.

ARTERY	COURSE AND STRUCTURES SUPPLIED
Obturator	Arises from internal iliac artery (pelvis); has anterior and posterior branches; passes through obturator foramen
Femoral	Continuation of external iliac artery with numerous branches to perineum, hip, thigh, and knee
Deep artery of thigh	Arises from femoral artery; supplies hip and thigh

In the distal thigh, the **femoral artery** passes through the adductor hiatus of the adductor magnus muscle to reach the posterior aspect of the knee, where it becomes the **popliteal artery**. Just inferior to the knee, the popliteal artery divides into the anterior and **posterior tibial arteries**, which course down the leg in the anterior and posterior muscle compartments, respectively. The posterior tibial artery also gives rise to a small **fibular artery**, which courses in the lateral compartment of the leg.

In the foot the anterior tibial artery forms an anastomosis around the ankle joint and continues on the dorsum of the foot as the **dorsalis pedis artery**. The major blood supply to the muscles of the sole of the foot arise from the posterior tibial artery, which passes inferior to the medial malleolus and divides into the medial and lateral plantar arteries. The medial plantar divides into superficial and deep branches, whereas the lateral plantar forms a deep plantar arch and anastomoses with arteries on the dorsum of the foot.

COLOR the following arteries of the lower limb, using a different color for each artery:

- [ ] **1. Femoral**
- [ ] **2. Popliteal**
- [ ] **3. Anterior tibial**
- [ ] **4. Posterior tibial**
- [ ] **5. Dorsalis pedis**
- [ ] **6. Medial plantar**
- [ ] **7. Lateral plantar**

Clinical Note:

Pulse points in the lower limb include:

- Femoral: just inferior to the inguinal ligament where the femoral artery lies superficial
- Popliteal: behind the knee
- Posterior tibial: just superior to the medial malleolus as this artery begins to descend into the foot
- Dorsalis pedis: on the dorsum of the foot, this is the most distal pulse from the heart

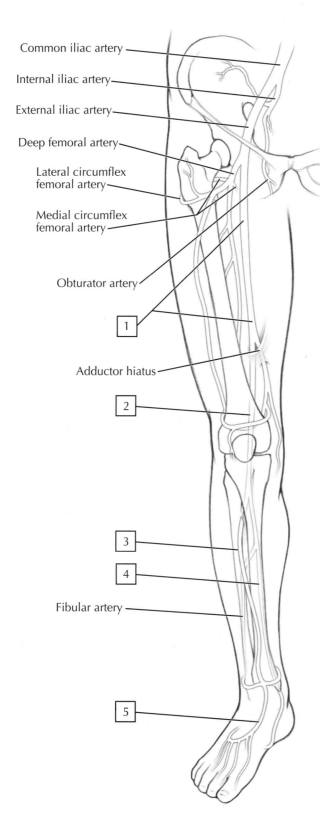

Common iliac artery

Internal iliac artery

External iliac artery

Deep femoral artery

Lateral circumflex femoral artery

Medial circumflex femoral artery

Obturator artery

1

Adductor hiatus

2

3

4

Fibular artery

5

A. Arteries of lower limb: anterior view

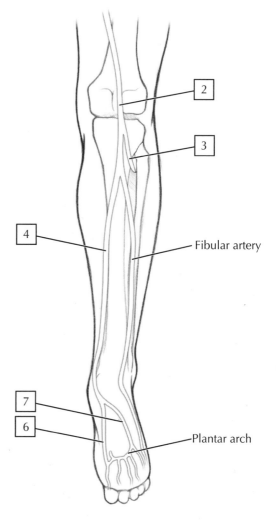

2

3

4

Fibular artery

7

6

Plantar arch

B. Arteries of leg and sole of foot: posterior view

The **thoracic aorta** gives rise to the following major arteries:
- Right and left coronary arteries to the heart
- Brachiocephalic trunk (divides into the right common carotid and subclavian)
- Left common carotid
- Left subclavian
- Right and left bronchial arteries, variable in number, to the primary bronchi and lungs
- Pericardial branches (small and variable in number)
- Intercostal arteries (course along the inferior margins of each rib)
- Esophageal arteries to supply the esophagus
- Superior phrenic arteries to the diaphragm

The **abdominal aorta** enters the abdomen via the aortic hiatus (T12 vertebral level) and divides into the common iliac arteries anterior to the L4 vertebra. Unpaired arteries to the gastrointestinal tract include the celiac, superior and inferior mesenteric arteries. Paired arteries to the other viscera include the suprarenal, renal, and gonadal (ovarian or testicular) arteries. Arteries to the musculoskeletal structures include paired inferior phrenic arteries, four to five pairs of lumbar arteries, and the unpaired median sacral artery. These arteries are summarized in the following table.

COLOR the following arteries arising from the aorta, using a different color for each artery:
- [ ] 1. **Brachiocephalic trunk**
- [ ] 2. **Celiac trunk (artery)**
- [ ] 3. **Superior mesenteric**
- [ ] 4. **Gonadals (ovarian or testicular)**
- [ ] 5. **Common iliacs**
- [ ] 6. **Inferior mesenteric**
- [ ] 7. **Aorta (color the entire aorta red)**
- [ ] 8. **Renals**
- [ ] 9. **Left subclavian**
- [ ] 10. **Left common carotid**

BRANCHES OF THE ABDOMINAL AORTA

ARTERY	ARISES FROM AORTA	SITE OF ORIGIN	SUPPLIES
Celiac trunk	Anterior	Just inferior to aortic hiatus of diaphragm	Abdominal foregut
Superior mesenteric artery	Anterior	Just inferior to celiac trunk	Abdominal midgut
Inferior mesenteric artery	Anterior	Inferior to gonadal arteries	Abdominal hindgut
Middle suprarenal arteries	Lateral	Just superior to renal arteries	Suprarenal glands
Renal arteries	Lateral	Just inferior to superior mesenteric artery	Kidneys
Gonadal (testicular or ovarian) arteries	Paired anterolateral	Inferior to the renal arteries	Testes or ovaries
Inferior phrenic arteries	Paired anterolateral	Just inferior to aortic hiatus	Diaphragm
Lumbar arteries	Posterior	Four pairs	Posterior abdominal wall and spinal cord
Median sacral artery	Posterior	Just superior to aortic bifurcation	Remnant of our caudal artery
Common iliac arteries	Terminal	Bifurcation L4 vertebra	Pelvis, perineum, gluteal region, and lower limb

Clinical Note:

Aneurysms (bulges in the arterial wall) usually involve larger arteries. The etiology includes family history, hypertension, a breakdown of collagen and/or elastin within the vessel wall that leads to inflammation and weakening of the wall, and atherosclerosis. The abdominal aorta (below the level of the renal arteries) and iliac arteries are most often involved. Surgical repair for large aneurysms is important, because a ruptured aneurysm can be fatal.

Plate 5-14   **Cardiovascular System**

Thoracic and Abdominal Aorta

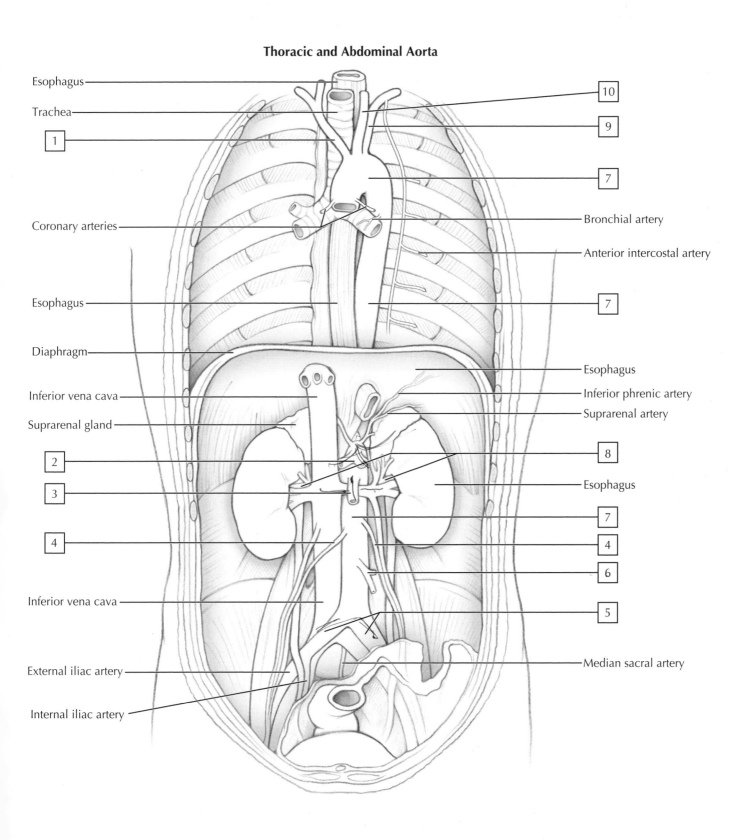

Esophagus

Trachea

1

Coronary arteries

Esophagus

Diaphragm

Inferior vena cava

Suprarenal gland

2

3

4

Inferior vena cava

External iliac artery

Internal iliac artery

10

9

7

Bronchial artery

Anterior intercostal artery

7

Esophagus

Inferior phrenic artery

Suprarenal artery

8

Esophagus

7

4

6

5

Median sacral artery

Arteries of the Gastrointestinal Tract

Arteries that supply the gastrointestinal (GI) tract include the three unpaired arteries that arise from the anterior aspect of the abdominal aorta and include the:

- **Celiac trunk**: supplies visceral structures derived from the embryonic foregut, and the spleen
- **Superior mesenteric (SMA)**: supplies visceral structures derived from the embryonic midgut
- **Inferior mesenteric (IMA)**: supplies visceral structures derived from the embryonic hindgut

These three GI tract arteries and their major branches are summarized in the tables below.

ARTERY	STRUCTURES SUPPLIED
Celiac	Supplies stomach, spleen, liver, gallbladder, and portions of pancreas and duodenum
Left gastric	Supplies proximal stomach and distal esophagus
Splenic	Supplies pancreas (dorsal branch), stomach (short gastrics and left gastro-epiploic), and spleen
Common hepatic	Divides into hepatic artery proper and gastroduodenal artery, which supply liver, gallbladder, stomach, duodenum, and pancreas
SMA	Supplies small intestine and proximal half of colon; arises from aorta posterior to neck of pancreas
Inferior pancreaticoduodenal	Supplies duodenum and pancreas
Middle colic	Supplies transverse colon
Intestinal	About 15 branches supply jejunum and ileum
Ileocolic	Supplies ileum, cecum, and appendix
Right colic	Supplies ascending colon
IMA	Supplies distal colon; arises from aorta about 2 cm superior to its bifurcation

ARTERY	STRUCTURES SUPPLIED
Left colic	Supplies distal transverse and descending colon
Sigmoid arteries	Three or four branches supply sigmoid colon
Superior rectal	Supplies proximal rectum (anastomoses with other rectal arteries)

The arterial supply of the GI tract in some senses mirrors the autonomic innervation of the GI tract. Thus, if one is familiar with the foregut, midgut, and hindgut embryonic derivatives of the GI tract, one can correlate the blood supply with the parasympathetic and sympathetic innervation of the same bowel regions. This relationship between the GI tract, its blood supply, and innervation is summarized in the bottom table arranged around the derivatives of the foregut, midgut, and hindgut embryonic bowel.

COLOR the following arteries supplying the GI tract, using a different color for each artery:

- [ ] 1. **Common hepatic branch of the celiac trunk**
- [ ] 2. **Left gastric branch of the celiac trunk**
- [ ] 3. **Splenic branch of the celiac trunk**
- [ ] 4. **Main portion of the superior mesenteric artery (SMA)**
- [ ] 5. **Middle colic branch of the SMA**
- [ ] 6. **Right colic branch of the SMA**
- [ ] 7. **Ileocolic branch of the SMA**
- [ ] 8. **Left colic branch of the inferior mesenteric artery (IMA)**
- [ ] 9. **Sigmoid branches of the IMA**
- [ ] 10. **Superior rectal branch of the IMA**

	FOREGUT	MIDGUT	HINDGUT
Organs	Stomach Liver Gallbladder Pancreas Spleen 1st half duodenum	2nd half duodenum Jejunum Ileum Cecum Ascending colon ⅔ of transverse colon	Left ⅓ of transverse colon Descending colon Sigmoid colon Rectum
Arteries	Celiac trunk: Splenic artery Left gastric Common hepatic	Superior mesenteric: Ileocolic Right colic Middle colic	Inferior mesenteric: Left colic Sigmoid branches Superior rectal
Ventral mesentery	Lesser omentum Falciform ligament Coronary/triangular ligaments	None	None
Dorsal mesentery	Gastrosplenic ligament Splenorenal ligament Gastrocolic ligament Greater omentum	Meso-intestine Meso-appendix Transverse mesocolon	Sigmoid mesocolon
Nerve supply: Parasympathetic Sympathetic	Vagus Thoracic splanchnic nerves (T5-T10)	Vagus Thoracic splanchnic nerves (T11-T12)	Pelvic splanchnic nerves (S2-S4) Lumbar splanchnic nerves (L1-L2)

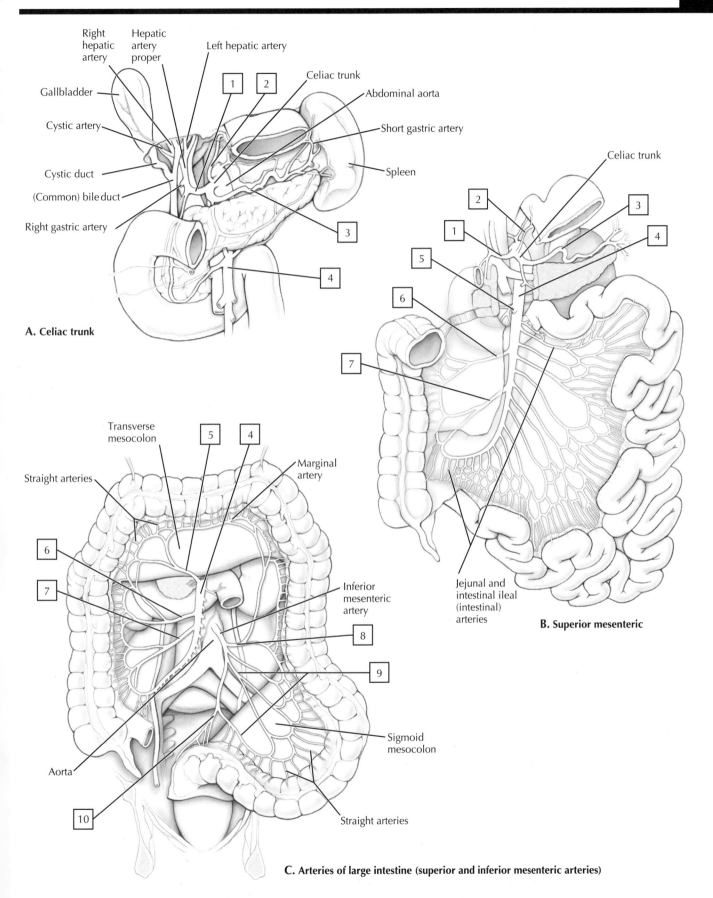

Right hepatic artery

Hepatic artery proper

Left hepatic artery

Gallbladder

Cystic artery

Celiac trunk

Abdominal aorta

Short gastric artery

Spleen

Cystic duct

(Common) bile duct

Right gastric artery

A. Celiac trunk

Celiac trunk

B. Superior mesenteric

Jejunal and intestinal ileal (intestinal) arteries

Transverse mesocolon

Straight arteries

Marginal artery

Inferior mesenteric artery

Aorta

Sigmoid mesocolon

Straight arteries

C. Arteries of large intestine (superior and inferior mesenteric arteries)

The abdominal aorta divides at the level of the L4 vertebra into the **right** and **left common iliac arteries**. The common iliac arteries then divide into the external iliac arteries, each of which passes forward and beneath the inguinal ligament to enter the thigh as the femoral arteries and the **internal iliac arteries**. The internal iliac arteries supply the pelvic viscera, its muscular walls, the muscles of the gluteal (buttock) region, and the perineum and external genitalia. The major branches of the pelvic arteries are summarized in the following table (note these are for the female).

ARTERY (DIVISION)	COURSE AND STRUCTURES SUPPLIED
Common iliac	Divides into external (to thigh) and internal (to pelvis) iliac
Internal iliac	Divides into posterior division (P) and anterior division (A)
Iliolumbar (P)	To iliacus muscle (iliac artery), psoas, quadratus lumborum, and spine (lumbar artery)
Lateral sacral (P)	Piriformis muscle and sacrum (meninges and nerves)
Superior gluteal (P)	Between lumbosacral trunk and S1 nerves, through greater sciatic foramen and into gluteal region
Inferior gluteal (A)	Between S1 or S2 and S2 or S3 to gluteal region
Internal pudendal (A)	To perineal structures
Umbilical (A)	Gives rise to superior vesical artery to bladder and becomes medial umbilical ligament when it reaches anterior abdominal wall
Obturator (A)	Passes into medial thigh via obturator foramen (with nerve)
Uterine (A)	Runs over levator ani and ureter to reach uterus
Vaginal (A)	From internal iliac or uterine, passes to vagina
Middle rectal (A)	To lower rectum and superior part of anal canal
Ovarian	From abdominal aorta, runs in suspensory ligament of ovary
Superior rectal	Continuation of inferior mesenteric artery (IMA) to rectum
Median sacral	From aortic bifurcation, unpaired artery to sacrum and coccyx

Arteries for the male are similar, except that the uterine, vaginal, and ovarian branches are replaced by arteries to the ductus deferens (from a vesical branch), prostate (from the inferior vesical), and testis (from the aorta). Significant variability exists for these arteries, so they are best identified by naming them for the structure they supply.

The blood supply to the perineum is via the **internal pudendal artery** from the internal iliac. The internal pudendal (pudendal means "shameful") artery gives rise to the following branches:
- **Inferior rectal**: to the external anal sphincter
- **Perineal**: arises from the pudendal and provides branches to the labia (scrotum in males)
- **Terminal portion of the pudendal**: terminates by providing branches to the erectile tissues (bulb of the vestibule in females and bulb of the penis in males) and branches to the clitoris (penis in male)

COLOR the following branches of the internal iliac artery, using a different color for each artery:
- [ ] 1. **Superior gluteal**
- [ ] 2. **Umbilical**
- [ ] 3. **Inferior gluteal**
- [ ] 4. **Internal pudendal**
- [ ] 5. **Inferior rectal**
- [ ] 6. **Superior vesical**
- [ ] 7. **Uterine**
- [ ] 8. **Obturator**
- [ ] 9. **Perineal**

Clinical Note:

Erectile dysfunction (ED) is an inability to achieve and/or maintain penile erection sufficient for sexual intercourse. Its occurrence increases with age. Normal erectile function occurs when a sexual stimulus causes the release of nitric oxide from nerve endings and the endothelial cells of the corpus cavernosum. This relaxes the vascular smooth muscle tone and increases the blood flow that simultaneously engorges the erectile tissues and compresses the veins that might otherwise drain the blood away. Available drugs to treat ED in males aid in relaxing the vascular smooth muscle of the small arteries that supply the penile erectile tissues (these arteries are branches of the internal pudendal). Realize that this same mechanism also functions in females, and is responsible for erectile tissue engorgement of the bulb of the vestibule and clitoris.

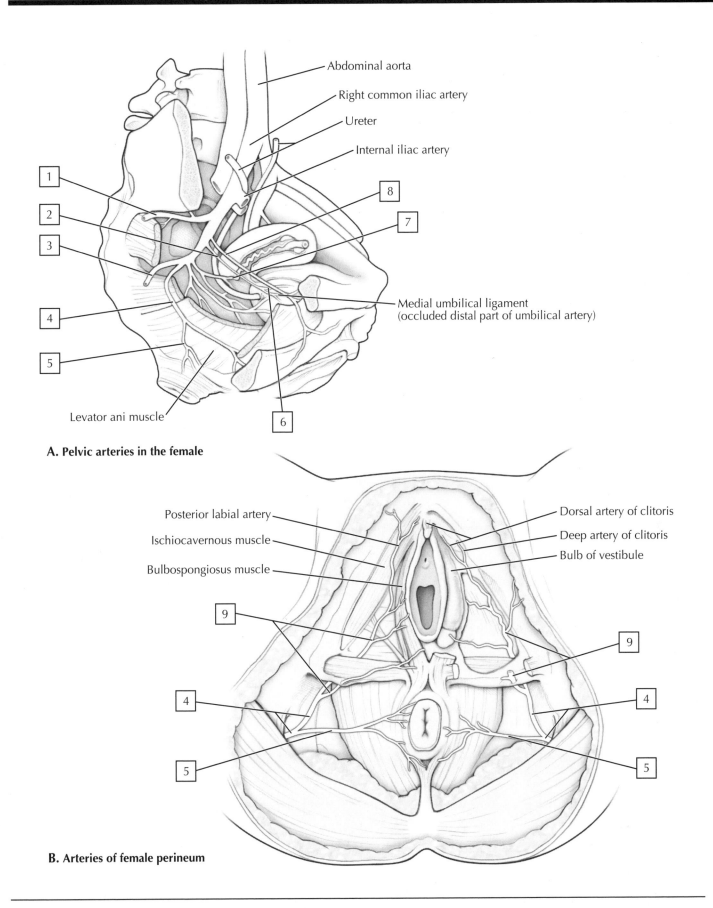

Abdominal aorta

Right common iliac artery

Ureter

Internal iliac artery

Medial umbilical ligament
(occluded distal part of umbilical artery)

Levator ani muscle

A. Pelvic arteries in the female

Posterior labial artery

Ischiocavernous muscle

Bulbospongiosus muscle

Dorsal artery of clitoris

Deep artery of clitoris

Bulb of vestibule

B. Arteries of female perineum

The venous system of the body cavities (thorax and abdominopelvic cavities) is composed of the:

- Caval system: superior and inferior vena cava and their tributaries
- Hepatic portal system: portal vein and its tributaries

The **caval system** drains:

- Body walls, including the musculoskeletal components and the overlying skin
- Head and neck regions, via the dural venous sinuses (brain), and the internal and external jugular system of veins
- Upper and lower limbs, via a set of deep and superficial veins that ultimately drain into the superior (upper limb) or inferior (lower limb) vena cava

The **portal system** drains the:

- GI tract in the abdominopelvic cavity and its accessory organs (liver, gallbladder, pancreas) via its superior and inferior mesenteric branches and their tributaries
- Spleen, an organ of the lymphoid system, via the splenic vein

In the thorax, the thoracic walls and visceral structures (lungs, esophagus, thymus) are drained by the **azygos system** of veins (the heart is drained by its own system of cardiac veins). The azygos venous blood ultimately drains into the superior vena cava (SVC) just before the SVC enters the right atrium of the heart. The azygos tributaries include the:

- Intercostal veins (posterior)
- Hemi-azygos vein (drains into azygos and often the accessory hemi-azygos)
- Accessory hemi-azygos vein
- Lumbar veins (ascending connections with azygos vein)
- Esophageal veins
- Mediastinal veins
- Pericardial veins
- Bronchial veins

The azygos system forms an important venous conduit between the inferior vena cava and the SVC. It is part of the deep venous drainage system but has connections with superficial veins that course in the subcutaneous tissues. The azygos system of veins does not possess valves (so the direction of blood flow is pressure dependent) and its branches can be variable, as is typical of the venous system in general.

COLOR the following veins, using a different color for each vein:

- [ ] 1. **Right brachiocephalic**
- [ ] 2. **Superior vena cava (SVC)**
- [ ] 3. **Azygos**
- [ ] 4. **Left brachiocephalic**
- [ ] 5. **Accessory hemi-azygos**
- [ ] 6. **Hemi-azygos**

Azygos System of Veins

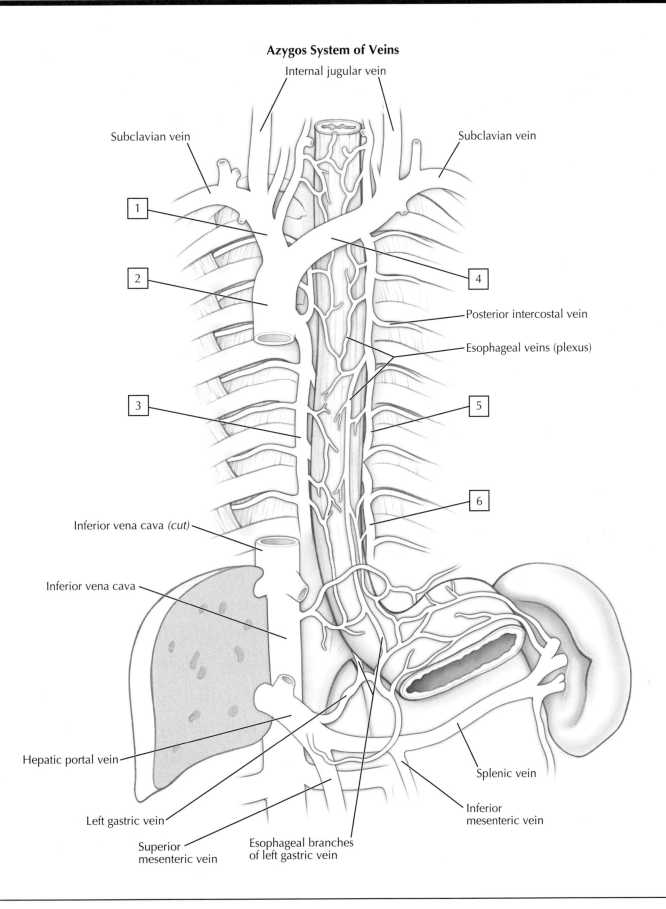

Internal jugular vein

Subclavian vein

Subclavian vein

1

4

2

Posterior intercostal vein

Esophageal veins (plexus)

3

5

6

Inferior vena cava *(cut)*

Inferior vena cava

Hepatic portal vein

Splenic vein

Inferior
mesenteric vein

Left gastric vein

Superior
mesenteric vein

Esophageal branches
of left gastric vein

Veins that drain everything in the abdominopelvic cavity except the GI tract, its accessory organs (liver, gallbladder, pancreas), and the spleen are tributaries that primarily drain into the **inferior vena cava** (IVC).

Venous drainage from the pelvis occurs primarily into tributaries that correspond to the arterial branches of the internal iliac artery, and are correspondingly given the same names. Ultimately, this venous blood collects in the common iliac veins, which then drain into the IVC. The perineum and external genitalia are largely drained by the **internal pudendal vein**, which corresponds to the artery of the same name that supplies this region. The IVC runs superiorly and pierces the dome of the diaphragm anterior to the T8 vertebra to drain into the right atrium of the heart.

The major tributaries of the IVC include the:
- Common iliac veins
- Lumbar veins (the upper lumbar veins usually form connections to the azygos system of veins via ascending lumbar veins)
- Right gonadal (ovarian or testicular) vein (the left gonadal vein drains into the left renal vein)
- Renal veins
- Right suprarenal vein (left suprarenal drains into the left renal vein)
- Inferior phrenic veins
- Hepatic veins

These abdominopelvic veins do not possess valves, so blood flow direction is dependent upon the pressure gradient in the vessels. As with the azygos system in the thorax, connections with superficial veins in the subcutaneous tissues occur with the veins draining the interior body walls.

COLOR the following veins, using a different color for each vein:

- [ ] **1. IVC**
- [ ] **2. External iliac**
- [ ] **3. Internal iliac**
- [ ] **4. Inferior rectal**
- [ ] **5. Hepatic**
- [ ] **6. Renal**
- [ ] **7. Right and left gonadal (ovarian or testicular veins)***

*Note that the left gonadal vein drains into the left renal vein, not the IVC

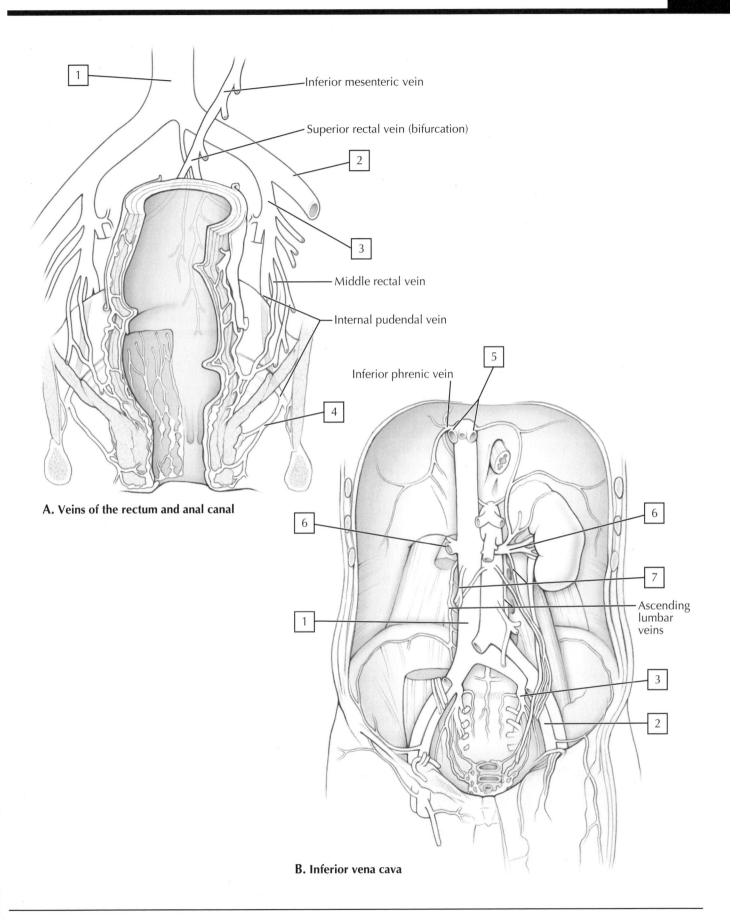

Inferior mesenteric vein

Superior rectal vein (bifurcation)

Middle rectal vein

Internal pudendal vein

A. Veins of the rectum and anal canal

Inferior phrenic vein

Ascending lumbar veins

B. Inferior vena cava

The GI tract, its accessory organs (gallbladder, liver, pancreas), and the spleen are drained by the portal system of veins. Four major veins make up this system:

- **Inferior mesenteric**: drains the hindgut derivatives of the GI tract, including the distal transverse colon, descending colon, sigmoid colon, and proximal rectum
- **Superior mesenteric**: drains the midgut derivatives of the GI tract, including the distal duodenum, small intestine, ascending colon, and proximal transverse colon, as well as the pancreas
- **Splenic**: drains the spleen, stomach, and pancreas
- **Portal**: formed by the union of the **splenic** and **superior mesenteric veins**, this large vein drains the stomach and gallbladder and receives all the venous drainage from the three veins just mentioned

All of the blood from the visceral structures listed previously drains ultimately into the portal vein and then into the liver. The liver processes important products and energy sources (glucose, fat, protein, vitamins) from the GI tract, produces cellular fuels, produces plasma proteins and clotting factors, metabolizes toxins and drugs, excretes substances like bilirubin, and produces bile acids. From the liver the venous blood flows into several hepatic veins, which immediately drain into the inferior vena cava just before it pierces the diaphragm and enters the right atrium of the heart.

Various conditions, such as cirrhosis, can damage the liver and impede venous blood flow through this vital organ. However, blood must return to the heart for gas exchange in the lungs, so it will bypass the liver via important portosystemic anastomoses to gain access to the caval system (SVC, IVC, and azygos veins) and its tributaries, which can then return the blood to the heart. The impeded venous return raises the blood pressure in the portal system causing portal hypertension; because the veins of the portal system lack valves, the venous blood can reverse flow and seek alternative routes back to the heart. Clinically, these portosystemic anastomoses are lifesaving and include the following major routes:

- **Esophageal**: blood will shunt from the portal and splenic veins into gastric veins of the stomach and then into esophageal veins that are connected to the azygos system of veins, ultimately draining into the SVC and the heart (see part A)
- **Rectal**: blood will drain inferiorly in the inferior mesenteric vein to the superior rectal vein and then into the middle and inferior rectal veins (anastomosis around the rectum) to access the IVC and the heart (see part B)

- **Para-umbilical**: blood from the portal vein will drain into the para-umbilical veins and fill the subcutaneous veins of the abdominal wall (forms a tortuous tangle of veins visible on the abdominal surface called the caput medusae), which then may drain into tributaries of the SVC, IVC, and azygos system (see part C)
- **Retroperitoneal**: least important of the pathways; some blood will drain from retroperitoneal GI viscera into parietal veins in the body wall to access the caval tributaries (not shown)

COLOR the following veins that contribute to the portocaval anastomotic system, using the colors suggested for each vein:

- ☐ 1. **Portal (dark blue)**
- ☐ 2. **Superior mesenteric (purple)**
- ☐ 3. **Splenic (dark red)**
- ☐ 4. **Inferior mesenteric (light blue)**

Clinical Note:

Cirrhosis, a largely irreversible disease, is characterized by diffuse fibrosis, parenchymal nodular regeneration, and a disturbed hepatic architecture that progressively disrupts portal blood flow through the liver (leading to portal hypertension). Major causes of cirrhosis include:

- Alcoholic liver disease: 60% to 70%
- Viral hepatitis: 10%
- Biliary diseases: 5% to 10%
- Other: 5% to 15%

Portal hypertension, a result of the increased resistance to venous blood flow through the diseased liver, has the following clinical consequences:

- Ascites (abnormal accumulation of fluid in the abdominal cavity)
- Formation of portosystemic venous shunts via the anastomoses previously noted
- Congestive splenomegaly (engorgement of the spleen with blood)
- Hepatic encephalopathy (toxins in the blood, not removed by the diseased liver, cause brain disease)

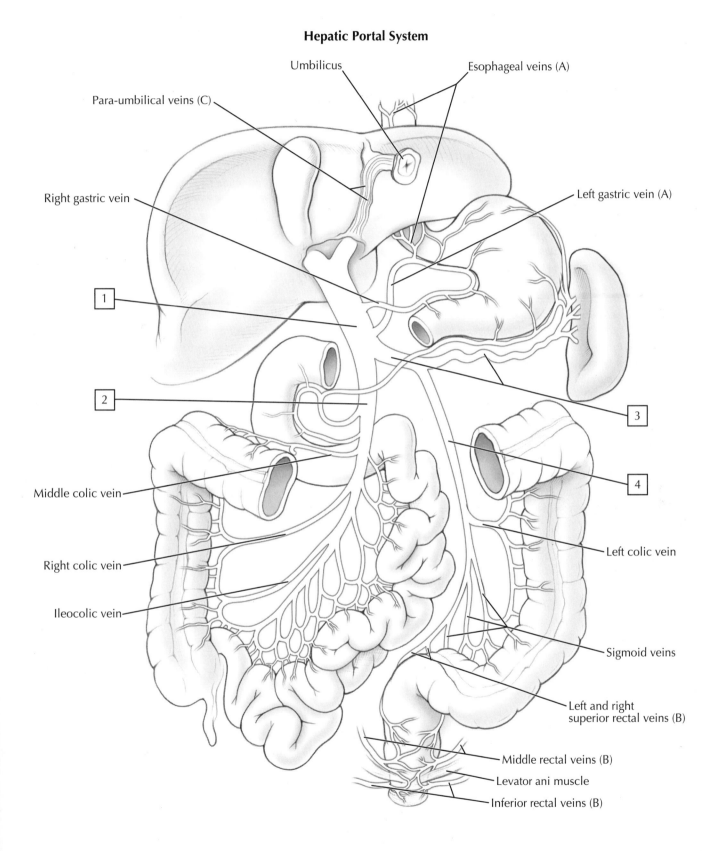

Hepatic Portal System

Umbilicus

Esophageal veins (A)

Para-umbilical veins (C)

Right gastric vein

Left gastric vein (A)

1

2

3

4

Middle colic vein

Right colic vein

Ileocolic vein

Left colic vein

Sigmoid veins

Left and right
superior rectal veins (B)

Middle rectal veins (B)

Levator ani muscle

Inferior rectal veins (B)

Similar to the rest of the body, the upper limb is drained by a set of deep and superficial veins. However, the veins of the upper (and lower) limb contain valves, which assist, largely by the action of adjacent muscle contraction, to return venous blood to the heart against gravity.

The **deep set of veins** of the upper limb parallel the arteries and include the following major veins:
- **Radial**: parallels the deep radial artery in the lateral forearm
- **Ulnar**: parallels the ulnar artery in the medial forearm
- **Brachial**: formed by the union of the radial and ulnar veins in the cubital fossa; this vein parallels the brachial artery in the medial aspect of the arm
- **Axillary**: in the armpit, it parallels the axillary artery in the axillary sheath (surrounded by the cords of the brachial nerve plexus)
- **Subclavian**: parallels the subclavian artery but passes anterior to the anterior scalene muscle rather than posterior to it (artery lies posterior)

The **superficial set of veins** of the upper limb are connected by communicating veins to the deep set of veins and provide an additional route for venous return to the heart. These veins can vary considerably from person to person and have extensive tributaries. The veins also have valves to assist in venous return and include the following major veins:
- **Dorsal venous network**: most of the blood from the palm will drain into these veins (especially when the hand is squeezed)
- **Cephalic**: runs in the subcutaneous tissue along the lateral forearm and arm to ultimately drain into the axillary vein
- **Basilic**: runs in the subcutaneous tissue along the medial forearm and distal arm to ultimately dive deep into the medial arm and drain into the axillary vein
- **Median cubital**: passes from the cephalic to the basilic vein in the cubital fossa and is a common site for venipuncture to withdraw a blood sample or administer fluids intravenously

COLOR the following veins of the upper limb, using a different color for each vein:
- [ ] 1. Subclavian
- [ ] 2. Axillary
- [ ] 3. Cephalic (superficial)
- [ ] 4. Brachial
- [ ] 5. Median cubital (superficial)
- [ ] 6. Radial
- [ ] 7. Ulnar
- [ ] 8. Basilic (superficial)

Clinical Note:

In general, veins are more numerous than arteries, more variable in their location, and often parallel arteries, especially deep within the body or extremities. Veins of the limbs and those in the lower neck (internal jugular veins) contain valves, whereas most other veins in the body are valveless. Often, when a vein such as the brachial or axillary vein parallels the artery of the same name, the vein actually forms "venae comitantes" (accompanying veins), or a network of veins that entwines the parallel artery like vines entwine a tree trunk. With several major exceptions, many veins may be sacrificed during surgery because so many alternative venous channels exist to return blood from a region back to the heart (of course, if venous repair is feasible, it is preferred). Additionally, the body will usually "sprout" new veins from adjacent tributaries to drain an area denuded of its venous drainage.

Plate 5-20   **Cardiovascular System**

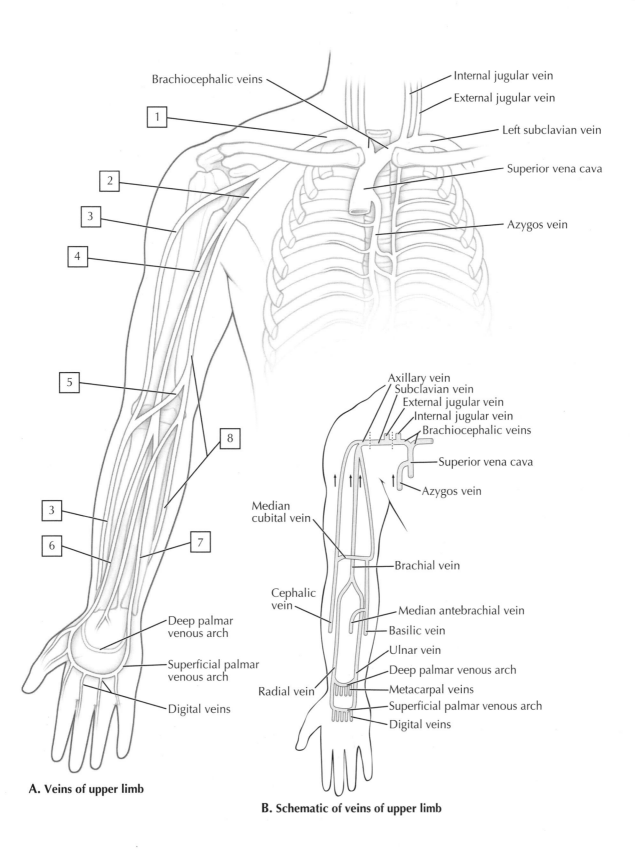

Brachiocephalic veins

Internal jugular vein

External jugular vein

Left subclavian vein

Superior vena cava

Azygos vein

1

2

3

4

5

8

3

6

7

Deep palmar venous arch

Superficial palmar venous arch

Digital veins

A. Veins of upper limb

Axillary vein

Subclavian vein

External jugular vein

Internal jugular vein

Brachiocephalic veins

Superior vena cava

Azygos vein

Median cubital vein

Brachial vein

Cephalic vein

Median antebrachial vein

Basilic vein

Ulnar vein

Deep palmar venous arch

Metacarpal veins

Superficial palmar venous arch

Radial vein

Digital veins

B. Schematic of veins of upper limb

Similar to the rest of the body, the lower limb is drained by a set of deep and superficial veins. However, the veins of the lower (and upper) limb contain valves, which assist, largely by the action of adjacent muscle contraction, to return venous blood to the heart against gravity.

The **deep set of veins** of the lower limb parallel the arteries and include the following major veins:

• **Posterior tibial**: drains from the sole of the foot and medial ankle superiorly up the leg, paralleling the posterior tibial artery in the posterior compartment of the leg

• **Anterior tibial**: begins as the dorsalis pedis vein on the dorsum of the foot and parallels the anterior tibial artery in the anterior compartment of the leg

• **Fibular**: small vein that parallels the artery of the same name in the lateral compartment of the leg and drains into the posterior tibial vein

• **Popliteal**: lies behind the knee and is formed by the anterior and posterior tibial veins

• **Femoral**: the popliteal becomes the femoral in the distal thigh and then the femoral drains deep to the inguinal ligament to become the external iliac vein in the pelvis

The **superficial set of veins** of the lower limb are connected by communicating veins to the deep set of veins and provide an additional route for venous return to the heart. These veins can vary considerably from person to person and have extensive tributaries. The veins also have valves to assist in venous return and include the following major veins:

• **Dorsal venous arch**: drains blood from the foot into the small and large saphenous veins at the lateral and medial aspect of the ankle, respectively

• **Small saphenous**: courses superiorly in the subcutaneous tissue of the calf (posterior aspect of the leg) and then dives deeply to drain into the popliteal vein behind the knee

• **Great saphenous**: courses superiorly from the medial side of the ankle to run up the medial leg and thigh, draining into the femoral vein just inferior to the inguinal ligament

Note that the great saphenous vein and the cephalic vein of the upper limb are analogous veins, as are the small saphenous and the basilic vein of the upper limb (both dive deeply to join a deeper vein).

COLOR the following veins of the lower limb, using a different color for each vein:

☐ 1. Femoral

☐ 2. Great saphenous (superficial)

☐ 3. Anterior tibial

☐ 4. Popliteal

☐ 5. Small saphenous (superficial)

☐ 6. Posterior tibial

Clinical Note:

Veins of the extremities and those in the lower neck contain valves. The valves are an extension of the tunica intima of the venous wall, project into the vein's lumen, and are similar in appearance to the semilunar valves of the heart. Venous valves assist in venous return against gravity by preventing the backflow of blood. The blood in the veins of the extremities is propelled along, in part, by the contraction of adjacent skeletal muscle. The walls of veins adjacent to the valves can become weakened and distended, thus compromising the ability of the valve to work properly and affecting venous return. Such veins are called **varicose** (enlarged and tortuous) **veins**, and this condition is most common in the veins of the lower limb.

Plate 5-21 **Cardiovascular System**

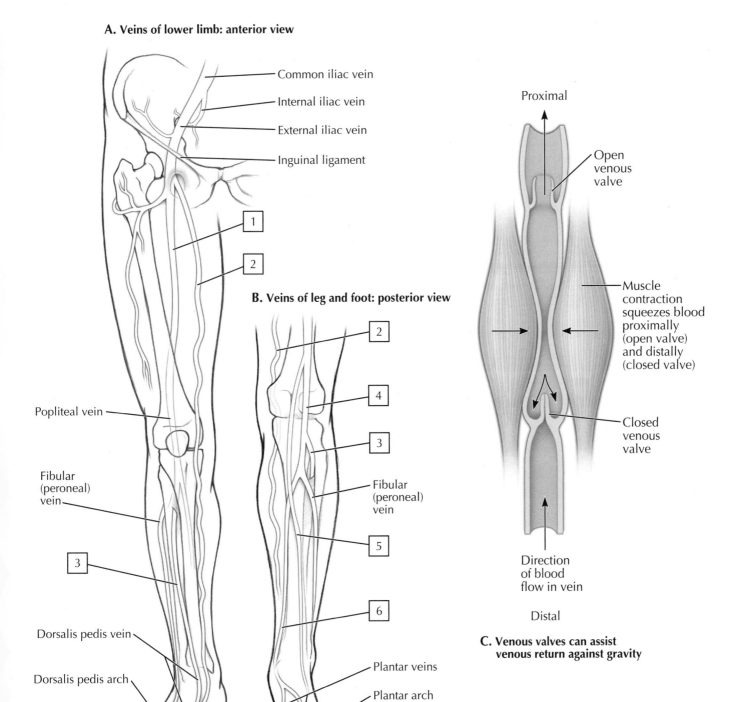

A. Veins of lower limb: anterior view

Common iliac vein

Internal iliac vein

External iliac vein

Inguinal ligament

1

2

Popliteal vein

Fibular
(peroneal)
vein

3

Dorsalis pedis vein

Dorsalis pedis arch

Metatarsal veins

B. Veins of leg and foot: posterior view

2

4

3

Fibular
(peroneal)
vein

5

6

Plantar veins

Plantar arch

Digital veins

Proximal

Open
venous
valve

Muscle
contraction
squeezes blood
proximally
(open valve)
and distally
(closed valve)

Closed
venous
valve

Direction
of blood
flow in vein

Distal

**C. Venous valves can assist
venous return against gravity**

The pattern of fetal circulation is one of gas exchange and nutrient/metabolic waste exchange across the placenta with the maternal blood (but not the exchange of blood cells) and distribution of oxygen and nutrient-rich blood to the tissues of the fetus. Various shunts allow fetal blood to largely bypass the liver, which is not needed for metabolic processing in utero, and the lungs, also not needed in utero for gas exchange. The mother takes care of this for the fetus. Therefore, the blood in the fetus needs to bypass the liver and lungs and gain direct access to the left side of the heart so that it may be pumped into the fetal systemic circulation. Several fetal shunts allow this to happen and include the following:

• **Ductus venosus** (bypasses the liver)
• **Foramen ovale** (shunts blood from the right atrium to the left atrium, thus bypassing the lungs)
• **Ductus arteriosus** (shunts any blood in the pulmonary trunk into the aorta, also bypassing the lungs)
• **Umbilical arteries and vein** (placental vessels that return blood to the placenta or convey blood from the placenta to the heart)

These shunts close at birth or shortly thereafter, and the newborn infant begins gas exchange through his or her own lungs and processes ingested liquids, and ultimately solid food, through his or her own liver. These changes at birth include the following:

• Ductus venosus becomes a ligament (ligamentum venosum)
• Foramen ovale becomes the fossa ovalis
• Ductus arteriosus becomes the ligamentum arteriosum
• Umbilical arteries and veins become ligaments

COLOR the following features of the prenatal and postnatal circulation:

☐ 1. **Umbilical arteries (carries blood from fetus to placenta)**

☐ 2. **Umbilical vein (carries blood from placenta to fetal heart)**

☐ 3. **Ductus venosus (shunt to bypass fetal liver)**

☐ 4. **Foramen ovale (shunt from fetal right atrium to left atrium to bypass fetal lungs)**

☐ 5. **Ductus arteriosus (shunt from pulmonary trunk to aorta to bypass fetal lungs)**

☐ 6. **Ligamentum arteriosum (obliterated ductus arteriosus)**

☐ 7. **Fossa ovalis (obliterated foramen ovale)**

☐ 8. **Ligamentum venosum (obliterated ductus venosus)**

☐ 9. **Ligamentum teres of liver (obliterated umbilical vein)**

☐ 10. **Medial umbilical ligaments (occluded part of umbilical arteries)**

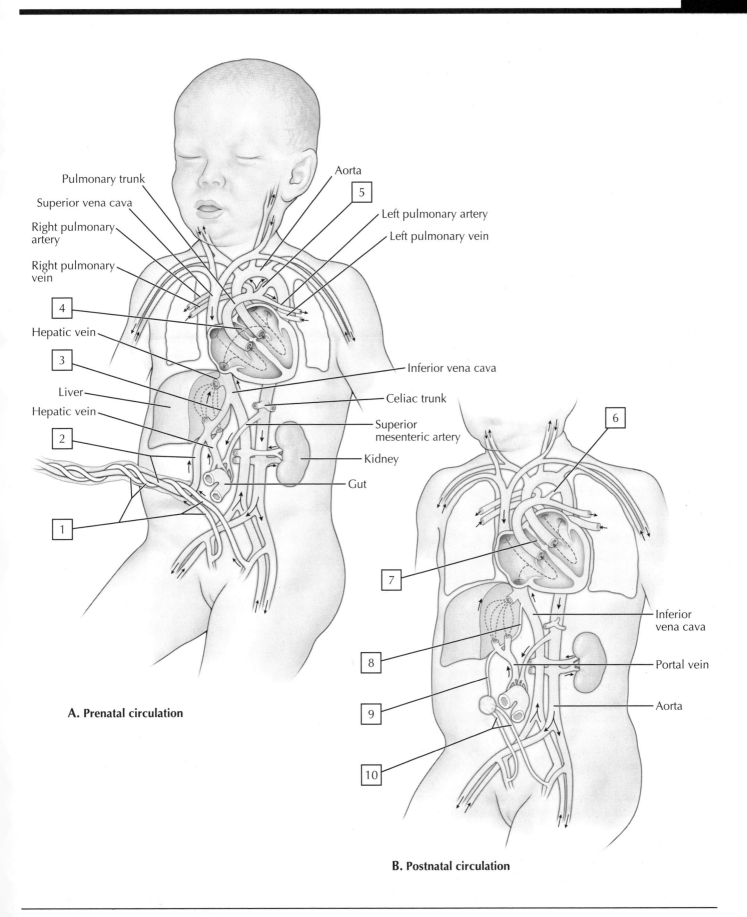

Pulmonary trunk

Superior vena cava

Right pulmonary artery

Right pulmonary vein

4

Hepatic vein

3

Liver

Hepatic vein

2

1

Aorta

5

Left pulmonary artery

Left pulmonary vein

Inferior vena cava

Celiac trunk

Superior mesenteric artery

Kidney

Gut

A. Prenatal circulation

6

7

8

9

10

Inferior vena cava

Portal vein

Aorta

B. Postnatal circulation

For each description below, color that feature in the image of the sectioned heart

1. This muscle extends into the ventricles and prevents prolapse of the valve leaflets.

2. Blood passing from the left ventricle passes through this valve.

3. Blood from the left atrium passes through this valve to enter the left ventricle.

4. Blood returning from the lower portion of the body enters the right atrium via this vein.

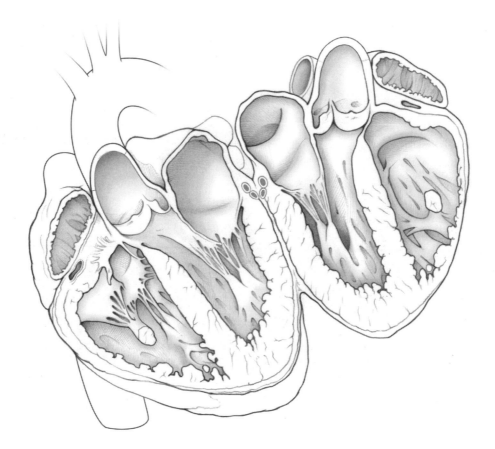

5. An atrial septal defect often occurs at the site of this interatrial septal shunt in the fetal heart. Which of the following structures or features of the fetal heart are involved in this defect?
   A. Ductus arteriosus
   B. Ductus venosus
   C. Foramen ovale
   D. Ligamentum arteriosum
   E. Ligamentum venosum

6. A gunshot wound to the anterior shoulder region traumatizes the cords of the brachial plexus and most likely would also involve damage to which of the following arteries?
   A. Axillary
   B. Brachial
   C. Brachiocephalic
   D. Common carotid
   E. Subclavian

7. The left ovarian vein drains into which of the following veins?
   A. Inferior mesenteric
   B. Inferior vena cava
   C. Left external iliac
   D. Left renal
   E. Portal

8. What three unpaired arteries provide the major blood supply to the abdominal gastrointestinal tract?
   A. _____
   B. _____
   C. _____

9. A laceration to the perineal region would most likely involve bleeding from branches of which major artery supplying this region?
   _____

10. Which artery is responsible for the most distal pulse in the body that is frequently assessed by clinicians? _____
   _____

ANSWER KEY

1. Papillary muscle(s) in either ventricle

2. Aortic valve

3. Mitral valve

4. Inferior vena cava

5. C

6. A

7. D

8. Celiac trunk, superior mesenteric artery, and inferior mesenteric artery

9. Internal pudendal artery

10. Dorsalis pedis pulse on the dorsum of the foot

Chapter 6 Lymphatic System

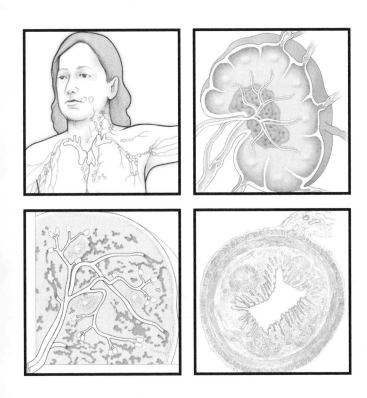

The lymphatic system is intimately associated with the cardio-vascular system, both in the development of its lymphatic vessels and in its immune function. The lymphatic system functions to:

- Protect the body against infection by activating defense mechanisms that make up our immune system
- Collect tissue fluids, solutes, hormones, and plasma proteins and return them to the circulatory system (bloodstream)
- Absorb fat (chylomicrons) from the small intestine into the lymphatic lacteals

Components of the lymphatic system include:

- **Lymph**: a watery fluid that resembles plasma but contains fewer proteins and may contain fat together with cells (mainly lymphocytes and a few red blood cells)
- **Lymphocytes**: cellular components of lymph, which include T cells, B cells
- **Lymph vessels**: an extensive network of vessels and capillaries in peripheral tissues that transport lymph and lymphocytes
- **Lymphoid organs**: collections of lymphoid tissue that include lymph nodes, aggregates of lymphoid tissue along the respiratory and gastrointestinal (GI) passageways, tonsils, thymus, spleen, and bone marrow

COLOR the lymphoid organs, using a different color for each organ:

- [ ] **1. Tonsils**
- [ ] **2. Thymus gland**
- [ ] **3. Spleen**
- [ ] **4. Bone marrow**

The body is about 60% fluid by weight, with 40% intracellular fluid and 20% extracellular fluid (ECF). The lymphatics are essential for returning ECF, solutes, and protein (lost via the capillaries into the ECF compartment) back to the bloodstream. The lymphatics return about 3.5 to 4.0 L of fluid per day back to the bloodstream and also distribute hormones, nutrients (fats from the bowel and proteins from the interstitium), and waste products from the ECF to the bloodstream.

Lymphatic vessels transport lymph from everywhere in the body, except the central nervous system, to major lymphatic channels, with the majority of the lymph collecting in the **thoracic lymphatic duct** (joins the veins at the union of the left internal jugular and left subclavian veins). A much smaller **right lymphatic duct** drains lymphatics from the right upper quadrant of the body to a similar site on the right side. Encapsulated **lymph nodes** are strategically placed to act as "filters" of the lymph as it moves toward the venous system.

COLOR the following features of a lymph node, using the colors indicated for each feature:

- [ ] **5. Vein (blue)**
- [ ] **6. Artery (red)**
- [ ] **7. Efferent lymph vessel (yellow)**
- [ ] **8. Afferent lymph vessels (green)**

Cells associated with the lymphatic system and its immune responses include:

- **Lymphocytes**: B cells (bone marrow–derived cells, comprising about 10% to 15% of the circulating lymphocytes; can differentiate into **plasma cells**, which secrete antibodies that can bind to foreign antigens), T cells (thymus-dependent cells, comprising about 80% of circulating lymphocytes; attack foreign cells and virus-infected cells, and can be cytotoxic, helper, or suppressor T cells), and NK cells (natural killer cells, comprising about 5% to 10% of circulating lymphocytes; attack foreign cells, cancer cells, or virus-infected cells, and constantly provide immunologic surveillance of the body)
- **White blood cells**: monocytes, neutrophils, basophils, and eosinophils (see Plate 5-1).
- **Macrophages**: phagocytic cells that act as scavengers and are antigen-presenting cells, which initiate immune responses
- **Reticular cells**: similar to fibroblasts, these cells can attract T and B cells and dendritic cells
- **Dendritic cells**: bone marrow–derived cells that are potent antigen-presenting cells to T cells and are found mainly in the skin, nose, lungs, stomach, and intestines
- **Follicular dendritic cells**: highly branching cells that mingle with B cells in the germinal center of the lymph node and contain antigen-antibody complexes for months or years, but are not antigen-presenting cells

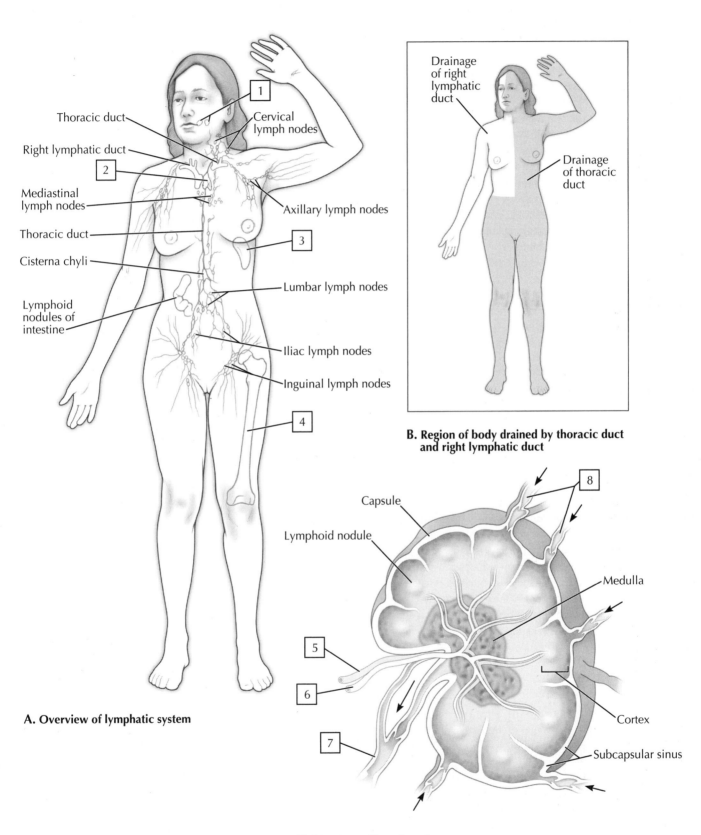

Thoracic duct

Cervical lymph nodes

Right lymphatic duct

Mediastinal lymph nodes

Thoracic duct

Cisterna chyli

Lymphoid nodules of intestine

Axillary lymph nodes

Lumbar lymph nodes

Iliac lymph nodes

Inguinal lymph nodes

A. Overview of lymphatic system

Drainage of right lymphatic duct

Drainage of thoracic duct

B. Region of body drained by thoracic duct and right lymphatic duct

Capsule

Lymphoid nodule

Medulla

Cortex

Subcapsular sinus

C. Structure of lymph node

When a foreign microorganism, virus-infected cell, or a cancer cell is detected within the body, the lymphatic system mounts what is called an **immune response**. The detected pathogens are distinguished from the body's own normal cells, and then a response is initiated to neutralize the pathogen. The human body has evolved three major responses to protect against foreign invaders:

- **Nonspecific barriers**: a first line of defense composed of **physical barriers** to invasion that include the skin and mucous membranes that line the body's exterior (skin) or line its respiratory, GI, urinary, and reproductive systems (additional barriers: mucosae and their secretions, which may include enzymes and acidic secretions; flushing mechanisms such as tear secretion or the voiding of urine; sticky mucus to sequester pathogens; and physical coughing and sneezing to remove pathogens and irritants)
- **Innate immunity**: a second line of defense if the nonspecific barrier is breached; composed of a variety of cells, antimicrobial secretions, inflammation, and fever
- **Adaptive immunity**: a third line of defense characterized by **specific pathogen recognition**, immunological memory, amplification of immune responses, and rapid response against pathogens that reinvade

The hallmark of innate immunity is **inflammation**, a relatively nonspecific response with symptoms of redness, heat, swelling, and pain. The key elements of inflammation include:

- **Tissue injury**: the physical nonspecific barriers are breached by a pathogen
- **Leukocytosis**: significant increase in white blood cells in the bloodstream, primarily neutrophils, which flow to and migrate from the vasculature (diapedesis) into the site of inflammation
- **Release of chemical inflammatory mediators**: histamine (mast cells and basophils), kinins (neutrophils and other sources), prostaglandins (neutrophils and other cells), cytokines (leukocytes, fibroblasts, endothelial cells, lymphocytes), and complement (normally inactive, circulating plasma proteins—the humoral component of the innate immune response) are released by various cells that cause vasodilation, increased capillary permeability, and chemotaxis

- **Phagocytosis**: pathogens, dead cells, and debris are phagocytosed, usually forming pus at the site of injury
- **Healing**: the area is walled off, clots may form, and debris is removed as the healing process begins

The inflammation associated with the innate immune response is **genetically determined** and does not involve prior exposure to antigens, but does involve both cells and various chemical inflammatory mediators. Moreover, it appears the innate response activates the elements of the adaptive immune response.

COLOR the following elements of the innate immune response that lead to inflammation, using the suggested colors for each element:

- ☐ 1. **Pathogens (yellow)**
- ☐ 2. **Dendritic cell and its cytokines and inflammatory mediators (green)**
- ☐ 3. **Macrophages (blue)**
- ☐ 4. **Neutrophils (purple)**
- ☐ 5. **Blood vessel (red)**
- ☐ 6. **Monocytes (light blue)**

Plate 6-2   **Lymphatic System**

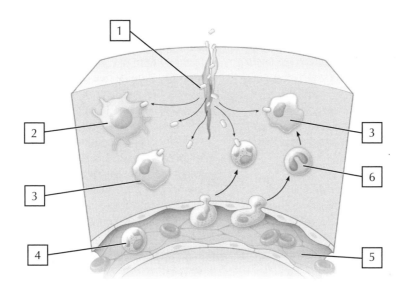

Physical barriers

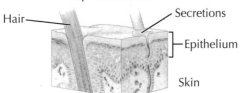

Hair

Secretions

Epithelium

Skin

Phagocytes

| Fixed macro-phage | Neutrophil | Free macro-phage | Eosinophil | Monocyte |

Immunological surveillance
Killer cells: destroy abnormal cells

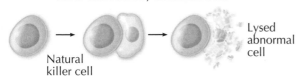

Natural killer cell

Lysed abnormal cell

Interferons
Protect cells by increasing their resistance to disease

Interferons are released after activation of lymphocytes or virus-infected cells

Complement system
Lyses cells: stimulates inflammatory response

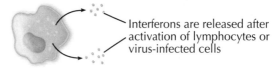

Complement

Lysed pathogen

Inflammatory response

- Increases blood flow
- Activates phagocytes
- Increases capillary permeability
- Activates the complement system
- Infected region is sequestered by clotting
- Fever
- Systemic defenses activated

Mast cells

Fever
Reduces pathogens, facilitates tissue repair, activates defenses

Body temperature rises above 37° C in response to pyrogens

The adaptive immune response is a specific response that is characterized by the following features:

- **Specificity**: a response that is directed toward a specific pathogen
- **Passive or active forms**: immunity that can be passed from another individual via antibodies (passive) or produced by antibodies that develop in response to antigens (active)
- **Systemic**: a response that is not confined simply to the site of inflammation; it is a slower response than the innate response but lasts much longer
- **Memory**: once antibodies are developed in response to a foreign antigen, the body "remembers" the response and can mount an even stronger response upon second exposure to the same antigen

The cells of the adaptive response are **lymphocytes** (B and T cells), derived from the pluripotent hemopoietic stem cells of the bone marrow. B cells are involved in the **humoral (chemical attack) response**, which can be summarized as follows:

- B cell recognizes a pathogen by the binding of its surface antibodies to a foreign antigen and becomes sensitized
- B cells then become activated when an inactive helper T cell recognizes the same antigens, binds to the B cell, and secretes lymphokines that cause activated B cells to divide
- B cell division yields millions of B cells, which then become plasma cells that secrete antibodies (immunoglobulins) to the antigen into the circulating blood and lymph
- These circulating antibodies bind to the specific antigens on pathogens and label them for destruction by phagocytes; the antibodies also may bind directly to bacterial toxins or receptors used by bacterial and viruses such that they directly neutralize the invader
- B cell division also yields memory B cells that remain in reserve should the body be re-exposed to the same foreign antigen

T cells are of several types and are involved in **cell-mediated responses**:

- **Helper T cells**: although not directly involved in killing pathogens or infected cells, these T cells control the immune response by directing the activities of other cells of the immune system; they recognize antigens presented by B cells, become activated, and secrete cytokines that promote humoral- and cell-mediated immunity
- **Memory T cells**: derived from helper and killer (cytotoxic) T cells, they remain in reserve in case of re-infection
- **Suppressor T cells**: activated later than other B and T cells, they suppress the immune response, thus limiting the overall intensity of any single response
- **Killer (cytotoxic) T cells**: respond to antigen on cell surfaces (other than B cells), become activated and divide, and produce memory T cells and killer T cells, which then travel throughout the body to find and destroy virus-infected cells, cancer cells, bacteria, fungi, protozoa, and foreign cells (e.g., from tissue transplants)

COLOR the following cells involved in the adaptive immune response, using the colors recommended for each cell type:

- [ ] 1. Antigen (yellow)
- [ ] 2. Infected cell displaying antigen (brown)
- [ ] 3. B cell (blue)
- [ ] 4. Dying infected cell (gray/light black)
- [ ] 5. Antibodies (red)
- [ ] 6. Memory B cell (light blue)
- [ ] 7. Memory T cell (light green)
- [ ] 8. Killer T cell (orange)
- [ ] 9. Activated T cell (green)

Plate 6-3   **Lymphatic System**

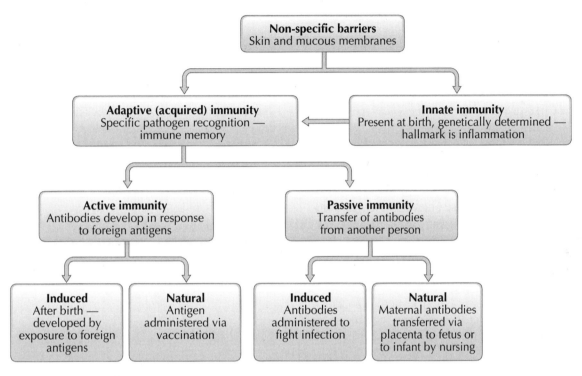

A. Different types of immunity

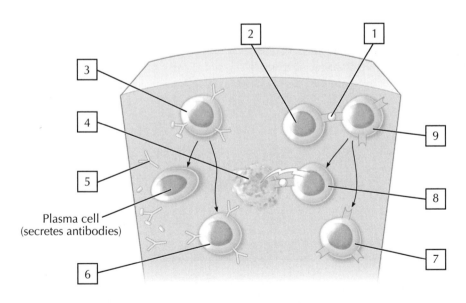

Plasma cell
(secretes antibodies)

B. Adaptive immune system

Lymphocytes are derived from the **pluripotent hemopoietic stem cells** of the bone marrow, but at this stage, all are immature cells, neither B nor T cells. This distinction occurs as part of the lymphocyte maturation process; B cells, so named for the bone marrow, mature in the red bone marrow and become immunocompetent (can recognize a specific antigen) and self tolerant (can recognize the body's own antigens as "self" and not "foreign"). Little is understood about the details of this process.

T cells, on the other hand, leave the **bone marrow** and travel to the **thymus** where they undergo immunocompetence. The thymus is a bilobed organ in the superior mediastinum that is quite large in neonates but involutes after puberty. In the thymus, T cells undergo rapid cell division, greatly increasing their numbers before their "education" as T cells. Positive selection occurs in the thymic cortex where T cells recognize self MHC (major histocompatibility complex) molecules; T cells that cannot are destroyed. Next, the surviving T cells must "learn" to recognize self-antigens by not binding too vigorously to self MHC or self-MHC–bound self-peptides; if they do, they are destroyed as a safety measure to ensure that T cells do not attack the body's own antigens. It is estimated that only about 2% of T cells survive this education process. While T cells undergo their education, they are sequestered from circulating antigens by the **blood-thymus barrier**, so they won't be "distracted" by any circulating antigens.

Lymphocytes are immunocompetent before encountering foreign antigens, and this process is entirely dependent upon our genes; our "endowed" genetic makeup for recognizing all of the possible antigens in our surrounding environment has been acquired through a process of natural selection during evolution. Many of the possible foreign antigens that we might encounter in our lifetime never invade our bodies, so those lymphocytes specifically selected to deal with those antigens will lie dormant.

Despite the fact that T and B cells are immunocompetent and have survived the rigorous "weeding out" process, they are still not mature until they have traveled to the spleen, lymph nodes, or other secondary lymphoid tissues and encountered their specific antigens, at which time they become antigen activated and are ready to initiate a response. Most of the T cells become helper and killer T cells once they reach the secondary lymphoid tissues; 60% to 80% of all circulating lymphocytes are T cells.

COLOR the following elements related to lymphocyte traffic from the bone marrow to the thymus and secondary lymph organs, using the colors suggested:

1. **Thymus (yellow)**
2. **Bone marrow (red)**
3. **Immature lymphocytes (blue with pink nuclei)**
4. **Lymph node (green)**
5. **Spleen (dark red)**

Plate 6-4   **Lymphatic System**

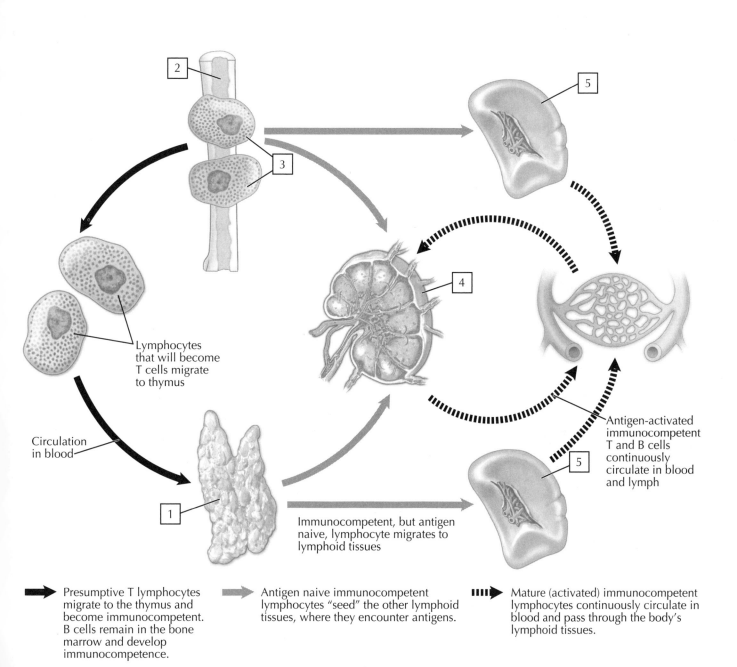

Lymphocytes that will become T cells migrate to thymus

Circulation in blood

Immunocompetent, but antigen naive, lymphocyte migrates to lymphoid tissues

Antigen-activated immunocompetent T and B cells continuously circulate in blood and lymph

Presumptive T lymphocytes migrate to the thymus and become immunocompetent. B cells remain in the bone marrow and develop immunocompetence.

Antigen naive immunocompetent lymphocytes "seed" the other lymphoid tissues, where they encounter antigens.

Mature (activated) immunocompetent lymphocytes continuously circulate in blood and pass through the body's lymphoid tissues.

6 | Spleen

The spleen is slightly larger than your clenched fist and lies in the upper left quadrant of the abdomen, tucked posterolateral to the stomach under the protection of the lower left rib cage. Simplistically, it is a large lymph node (and can become quite large during infections), although functionally it is much more involved in the following functions:
- Lymphocyte proliferation (B and T cells)
- Immune surveillance and response
- Blood filtration
- Destruction of old or damaged red blood cells (RBCs)
- Destruction of damaged platelets
- Recycles iron and globin
- Blood reservoir
- Production of RBCs in early fetal life

The spleen is an encapsulated organ with an extensive infrastructure composed of a trabecular network of connective tissue, which supports concentrations of lymphocytes in regions called the "**white pulp**." There are also regions of venous sinusoids rich in macrophages and red bloods cells called the "**red pulp**."

The white pulp is organized as an aggregation of lymphocytes that surround a **central artery**, forming a periarterial lymphatic sheath (PALS). The PALS gives the appearance of lymph nodules consisting largely of B cells surrounded by a more diffuse collection of T cells. The nodules contain a germinal center where B cells proliferate and become activated. The immune functions of the spleen include:
- Antigen presentation by macrophages and dendritic cells
- Proliferation and activation of B and T cells
- Production of antibodies directed against circulating antigens
- Removal of antigens from the blood

The red pulp is organized into regions of **splenic (venous) sinuses** separated by splenic cords (of Billroth) that consists of a meshwork of reticular fibers and cells, including:
- RBCs
- Macrophages
- Dendritic cells
- Lymphocytes
- Plasma cells
- Granulocytes

Macrophages associated with the splenic sinuses phagocytose damaged RBCs, break down the hemoglobin (heme is broken down to bilirubin), and recycle the iron (stored as ferritin or hemosiderin for recycling). Blood from the central artery flows into the white pulp and the splenic sinuses, with the blood cells percolating through the splenic cords before squeezing back into the collecting splenic venous sinuses. This "open circulatory" pattern exposes the RBCs to macrophages, which remove old or damaged cells from the circulation. Thus the primary function of the red pulp is to filter the blood.

COLOR the features of the splenic architecture, using a different color for each feature:
- [ ] 1. **Lymph vessel in the splenic capsule**
- [ ] 2. **Central artery**
- [ ] 3. **Splenic venous sinuses of the red pulp**
- [ ] 4. **White pulp (splenic nodule)**

Clinical Note:
The spleen, despite its protective position under the lower left rib cage, is the most commonly injured abdominal organ. Trauma to the abdominal wall (playground accidents in children, automobile accidents, and falls) can lacerate or **rupture the spleen**. This is serious because the rich blood supply to the spleen means that intraperitoneal hemorrhage and possible shock can result if the spleen's capsule and parenchyma are damaged by trauma. Surgical removal of the spleen generally is not problematic, because we can live without our spleen. Other lymphatic tissues and the bone marrow can take over the functions of the spleen.

Plate 6-5   **Lymphatic System**

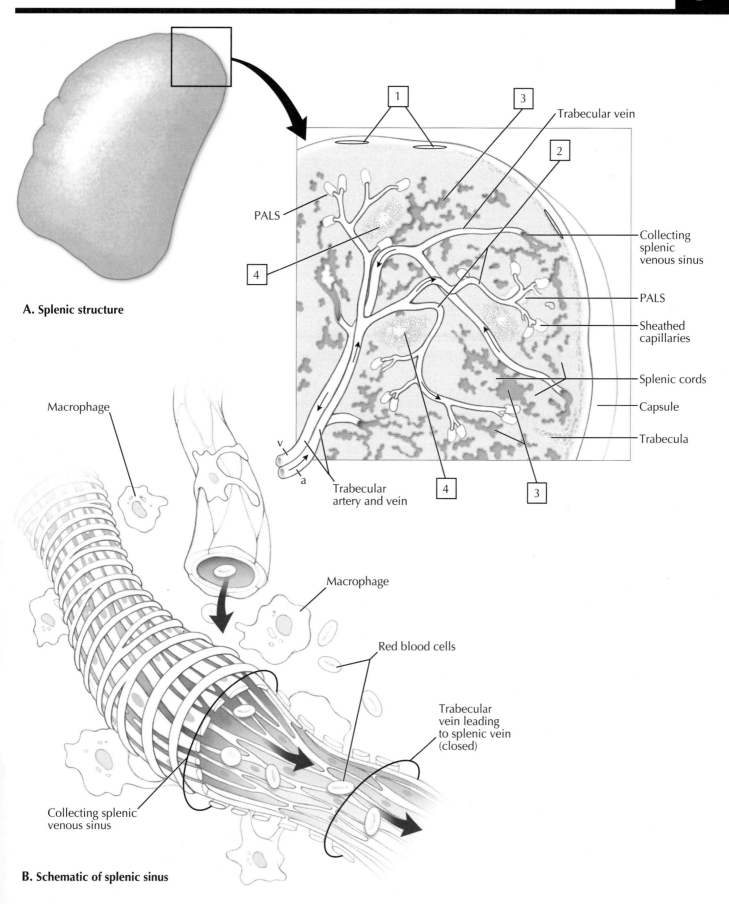

A. Splenic structure

PALS

Trabecular vein

1

3

2

4

Collecting
splenic
venous sinus

PALS

Sheathed
capillaries

Splenic cords

Capsule

Trabecula

v

a

Trabecular
artery and vein

4

3

Macrophage

Macrophage

Red blood cells

Trabecular
vein leading
to splenic vein
(closed)

Collecting splenic
venous sinus

B. Schematic of splenic sinus

In addition to the lymph nodes and vessels, bone marrow, thymus, and spleen, a number of other **diffuse lymphatic tissues** exist in the body and play a regional and systemic role in immune function. These accumulations include the:

- Tonsils
- Bronchus-associated lymphatic tissue (BALT)
- Vermiform appendix and gut-associated lymphatic tissue (GALT)
- Mucus-associated lymphatic tissue (MALT)

Tonsils

The tonsils include collections of lymphatic tissue in the oral cavity (palatine tonsils, visible when you open your mouth and say "ah"), lingual tonsils on the base of the tongue, pharyngeal tonsils (when enlarged and inflamed they are called adenoids) in the roof of the nasopharynx, and tubal tonsils around the opening of the auditory (eustachian) tube. Together, these lymphatic aggregations form "**Waldeyer's lymphatic ring**." They play an important immune role by protecting the nasal and oral passages from invading pathogens, especially during childhood. Some of these tissues atrophy with advancing age and become less important.

BALT

Accumulations of lymphoepithelial cells are diffusely located around the bronchi and the bronchial tree as they pass into the lung. BALT appears similar to the Peyer's patches that line the GI tract and provides immune responses against pathogens that may enter the airways and lungs.

Vermiform Appendix and GALT

The vermiform (wormlike) appendix is attached to the cecum (first portion of the colon) and contains a small lumen lined with mucosa and rich in lymphatic nodules. The amount of lymphatic tissue tends to decrease with advancing age.

Likewise, numerous aggregations of lymphatic tissue containing B and T cells reside in the lamina propria and submucosa of the ileum, which are called **Peyer's patches**. Diffuse lymphatic tissue (lymphocytes and plasma cells) also reside in the lamina propria and, together, these accumulations are referred to as the GALT. As one proceeds from proximal to distal in the bowel (including the colon), one tends to encounter a greater accumulation of lymphatic cells and nodules associated with the lamina propria; their primary function is to protect against pathogens and antigenic molecules that might invade the body.

MALT

The term MALT really refers to all of the mucosal-associated lymph nodules and diffuse lymphatic cells that encompass the BALT and GALT, but also include lymphatic accumulations in other organ systems, such as the female reproductive tract. Essentially the lymphatic tissues of the lamina propria of the digestive system, the respiratory lymphatics, and the genitourinary tract would be included as MALT.

COLOR the tissues associated with the lymphatic accumulations listed below:

- ☐ 1. Tonsils
- ☐ 2. BALT
- ☐ 3. GALT and Peyer's patches of the ileum
- ☐ 4. Lymph nodules of the vermiform appendix

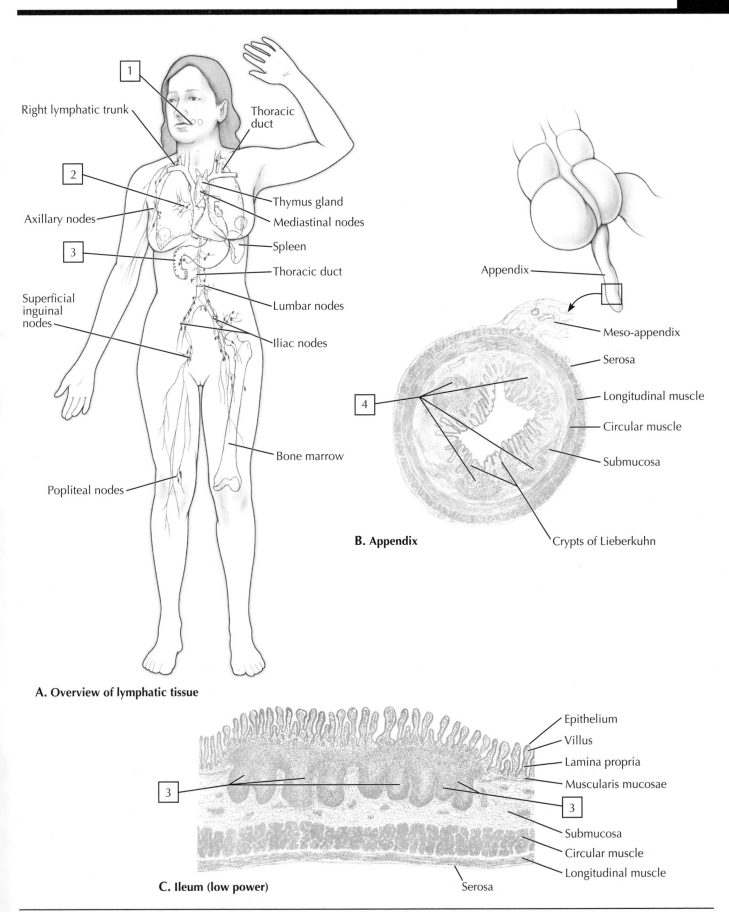

Right lymphatic trunk

1

Thoracic duct

Thymus gland

2

Mediastinal nodes

Axillary nodes

Spleen

3

Thoracic duct

Lumbar nodes

Superficial inguinal nodes

Iliac nodes

Bone marrow

Popliteal nodes

A. Overview of lymphatic tissue

Appendix

Meso-appendix

Serosa

Longitudinal muscle

4

Circular muscle

Submucosa

Crypts of Lieberkuhn

B. Appendix

Epithelium

Villus

Lamina propria

Muscularis mucosae

3

3

Submucosa

Circular muscle

Longitudinal muscle

C. Ileum (low power)

Serosa

The lymphatic and immune system are involved in a number of clinical disorders, coincident with the importance of this system in fighting pathogens and cancer.

Lymphatic Metastases

Cancer spreads from its primary site in one of three ways:
- Direct contact with adjacent tissues
- Via the venous system
- Via the lymphatic vessels

The lymphatics are especially important because cancer cells can easily access the lymphatic system. Once in the lymphatic vessels, the cancer cells encounter lymph nodes, where they are filtered from the lymph, seed the node and may grow, causing the nodes to enlarge, become fixed (immobile to palpation) but non-tender (as opposed to inflamed, noncancerous enlarged nodes, which are mobile and tender to the touch). Because of the predictable lymphatic drainage pattern, clinicians can usually trace the spread of cancer from one set of lymph nodes to the next set up the line. The first major lymph node that is enlarged because of metastasis is referred to as the "**sentinel node.**" Major lymph node accumulations exist in humans and include both a paired set of palpable nodes near the surface of the body and a deeper set of nodes that cannot be palpated, except by selective imaging techniques.

COLOR the major lymph node accumulations using the suggested colors for each set of nodes:

1. **Jugulodigastric nodes of the deep cervical chain: lie along the internal jugular vein, drain the head and neck, and are palpable when enlarged (orange)**

2. **Axillary nodes: drain the upper limb, shoulder, and chest region and are palpable when enlarged (red)**

3. **Mediastinal nodes: clustered around the tracheal bifurcation and hilum of the lungs, drain the lungs and thorax, and are deep nodes that cannot be palpated when enlarged (purple)**

4. **Para-aortic (lumbar) nodes: receive lymph from the abdominal cavity and lower half of the body, are clustered around the aorta near to the renal arteries, and are not palpable when enlarged; they drain into the cisterna chyli and thoracic duct (brown)**

5. **Iliac nodes: lie along the iliac vessels, receive lymph from the lower limbs and pelvic viscera, and drain toward the para-aortic nodes; they are deep and cannot be palpated when enlarged (blue)**

6. **Superficial inguinal nodes: drain the lower limb and external genitalia and are palpable when enlarged (yellow)**

Vaccination (Immunization)

Immunity can be artificially induced through the process of vaccination. This is done by injecting an antigen from the pathogen being immunized against that will stimulate the body's immune system. Most bacterial vaccines are designed to expose the body to antigens derived from acellular components of the bacterium or one of its harmless toxins. These antigens often produce a weak response in the body, so **adjuvants** are co-injected with the antigens to further activate the cells of the immune system. Most viral vaccines are **live attenuated** (diminished virulence) viruses that activate an immune response without infection.

Autoimmunity

When the immune system cannot distinguish self from nonself, it can mount an immune reaction against the body's own cells. Some autoimmune disorders include:
- Systemic lupus erythematosus, which largely affects the skin, kidneys, lungs, and heart
- Multiple sclerosis, which affects the normal myelination in the CNS
- Myasthenia gravis, which affects communication between nerves and skeletal muscle
- Type I diabetes mellitus, which affects the insulin-producing cells of the pancreatic islets
- Rheumatoid arthritis, which affects many of the body's joints

Immunodeficiencies

Immunodeficiencies occur when components of the immune system do not respond to pathogens and remain inactive. Common causes are genetic (congenital) or acquired (e.g., HIV), but can also include poor nutrition, alcoholism, and illicit drug use.

Hypersensitivity

Hypersensitivity occurs when the body's immune system battles a pathogen in such an aggressive manner that it damages its own tissues. Four types are recognized:
- **Type I**: acute, such as an anaphylactic reaction; allergy is a good example
- **Type II**: antibodies bind to antigens on the body's own cells (called antibody-dependent or cytotoxic hypersensitivity); a reaction to transfusion with the wrong blood type is an example
- **Type III**: an abundance of antibody-antigen complexes in the body causes an inflammatory reaction, initiating a robust hypersensitivity reaction; chronic infection or allergic reactions are examples
- **Type IV**: cell-mediated or delayed hypersensitivity reactions that usually take several days to develop and include allergic skin reactions (poison ivy and contact dermatitis) as well as protective reactions to infections, cancer cells, or the rejection of foreign tissue grafts

Lymph Node Accumulations

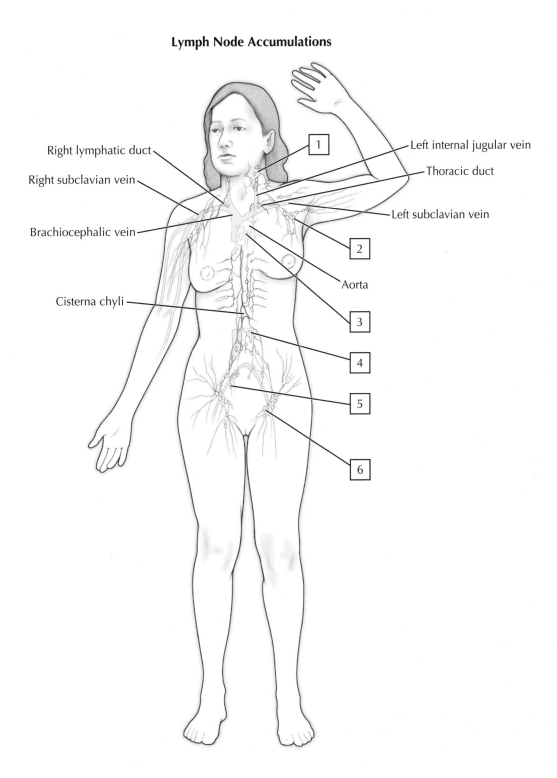

Right lymphatic duct

Right subclavian vein

Brachiocephalic vein

Cisterna chyli

Left internal jugular vein

Thoracic duct

Left subclavian vein

Aorta

1

2

3

4

5

6

1. T cells are part of the adaptive immune response and come in several different types. Which type of T cell responds to antigen on the cell surface and can become activated, destroy many viral and bacteria-infected cells, and divide to produce other types of T cells?
   A. Helper T cells
   B. Killer T cells
   C. Memory T cells
   D. Suppressor T cells

2. When a T cell leaves the bone marrow it travels to which organ to undergo immunocompetence?
   A. Lymph nodes
   B. Spleen
   C. Thymus
   D. Thyroid
   E. Tonsil

3. Which organ is important in recycling iron and globin?
   A. Colon
   B. Gallbladder
   C. Kidney
   D. Spleen
   E. Thymus

4. Many cells of the immune system are phagocytic. Which immune cells are especially important in the allergic response (hint: see Plate 5-1)?
   A. Eosinophils
   B. Fixed macrophages
   C. Free macrophages
   D. Monocytes
   E. Neutrophils

For each description below (5-8), color the appropriate area of the spleen

5. This splenic region is important in phagocytosis of damaged red blood cells.

6. This region is organized around a central artery.

7. This feature of the spleen is thin and fragile and damage to it can result in significant blood loss.

8. This is the site of the splenic red pulp and splenic sinuses.

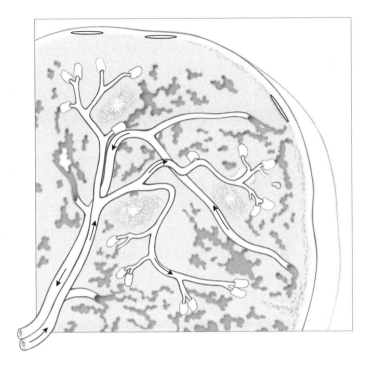

9. The thoracic duct begins in the upper abdomen, where numerous lymphatic vessels coalesce to form the beginning of the duct. What is this feature called? _____

10. Where does the thoracic duct ultimately end?_____

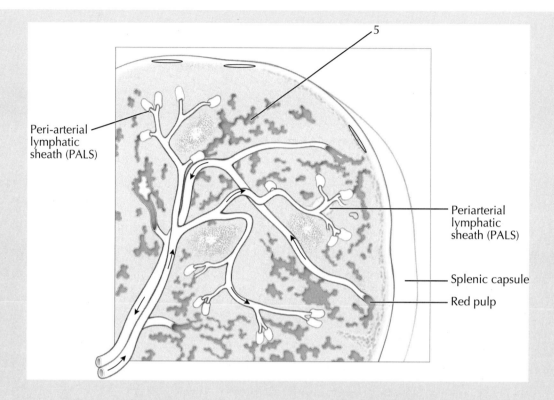

Peri-arterial
lymphatic
sheath (PALS)

5

Periarterial
lymphatic
sheath (PALS)

Splenic capsule

Red pulp

9. Cisterna chyli

10. In the venous system at the junction of the left subclavian and left internal jugular veins.

Chapter 7 **Respiratory System**

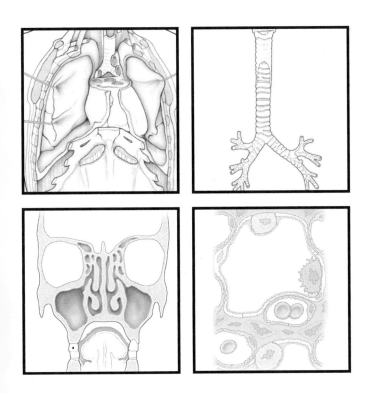

The respiratory system provides the body with oxygen for its metabolic needs and eliminates carbon dioxide. Structurally, the respiratory system includes the:
• Nose and paranasal sinuses
• Pharynx and its subdivisions, the nasopharynx, oropharynx, and laryngopharynx
• Larynx
• Trachea
• Bronchi, bronchioles, alveolar ducts and sacs, and alveoli
• Lungs

Functionally, the respiratory system performs five basic functions:
• Filters and humidifies the air and moves air into and out of the lungs
• Provides a large surface area for gas exchange with the blood
• Helps to regulate the pH of the body fluids
• Participates in vocalization
• Assists the olfactory system with the detection of smells

Histologically, the respiratory epithelium largely is ciliated, pseudostratified columnar epithelium with a few exceptions (vocal folds and epiglottis are stratified squamous epithelium, and the transition to small bronchioles is from respiratory to simple cuboidal epithelium). Alveoli are lined with thin squamous cells (**type I pneumocytes**) and simple cuboidal cells (**type II pneumocytes** that secrete surfactant).

The epithelial lining of the respiratory tract is important in warming, humidifying, and filtering the air before it reaches the sensitive lung alveoli. A rich vascular network helps to warm the air, while the ciliated epithelium and presence of mucous cells (goblet cells) helps humidify the air and capture particulate material that is then "swept" away by the cilia, to be swallowed or expectorated.

COLOR each of the following features of the respiratory system, using a different color for each feature:
☒ 1. Laryngopharynx
☐ 2. Oropharynx
☐ 3. Nasopharynx
☐ 4. Nasal cavity
☒ 5. Larynx
☐ 6. Trachea
☒ 7. Lungs

Clinical Note:
Asthma can be intrinsic (no clearly defined environmental trigger) or extrinsic (has a defined trigger). Asthma usually results from a hypersensitivity reaction to an allergen (dust, pollen, mold), which leads to irritation of the respiratory passages, smooth muscle contraction (narrowing of the passages), swelling (edema) of the epithelium, and increased production of mucus. Presenting symptoms are often wheezing, shortness of breath, coughing, tachycardia, and feelings of chest tightness. Asthma is a pathological inflammation of the airways and occurs in both children and adults.

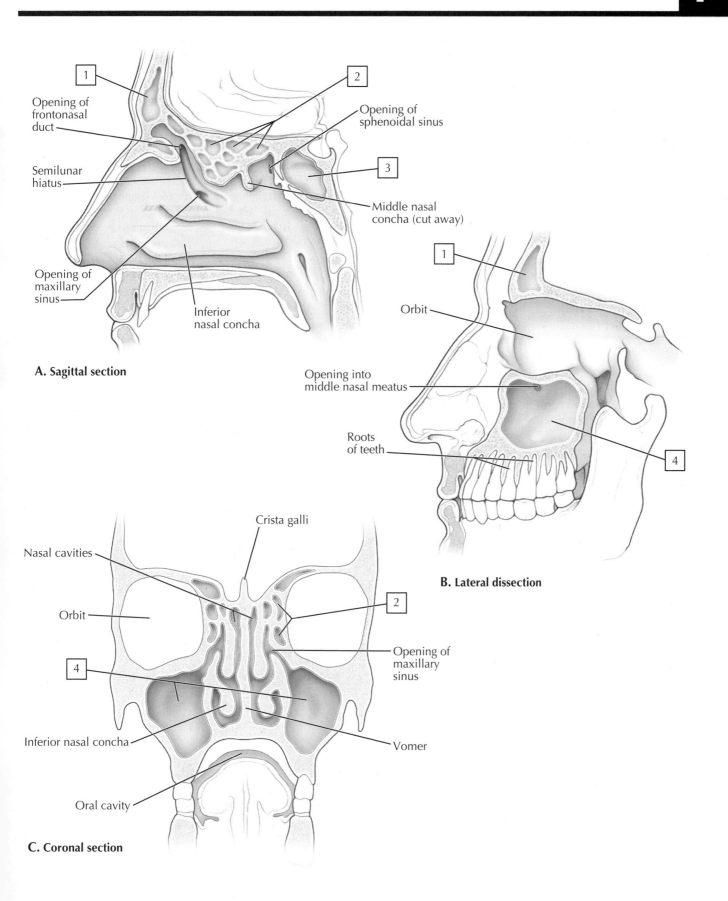

A. Sagittal section

1

Opening of
frontonasal
duct

Semilunar
hiatus

Opening of
maxillary
sinus

Inferior
nasal concha

2

Opening of
sphenoidal sinus

3

Middle nasal
concha (cut away)

B. Lateral dissection

1

Orbit

Opening into
middle nasal meatus

Roots
of teeth

4

Crista galli

Nasal cavities

Orbit

4

Inferior nasal concha

Oral cavity

2

Opening of
maxillary
sinus

Vomer

C. Coronal section

The pharynx (throat) is subdivided into three regions:
- **Nasopharynx**: lies posterior to the nasal cavities and above the soft palate (already discussed)
- **Oropharynx**: extends from the soft palate to the superior tip of the epiglottis, and lies posterior to the oral cavity
- **Laryngopharynx**: extends from the tip of the epiglottis to the inferior aspect of the cricoid cartilage (often referred to by clinicians as the "hypopharynx"), lying posterior to the larynx

The oropharynx and laryngopharynx provide a passageway for both air and food (solid and liquids) and are essentially fibromuscular tubes lined with stratified squamous epithelium to protect the lining from abrasion. The muscular walls of the pharynx are formed largely by the three pharyngeal constrictors discussed previously (see Plate 3-5). **Waldeyer's lymphatic ring**, composed of the tubal tonsils, nasopharyngeal tonsils, lingual tonsils, and the palatine tonsils, "guard" the openings into the pharynx and provide an important lymphatic immunologic defense mechanism, especially in children and adolescents (see Plate 6-6).

The larynx lies anterior to the laryngopharynx and proximal esophagus, at about the level of the C3-C6 vertebrae and superior to the trachea. Structurally, the larynx consists of nine cartilages joined by ligaments and membranes.

CARTILAGE	DESCRIPTION
Thyroid	Two hyaline laminae and the laryngeal prominence (Adam's apple)
Cricoid	Signet ring–shaped hyaline cartilage just inferior to thyroid
Epiglottis	Spoon-shaped elastic cartilage plate attached to thyroid
Arytenoid	Paired pyramidal cartilages that rotate on cricoid cartilage
Corniculate	Paired cartilages that lie on apex of arytenoid cartilages
Cuneiform	Paired cartilages in ary-epiglottic folds that have no articulations

The laryngeal cavity includes the following subdivisions:
- **Vestibule**: lies between the laryngeal inlet (just posterior to the epiglottis) and the vestibular folds
- **Rima glottidis**: the space or "slit" between the vocal folds

- **Ventricle**: the recesses that extend laterally between the vestibular and vocal folds
- **Infraglottic cavity**: the space below the vocal folds to the level of the cricoid cartilage; below the cricoid cartilage the infraglottic cavity becomes the proximal trachea

The **vestibular (false) folds** are protective in nature but the **vocal (true) folds** control phonation much like a reed instrument. Vibrations of the folds produce sounds as air passes through the rima glottidis; the pitch produced by these vibrations is dependent upon the diameter, length, thickness, and tension of the vocal folds. The size of the rima glottidis and tension on the folds is determined by the laryngeal muscles, but the amplification, resonance, and quality of the sound is a product of the shape and size of the pharynx, oral cavity, nasal and paranasal cavities, and movements of the tongue, lips, cheeks, and soft palate.

COLOR the following features of the larynx, using a different color for each feature:
- [ ] 1. Epiglottis
- [ ] 2. Thyroid cartilage
- [ ] 3. Infraglottic cavity
- [ ] 4. Cricoid cartilage
- [ ] 5. Trachea
- [ ] 6. Vestibular folds
- [ ] 7. Vocal folds
- [ ] 8. Laryngeal vestibule
- [ ] 9. Ventricle

Clinical Note:

Hoarseness can be due to any condition that results in improper vibration or coaptation of the vocal folds. **Acute laryngitis** is an inflammation of the vocal folds that results in edema (swelling) of the vocal fold mucosa and usually is a result of smoking, gastroesophageal reflux disease, chronic rhinosinusitis, cough, overuse of the voice (loud yelling, talking, or singing for extended periods), myxedema, and infections.

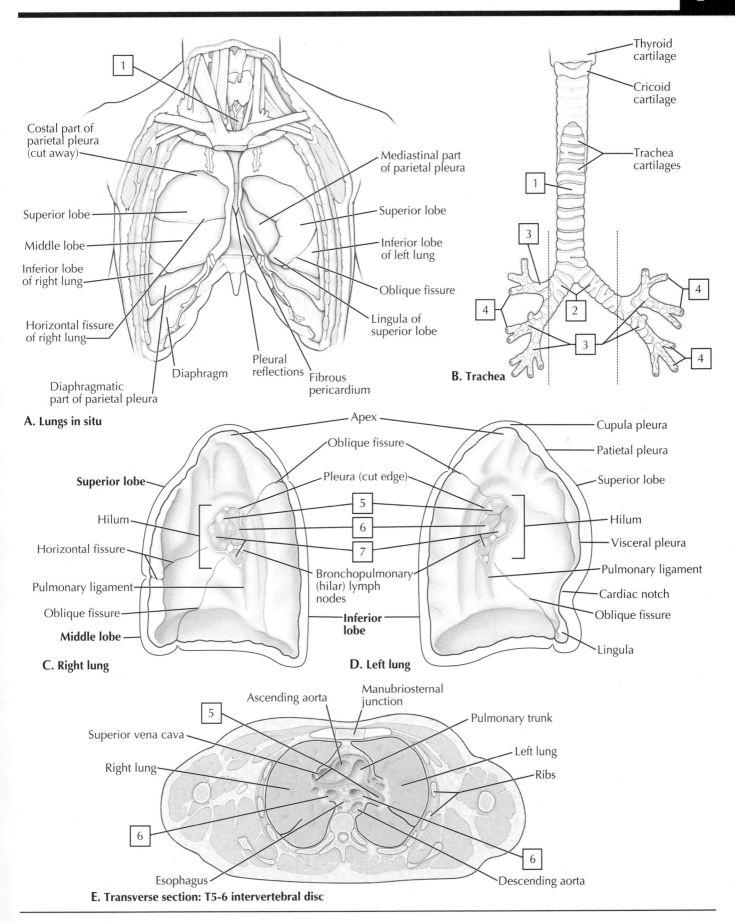

A. Lungs in situ

1

Costal part of parietal pleura (cut away)

Superior lobe

Middle lobe

Inferior lobe of right lung

Horizontal fissure of right lung

Diaphragmatic part of parietal pleura

Diaphragm

Pleural reflections

Fibrous pericardium

Mediastinal part of parietal pleura

Superior lobe

Inferior lobe of left lung

Oblique fissure

Lingula of superior lobe

B. Trachea

Thyroid cartilage

Cricoid cartilage

Trachea cartilages

1

3

4

2

3

4

4

C. Right lung

Superior lobe

Hilum

Horizontal fissure

Pulmonary ligament

Oblique fissure

Middle lobe

D. Left lung

Apex

Oblique fissure

Pleura (cut edge)

5

6

7

Bronchopulmonary (hilar) lymph nodes

Inferior lobe

Cupula pleura

Patietal pleura

Superior lobe

Hilum

Visceral pleura

Pulmonary ligament

Cardiac notch

Oblique fissure

Lingula

E. Transverse section: T5-6 intervertebral disc

Ascending aorta

Manubriosternal junction

Pulmonary trunk

5

Superior vena cava

Right lung

Left lung

Ribs

6

6

Esophagus

Descending aorta

The mechanics of ventilation involve the dynamic interaction of the lungs, chest wall, and diaphragm.

During quiet respiration, contraction of the diaphragm alone accounts for about 75% of inspiration. The external intercostal muscles of the thoracic wall (see Plate 3-11) and selected muscles of the neck (scalenes) also can assist in inspiration, especially during active exercise. Expiration involves the elastic recoil of the lungs themselves and is assisted by relaxation of the diaphragm and contraction of some of the intercostal and abdominal muscles (rectus abdominis and abdominal obliques).

Blood from the right ventricle of the heart perfuses the lungs (via the pulmonary arteries) at a resting rate of about 5 L/min under low pressure (normally about 6 mm Hg). Pulmonary capillary plexuses envelop the alveolar sacs, where most of the gas exchange occurs. Pulmonary veins collect the oxygenated blood and return it to the left side of the heart for distribution throughout the systemic circulation.

Gas exchange occurs at the level of the alveoli and capillaries and involves the following:
• Across the type I alveolar cells
• Across the fused basement membranes of the type I cells and endothelial cells
• Across the capillary endothelial cell

COLOR the following features of the intrapulmonary circulation, using the colors suggested:

☐ 1. Pulmonary artery (lower oxygen content) (blue)

☐ 2. Pulmonary vein (saturated with oxygen) (red)

☐ 3. Type II alveolar cell (secretes surfactant) (orange)

☐ 4. Type I alveolar cell (yellow)

☐ 5. Capillary endothelial cell (purple)

☐ 6. Type I alveolar cell and endothelial cell fused basement membranes (light blue)

☐ 7. Interstitial cells (green)

☐ 8. Red blood cell (red)

☐ 9. Alveolar macrophage (brown) (in alveolar airspace)

Type II alveolar cells secrete **surfactant**, which forms a thin film over the fluid that normally coats the surface of the alveolus, thus reducing the surface tension of the fluid-lined alveoli and helping to lower the pressure needed to inflate the alveoli.

As blood flows through the alveolar capillaries, oxygen diffuses from the alveolus into the red blood cell, where it binds to hemoglobin. At the same time, carbon dioxide diffuses out of the red blood cell and into the alveolus. Normally, blood traverses the entire capillary length in 0.75 second, and even faster when the cardiac output is increased. However, gas exchange is so efficient that it normally occurs in about 0.5 second. Almost all of the oxygen carried to the body's tissues by the blood is bound to hemoglobin; only a small fraction is dissolved and transported in the plasma. The interalveolar septum (separates the alveolar air space from the capillary lumen) is the **blood-air barrier** and is very thin, allowing for the rapid diffusion of gases across this septum. The septum consists of three layers:
• Type I pneumocyte and its surfactant layer in the alveolar air space
• Fused basal lamina of the type I pneumocyte and the capillary endothelial cell
• Endothelium of the continuous capillaries

Clinical Note:

Failure to produce sufficient amounts of **surfactant**, as can occur in premature infants because of the underdevelopment of the type II alveolar cells, can result in an increase in the work of breathing and cause respiratory distress. Because the lungs are not needed in utero, they are among one of the last systems to functionally develop in the fetus and often the limiting factor in survival of a premature infant.

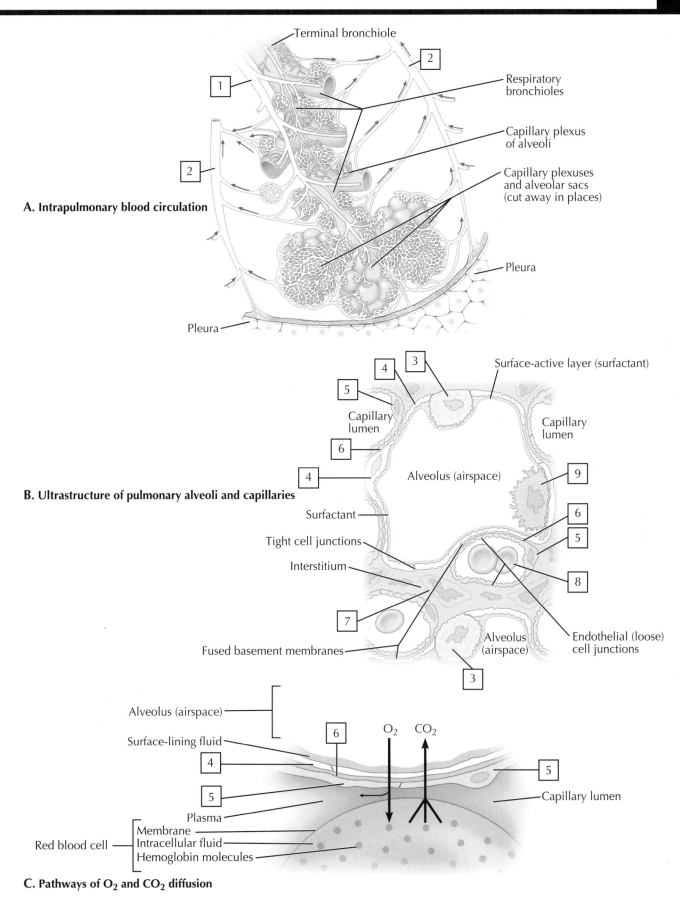

A. Intrapulmonary blood circulation

Terminal bronchiole

Respiratory bronchioles

Capillary plexus of alveoli

Capillary plexuses and alveolar sacs (cut away in places)

Pleura

Pleura

B. Ultrastructure of pulmonary alveoli and capillaries

Surface-active layer (surfactant)

Capillary lumen

Capillary lumen

Alveolus (airspace)

Surfactant

Tight cell junctions

Interstitium

Endothelial (loose) cell junctions

Alveolus (airspace)

Fused basement membranes

Alveolus (airspace)

Surface-lining fluid

Plasma

Membrane

Red blood cell — Intracellular fluid

Hemoglobin molecules

O_2 CO_2

Capillary lumen

C. Pathways of O_2 and CO_2 diffusion

1. A premature infant is having great difficulty breathing because of an incomplete coating of surfactant on the alveolar epithelium. Which of the following cells secrete surfactant?
   A. Alveolar endothelial cells
   B. Alveolar macrophages
   C. Simple ciliated columnar cells
   D. Type I pneumocytes
   E. Type II pneumocytes

2. A small child aspirates a peanut into her lung. Where in the lung is that peanut most likely to be found?
   A. Lower lobe of the left lung
   B. Primary bronchus of the left lung
   C. Primary bronchus of the right lung
   D. Tertiary bronchus of the left lung
   E. Tertiary bronchus of the right lung

3. A patient's frontal sinus appears to be blocked and infected. Where does the frontal sinus normally drain?
   A. Inferior meatus
   B. Middle meatus
   C. Nasopharynx
   D. Spheno-ethmoidal recess
   E. Superior meatus

4. A child bites into a very cold ice cream cone and immediately feels an intense pain, referred to as a "brain freeze." Which of the following regions is the most likely source of this pain?
   A. Hard palate
   B. Mandible
   C. Maxillary sinus
   D. Sphenoid sinus
   E. Soft palate

For each description below (5-7), color or highlight the relevant anatomy in the image

5. This cell possesses phagocytic characteristics and helps keep the alveolar sac free of debris.

6. This cell lines the alveolar sac but does not participate directly in gas exchange.

7. This cell does participate in gas exchange and is coated with surfactant.

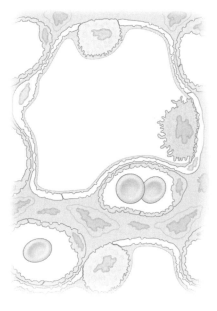

8. What type of epithelium normally lines the trachea? _____

9. Identify three important functions of the respiratory system _____

10. The lungs are contained within a pleural sac. What two layers of connective tissue comprise these sacs? _____
_____

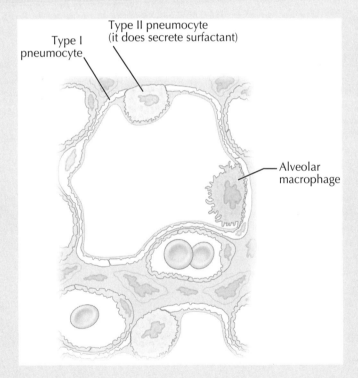

Type I pneumocyte

Type II pneumocyte (it does secrete surfactant)

Alveolar macrophage

Chapter 8 Gastrointestinal System

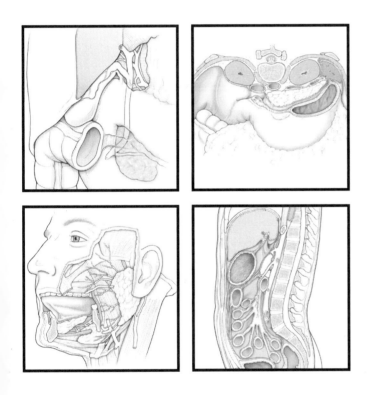

The gastrointestinal (GI) system consists of the epithelial-lined tube beginning with the **oral cavity** and extending to the **anal canal**, and also includes GI associated glands, such as the:

- **Salivary glands**: three major glands and thousands of microscopic minor salivary glands scattered throughout the oral mucosa
- **Liver**: the largest gland in the body
- **Gallbladder**: stores and concentrates bile needed for fat digestion
- **Pancreas**: an exocrine (digestive enzymes) and endocrine organ

The epithelial-lined tube that is the GI tract measures about 25 feet from mouth to anal canal and includes the following cavities and visceral structures:

- **Oral cavity**: tongue, teeth, and salivary glands
- **Pharynx**: throat, subdivided into the nasopharynx, oropharynx, and laryngopharynx
- **Esophagus**
- **Stomach**
- **Small intestine**: subdivided into the duodenum, jejunum, and ileum
- **Large intestine**: subdivided into the cecum, ascending colon, transverse colon, descending colon, sigmoid colon, rectum, and anal canal

COLOR each of the following visceral components of the thoracic and abdominal GI tract, using a different color for each component:

- [ ] 1. **Liver**
- [ ] 2. **Gallbladder**
- [ ] 3. **Duodenum (phantom in figure behind the transverse colon)**
- [ ] 4. **Ascending colon**
- [ ] 5. **Cecum**
- [ ] 6. **Ileum**
- [ ] 7. **Rectum**
- [ ] 8. **Anal canal**
- [ ] 9. **Sigmoid colon**
- [ ] 10. **Jejunum**
- [ ] 11. **Descending colon**
- [ ] 12. **Transverse colon**
- [ ] 13. **Stomach**
- [ ] 14. **Esophagus**

Clinically, because of the structural complexity of the abdominal viscera, it is important for students to know where underlying visceral structures lie in relationship to the surface of the abdominal wall. To facilitate this exercise, the abdomen can be divided into **four quadrants** or into **nine regions**, as shown in parts *B* and *C*. Additionally, various reference planes are used clinically in the physical exam to divide the abdomen into regions, as summarized below.

PLANES OF REFERENCE	DEFINITION
Median	Vertical plane from xiphoid process to pubic symphysis
Transumbilical	Horizontal plane across umbilicus (these two planes divide abdomen into quadrants)
Subcostal	Horizontal plane across inferior margin of 10th costal cartilage
Intertubercular	Horizontal plane across the tubercles of the ilium and the body of the L5 vertebra
Midclavicular	Two vertical planes through the midpoint of the clavicles (these two planes and the subcostal and intertubercular planes divide the abdomen into nine regions)

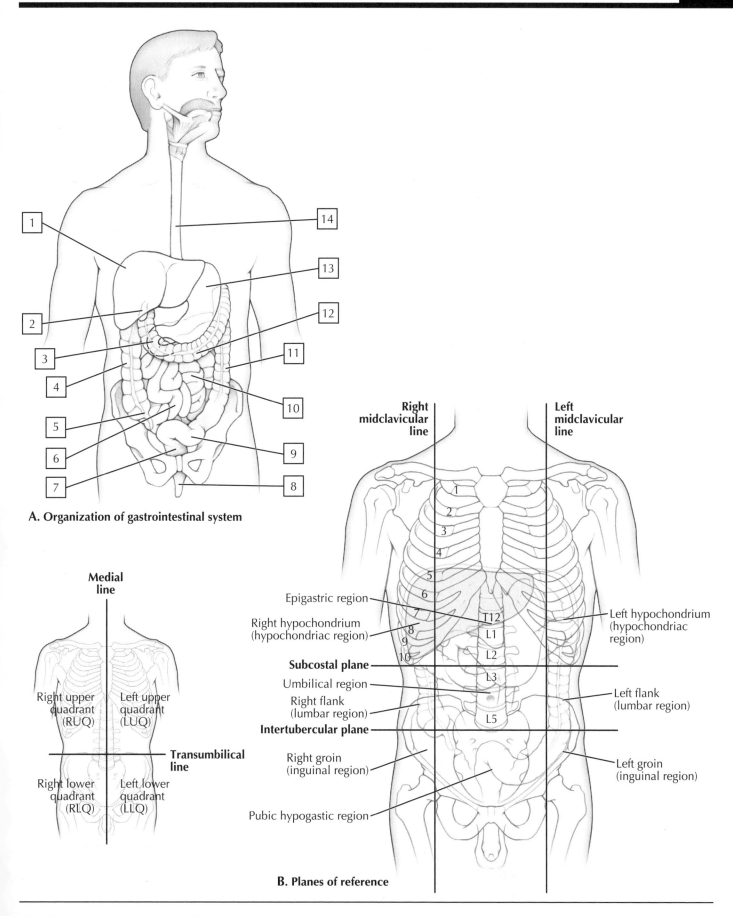

1	14
2	13
3	12
4	11
5	10
6	9
7	8

A. Organization of gastrointestinal system

Medial line

Right upper quadrant (RUQ) | Left upper quadrant (LUQ)

Transumbilical line

Right lower quadrant (RLQ) | Left lower quadrant (LLQ)

Right midclavicular line

Left midclavicular line

Epigastric region

Right hypochondrium (hypochondriac region)

Left hypochondrium (hypochondriac region)

Subcostal plane

Umbilical region

Right flank (lumbar region)

Left flank (lumbar region)

Intertubercular plane

Right groin (inguinal region)

Left groin (inguinal region)

Pubic hypogastic region

T12
L1
L2
L3
L5

B. Planes of reference

The oral cavity is the first portion of the GI tract and consists of the following:
- Mouth (oral vestibule), which is the narrow space between the lips or cheeks, and the teeth and gums
- Oral cavity proper, which includes the palate (hard and soft), teeth, gums (gingivae), salivary glands, and tongue

The mucosa of the palate, cheeks, tongue, and lips contain numerous **minor salivary glands** that secrete directly into the oral cavity. Additionally, three pairs of major salivary glands provide **saliva** to aid in the digestion, softening, and deglutition (swallowing) of food. Saliva also keeps the mucosal surfaces moist and lubricated to protect against abrasion, controls oral bacteria by secreting lysozyme, secretes calcium and phosphate for tooth formation and maintenance, and secretes amylase to begin the digestion of starches. The **serous acinar cells** of the salivary glands secrete the protein and enzymatic components of saliva, whereas the **mucous acinar cells** secrete a watery mucus. Finally, **lingual lipase**, secreted by the serous glands of the tongue, mixes with saliva and begins the digestion of fats. The major salivary glands are summarized in the table below.

GLAND	GLAND TYPE AND INNERVATION
Parotid	Serous gland innervated by CN IX parasympathetics that course to gland via auriculotemporal nerve (branch of CN V_3)
Submandibular	Serous and mucous gland innervated by CN VII parasympathetics that course to gland via lingual nerve (branch of CN V_3)
Sublingual	Largely mucous gland innervated by CN VII parasympathetics that course to gland via lingual nerve (branch of CN V_3)

See Plates 4-20 and 4-22 for the innervation of the salivary glands.

The parotid gland secretes saliva via its parotid (Stensen's) duct. The submandibular gland secretes saliva via its submandibular (Wharton's) duct, and the sublingual gland secretes saliva via numerous small ducts located at the base of the anterolateral tongue. As the saliva passes through the ducts, its electrolyte composition is modified such that the saliva entering the mouth is hypotonic to plasma and has a high bicarbonate concentration.

COLOR the following features of the oral cavity, using a different color for each feature:

- [ ] 1. Hard palate
- [ ] 2. Soft palate
- [ ] 3. Palatine tonsil
- [ ] 4. Tongue
- [ ] 5. Uvula
- [ ] 6. Sublingual glands
- [ ] 7. Submandibular gland
- [ ] 8. Parotid gland

Clinical Note:
Gingivitis is an inflammation of the gums caused by bacterial accumulation in the crevices between the teeth and gums. Both plaque and tartar buildup can cause irritation of the gums that leads to bleeding and swelling and, if left untreated, can result in damage to the bone and loss of teeth.

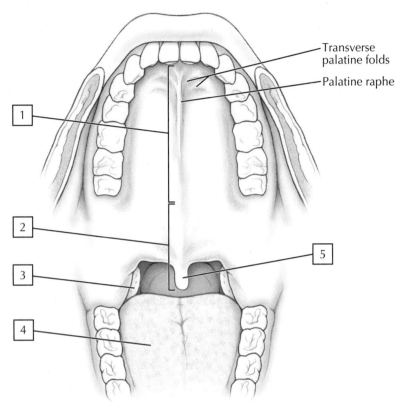

Transverse
palatine folds

Palatine raphe

1

2

3

5

4

A. Anterior view

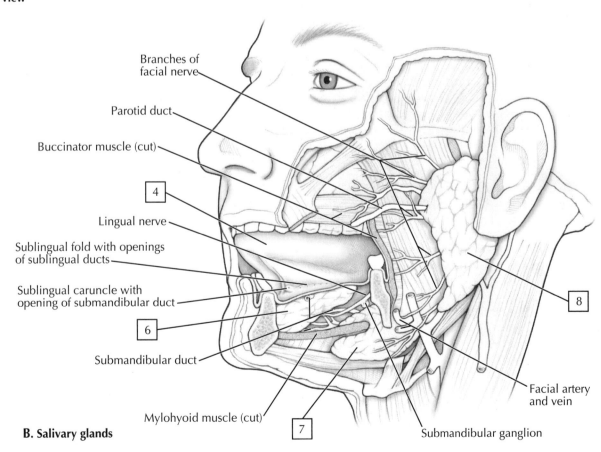

Branches of
facial nerve

Parotid duct

Buccinator muscle (cut)

4

Lingual nerve

Sublingual fold with openings
of sublingual ducts

Sublingual caruncle with
opening of submandibular duct

6

Submandibular duct

8

Facial artery
and vein

Mylohyoid muscle (cut)

7

Submandibular ganglion

B. Salivary glands

The teeth are hard structures set in the upper (maxilla) and lower (mandible) jaws in dental alveoli or sockets. The tooth has a crown, neck, and root, and these as well as other anatomical features of the tooth are summarized in the following table.

Crown	Anatomical crown: the portion of the tooth that has a surface of enamel
Root	Anatomical root: the portion of the tooth that has a surface of cementum
Apex of the root	The end tip of the root, which provides entrance of the neurovascular connective tissue into the pulp cavity
Enamel	The hard, shiny surface of the anatomical crown and the hardest part of the tooth.
Cementum	A thin dull layer on the surface of the anatomical root
Dentin	The hard tissue that underlies both the enamel and cementum and constitutes the majority of the tooth
Pulp cavity	Contains the dental pulp (highly neurovascular connective tissue)

Modified with permission from Norton N: *Netter's Head and Neck Anatomy for Dentistry*, Philadelphia, 2007, Elsevier, pp. 360-361.

Humans have two sets of teeth:
• **Deciduous teeth**: our primary dentition, it consists of 20 teeth that usually have all appeared by the age of 3 years (2 incisors, 1 canine, and 2 molars in each of the 4 quadrants of the jaws)
• **Permanent teeth**: our secondary dentition, that consists of 32 teeth that usually begin to appear around the age of 6 years (2 incisors, 1 canine, 2 premolars, and 3 molars in each quadrant), replacing the deciduous teeth. The third molars also are known as the "wisdom teeth" because they are normally the last teeth to erupt.

COLOR each of the following teeth and the features of a typical tooth, using a different color for each feature:

☐ 1. **Incisors**
☐ 2. **Canine**
☐ 3. **Premolars**
☐ 4. **Molars**
☐ 5. **Enamel**
☐ 6. **Dentin**
☐ 7. **Gingival (gum) epithelium (stratified squamous)**
☐ 8. **Cement**
☐ 9. **Root canals (containing vessels and nerves)**

Clinical Note:
Tooth decay (dental caries) can lead to cavities, which are caused by bacteria that convert food debris into acids that form plaque. The plaque adheres to the teeth and, if not removed in a timely fashion, can mineralize to form tartar. The acids in the plaque can erode into the enamel and form a cavity. Foods rich in sugars and starches promote cavity formation.

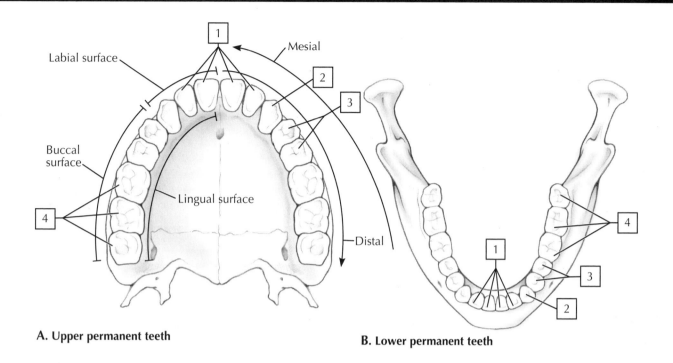

Labial surface

Mesial

Buccal
surface

Lingual surface

Distal

A. Upper permanent teeth

B. Lower permanent teeth

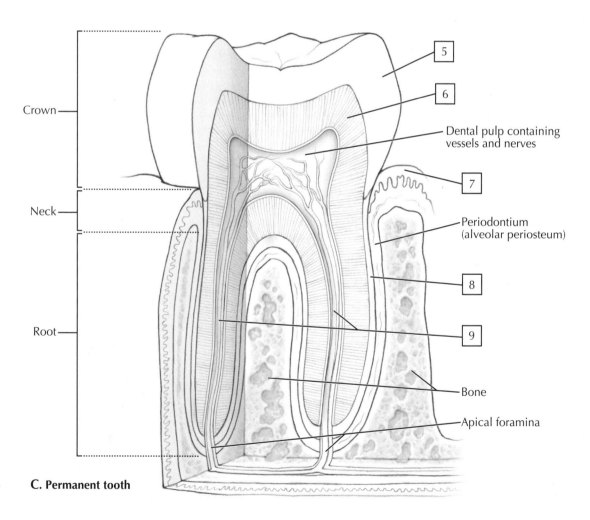

Crown

Neck

Root

Dental pulp containing
vessels and nerves

Periodontium
(alveolar periosteum)

Bone

Apical foramina

C. Permanent tooth

Pharynx

The pharynx is subdivided into the **nasopharynx**, **oropharynx**, and **laryngopharynx**, and has been previously reviewed in the muscular and respiratory system sections (see Plate 7-1). The mucosa of the oropharynx and laryngopharynx is stratified squamous, providing protection during swallowing, and is interspersed with mucous glands to keep the epithelium moist with a thin mucus covering. The laryngopharynx opens anteriorly into the laryngeal inlet and posteriorly is continuous with the esophagus. Deep to the mucosa lie the pharyngeal constrictor muscles (see Plate 3-5) that help propel the food into the esophagus.

Esophagus

The muscle of the upper third of the esophagus is skeletal, that of the lower third is smooth, and in the middle third it is mixed skeletal and smooth muscle. The muscular walls form an outer longitudinal and inner circular layer, and these layers participate in peristalsis, which moves the food toward the stomach. As the esophagus approaches the stomach, the smooth muscle thickens and forms the **lower esophageal sphincter (LES)**. Normally the resting tone of the LES is high, which prevents the reflux of gastric contents into the esophagus. As the peristaltic wave carries a bolus of food to the stomach, release of nitric oxide and vasoactive intestinal peptide from the myenteric (under vagal control) plexus causes a relaxation of the LES and food enters the stomach.

COLOR the following features of the pharynx and esophagus, using a different color for each feature:

- ☐ 1. Soft palate
- ☐ 2. Uvula
- ☐ 3. Epiglottis
- ☐ 4. Esophagus
- ☐ 5. Stomach

Clinical Note:

Gastroesophageal reflux disease (GERD) is a relatively common problem caused by a decreased tone of the LES or a sliding hiatal (stomach herniation into the thorax) hernia. Reflux of the acidic gastric contents can cause abdominal pain, dyspepsia, gas, heartburn, dysphagia, and other problems. The chronic inflammation of the lower esophageal wall may result in esophagitis, ulceration, or stricture.

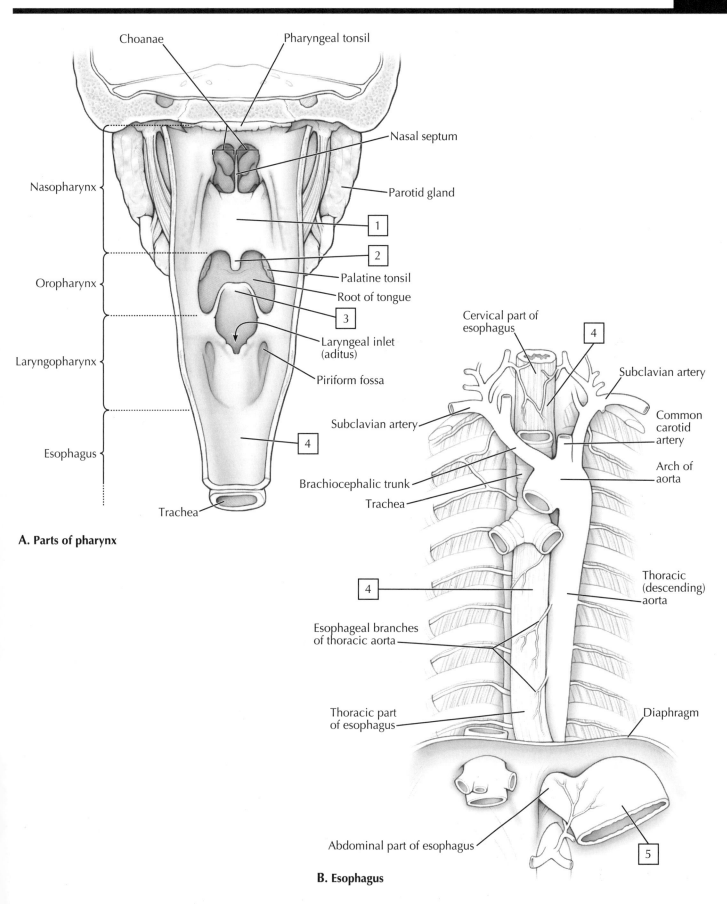

Choanae

Pharyngeal tonsil

Nasal septum

Nasopharynx

Parotid gland

1

2

Palatine tonsil

Oropharynx

Root of tongue

3

Laryngeal inlet
(aditus)

Laryngopharynx

Piriform fossa

Esophagus

4

Trachea

A. Parts of pharynx

Cervical part of
esophagus

4

Subclavian artery

Subclavian artery

Common
carotid
artery

Brachiocephalic trunk

Arch of
aorta

Trachea

4

Thoracic
(descending)
aorta

Esophageal branches
of thoracic aorta

Thoracic part
of esophagus

Diaphragm

Abdominal part of esophagus

5

B. Esophagus

The abdominal cavity is lined by muscles that assist in movements of the trunk, assist in respiration, and by increasing intra-abdominal pressure, facilitate micturition, defecation, and childbirth. The viscera of the abdominopelvic cavity lie within a potential space called the **peritoneal cavity** (not unlike the pleural and pericardial cavities), which has the following features:

- **Parietal peritoneum:** a serosal lining that covers the inner aspects of the walls of the abdominopelvic cavity
- **Visceral peritoneum:** a direct continuation of the parietal peritoneum, which reflects from the inner abdominal wall and covers the visceral structures of the abdomen
- **Mesenteries:** a double layer of visceral peritoneum that reflects from the inner wall of the abdomen and envelops portions of the abdominal viscera
- **Retroperitoneal viscera:** lie against the posterior abdominal wall and do not possess a suspending mesentery
- **Intraperitoneal viscera:** are suspended from the abdominal walls by a mesentery
- **Serous fluid:** secreted in small amounts by the peritoneum and lubricates the viscera, thus reducing friction during peristalsis and other movements of the abdominal viscera when they rub against one another

These features and several others are depicted in part *A* in a sagittal view and are summarized in the following table.

FEATURE	DESCRIPTION
Greater omentum	An "apron" of peritoneum hanging from greater curvature of stomach, folding back on itself to attach to transverse colon
Lesser omentum	Double layer of peritoneum extending from lesser curvature of stomach and proximal duodenum to liver (hepatoduodenal and hepatogastric ligaments)
Mesenteries	Double fold of peritoneum suspending parts of bowel and conveying vessels, lymphatics, and nerves of bowel
Peritoneal ligaments	Double layer of peritoneum attaching viscera to walls or to other viscera

The **omental bursa** is the cul-de-sac posterior to the stomach and anterior to the pancreas (see part B.) It also is known as the lesser sac, while the remainder of the abdominopelvic cavity is the greater sac.

As the simple gut tube of the embryo, which is suspended by a mesentery, begins to grow in length and breadth, it twists upon itself so that the significant length of bowel, necessary for complete digestion, can be accommodated in the confined space of the abdomen. As this twisting and growth occurs, portions of the bowel and its accessory digestive glands are pushed to the posterior abdominal wall and fuse to the parietal peritoneum, thus losing their mesentery and becoming **retroperitoneal** (sometimes referred to as "secondarily retroperitoneal" because at one time in human embryonic development they did have a mesentery). Other portions of the bowel retain their mesenteries and continue to be intraperitoneal. Summarized below are those portions of the bowel that are largely intraperitoneal (have a mesentery, which is listed) or retroperitoneal (have lost their mesentery).

INTRAPERITONEAL	RETROPERITONEAL
Stomach (lesser omentum)	Duodenum (most of it)
Jejunum and ileum (mesentery of the small intestine)	Ascending colon
Transverse colon (transverse mesocolon)	Descending colon
Sigmoid colon (sigmoid mesocolon)	Rectum

COLOR the following features of the peritoneal cavity, using a different color for each feature:

- [ ] 1. **Lesser omentum (mesentery suspending the stomach)**
- [ ] 2. **Transverse mesocolon (suspends the transverse colon)**
- [ ] 3. **Mesentery of the small intestine (suspends the jejunum and ileum)**
- [ ] 4. **Greater omentum (apron of peritoneum filled with fat)**

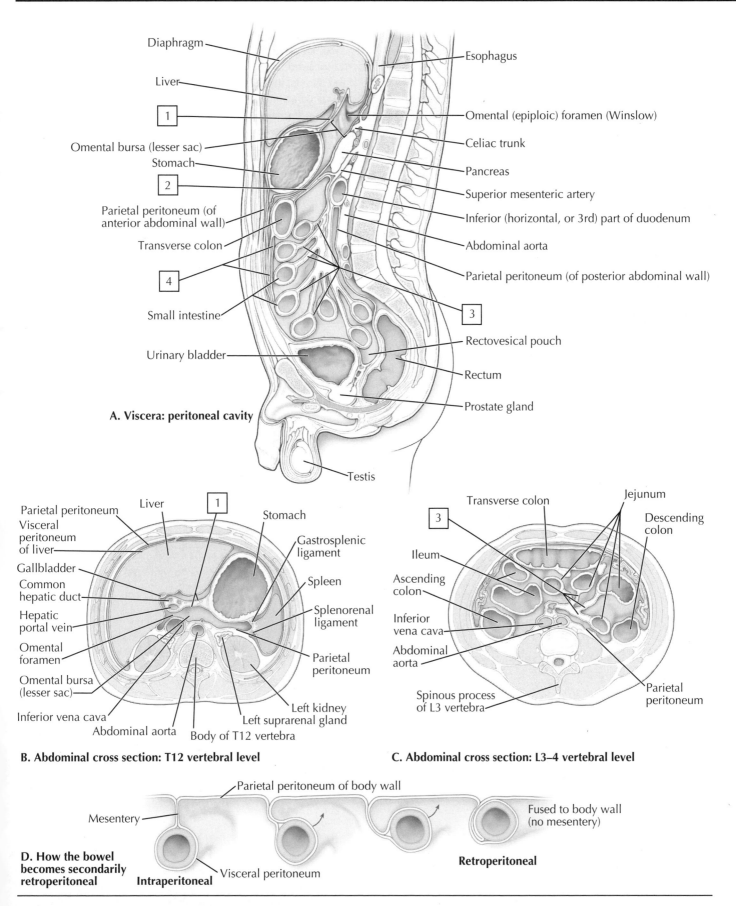

Diaphragm

Liver

1

Omental bursa (lesser sac)

Stomach

2

Parietal peritoneum (of anterior abdominal wall)

Transverse colon

4

Small intestine

Urinary bladder

Esophagus

Omental (epiploic) foramen (Winslow)

Celiac trunk

Pancreas

Superior mesenteric artery

Inferior (horizontal, or 3rd) part of duodenum

Abdominal aorta

Parietal peritoneum (of posterior abdominal wall)

3

Rectovesical pouch

Rectum

Prostate gland

Testis

A. Viscera: peritoneal cavity

Parietal peritoneum

Visceral peritoneum of liver

Gallbladder

Common hepatic duct

Hepatic portal vein

Omental foramen

Omental bursa (lesser sac)

Inferior vena cava

Abdominal aorta

Liver

1

Stomach

Gastrosplenic ligament

Spleen

Splenorenal ligament

Parietal peritoneum

Left kidney

Left suprarenal gland

Body of T12 vertebra

B. Abdominal cross section: T12 vertebral level

Transverse colon

3

Ileum

Ascending colon

Inferior vena cava

Abdominal aorta

Spinous process of L3 vertebra

Jejunum

Descending colon

Parietal peritoneum

C. Abdominal cross section: L3–4 vertebral level

Parietal peritoneum of body wall

Mesentery

D. How the bowel becomes secondarily retroperitoneal

Visceral peritoneum

Intraperitoneal

Fused to body wall (no mesentery)

Retroperitoneal

The stomach is a muscular bag, with its smooth muscle layers oriented in several different planes to one another that functions to blend the macerated bolus of food entering from the esophagus. The stomach begins the major enzymatic digestion of the food into a semiliquid mixture or slurry called **chyme,** that then passes on to the duodenum. Features of the stomach are summarized in the table below.

FEATURE	DESCRIPTION
Lesser curvature	Right border of stomach; lesser omentum attaches here and extends to liver (hepatogastric ligament)
Greater curvature	Convex border with greater omentum suspended from its margin
Cardiac part	Area of stomach that communicates with esophagus superiorly
Fundus	Superior part just under left dome of diaphragm
Body	Main part between fundus and pyloric antrum
Pyloric part	Portion that is divided into proximal antrum and distal canal
Pylorus	Site of pyloric sphincter muscle; joins first part of duodenum

The stomach is flexible and can assume a variety of configurations during digestion, depending upon the contractions of its smooth muscle walls and how full and distended it is. Despite this flexibility, it still is tethered superiorly to the esophagus and distally to the first portion of the duodenum. Both the stomach and this proximal portion of the duodenum are suspended in a mesentery called the **lesser omentum** (hepatogastric and hepatoduodenal ligaments). However, realize that most of the duodenum is retroperitoneal, having lost its mesentery along most of its length. Behind the stomach is the **lesser sac** or omental bursa, a space that communicates with the greater sac via the **epiploic foramen** (of Winslow). The greater sac is the entire rest of the peritoneal cavity. The omental bursa is a cul-de-sac that forms posterior to the stomach and anterior to the retroperitoneal pancreas as a result of the twisting of the stomach during differential growth in the embryo.

The mucosa of the stomach is thrown into large, longitudinal folds called **rugae** and into thousands of microscopic folds and gastric pits lined with a renewing epithelium (simple columnar). At the base of the gastric pit are the gastric or fundic glands, which contain the following four cell types:
- **Mucous neck cells**: secrete mucus to protect the stomach lining
- **Chief cells**: situated deep in the glands, these cells secrete primarily **pepsinogen**, which is converted to pepsin once it contacts the gastric juice and aids in the digestion of proteins

- **Parietal cells**: mostly found in the neck of the gastric glands and secrete **hydrochloric acid (HCl)** and **intrinsic factor** (complexes with vitamin B_{12} so it can be absorbed in the ileum)
- **Enteroendocrine cells**: concentrated more near the base of the glands, they secrete a host of hormones or hormonelike substances that regulate digestion

COLOR the following features of the stomach and its mucosa, using a different color for each feature:
- [ ] 1. **Fundus of stomach**
- [ ] 2. **Body of stomach**
- [ ] 3. **Pyloric antrum**
- [ ] 4. **Pyloric canal (contains the pyloric smooth muscle sphincter that releases measured amounts of chyme into the duodenum during digestion)**
- [ ] 5. **Mucous neck cells (mucus)**
- [ ] 6. **Parietal cells (HCl and intrinsic factor)**
- [ ] 7. **Chief cells (pepsinogen)**
- [ ] 8. **Enteroendocrine cells (gastric hormones and regulatory peptides)**

Clinical Note:

Hiatal hernia is a herniation of the stomach through the esophageal hiatus. Two anatomical types of hiatal hernias are recognized:
- Sliding, rolling, or axial hernia: comprise 95% of hiatal hernias
- Paraesophageal or nonaxial hernia: usually involves only the fundus of the stomach

Peptic ulcers are GI lesions that may extend through the muscularis mucosae and are remitting, relapsing lesions (can come and go). Exposure to gastric acid and pepsin, aspirin, alcohol, and *Helicobacter pylori* infection (about 70% of gastric ulcers) are common aggravating factors.

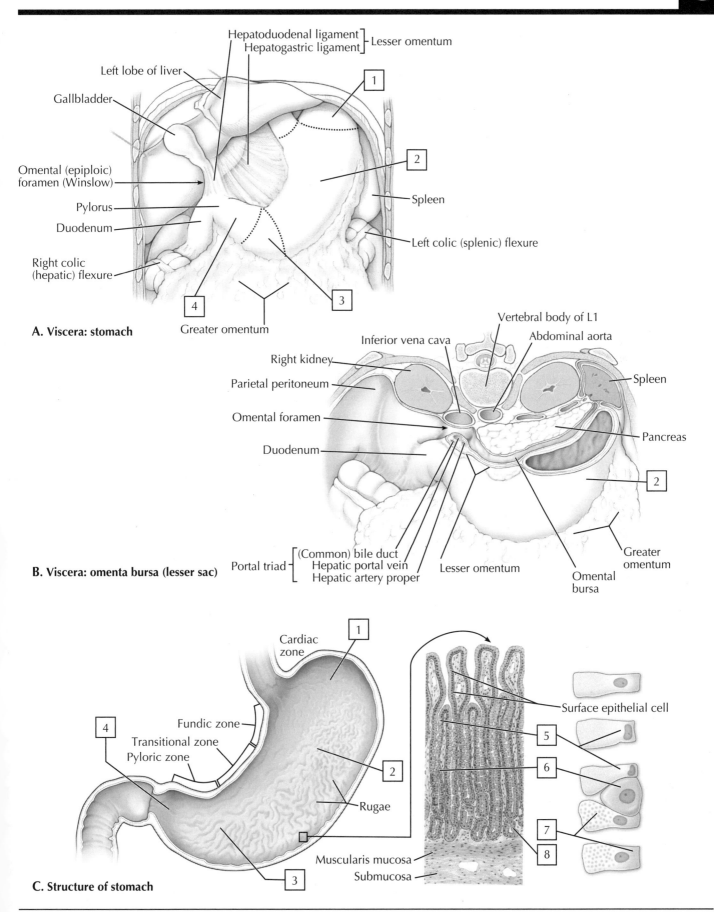

Hepatoduodenal ligament
Hepatogastric ligament ⎤ Lesser omentum

Left lobe of liver

Gallbladder

Omental (epiploic) foramen (Winslow)

Pylorus

Duodenum

Right colic (hepatic) flexure

1

2

Spleen

Left colic (splenic) flexure

4

3

A. Viscera: stomach

Greater omentum

Vertebral body of L1

Inferior vena cava

Abdominal aorta

Right kidney

Parietal peritoneum

Omental foramen

Duodenum

Spleen

Pancreas

2

(Common) bile duct
Portal triad ⎡ Hepatic portal vein
⎣ Hepatic artery proper

Lesser omentum

Greater omentum

Omental bursa

B. Viscera: omenta bursa (lesser sac)

Cardiac zone

1

Surface epithelial cell

Fundic zone

4

Transitional zone

Pyloric zone

2

5

6

Rugae

7

8

Muscularis mucosa

Submucosa

3

C. Structure of stomach

As an embryonic midgut structure, the small intestine is supplied with blood by the **superior mesenteric artery** and drained by the **hepatic portal system** (see Plate 5-19). The small intestine includes the:

- **Duodenum**: first part of the small intestine (about 25 cm long); it is largely retroperitoneal
- **Jejunum**: the proximal two fifths of the mesenteric small intestine (about 2.5 m long); this is primarily where most of the absorption takes place
- **Ileum**: the distal three fifths of the mesenteric small intestine (about 3.5 m long), which then opens via the ileocecal valve into the cecum of the large intestine

Duodenum

The duodenum is where bile and pancreatic enzymes are added to the chyme, which has just arrived from the stomach. The features of the duodenum are summarized below.

PART OF DUODENUM	DESCRIPTION
Superior	First part; attachment site for hepatoduodenal ligament of lesser omentum
Descending	Second part; site where bile and pancreatic ducts empty
Inferior	Third part; part that crosses inferior vena cava (IVC) and aorta and is crossed anteriorly by mesenteric vessels
Ascending	Fourth part; portion tethered by suspensory ligament at duodenojejunal flexure

Jejunum and Ileum

The jejunum has a larger diameter, thicker walls, greater vascularity, less fat in its mesentery, fewer lymph nodules, and larger and taller circular folds (**plicae circulares**) than the ileum. Both the jejunum and ileum are suspended in an elaborate mesentery (two folds of peritoneum that convey vessels, lymphatics, and nerves) that originates from the midposterior abdominal wall and tethers the approximately 6 m of small intestine.

The jejunum and ileum have a large surface area for secretion and absorption. The surface area is increased by the presence of **circular folds, villi**, and **microvilli** (brush border on the columnar epithelium). Simple columnar epithelium lines the bowel, and the lamina propria contains lymphatics, vessels, and connective tissue cells. Intestinal glands (crypts of Lieberkühn) extend into the lamina propria, and **aggregated lymphatic** nodules (Peyer's patches) increase in number as one moves toward the distal ileum.

COLOR the following features of the small intestine, using a different color for each feature:

- [ ] 1. **First (superior) part of the duodenum (tethered by the hepatoduodenal ligament containing the common bile duct, hepatic artery proper, and portal vein)**
- [ ] 2. **Second (descending) part of the duodenum**
- [ ] 3. **Third (horizontal) part of the duodenum**
- [ ] 4. **Fourth (ascending) part of the duodenum**
- [ ] 5. **Circular fold**
- [ ] 6. **Villi**
- [ ] 7. **Lymph nodule**

Clinical Note:

Crohn's disease is an idiopathic (thought to be an autoimmune disease with a genetic component), episodic, and chronic inflammatory bowel condition that usually involves the small intestine and colon. Often it occurs between the ages of 15 and 30 years and presents with abdominal pain, diarrhea, fever, and other signs and symptoms. The lumen of the bowel is narrowed, mucosal ulcerations are present, and the bowel wall is thick and rubbery; thus it affects the entire thickness of the bowel.

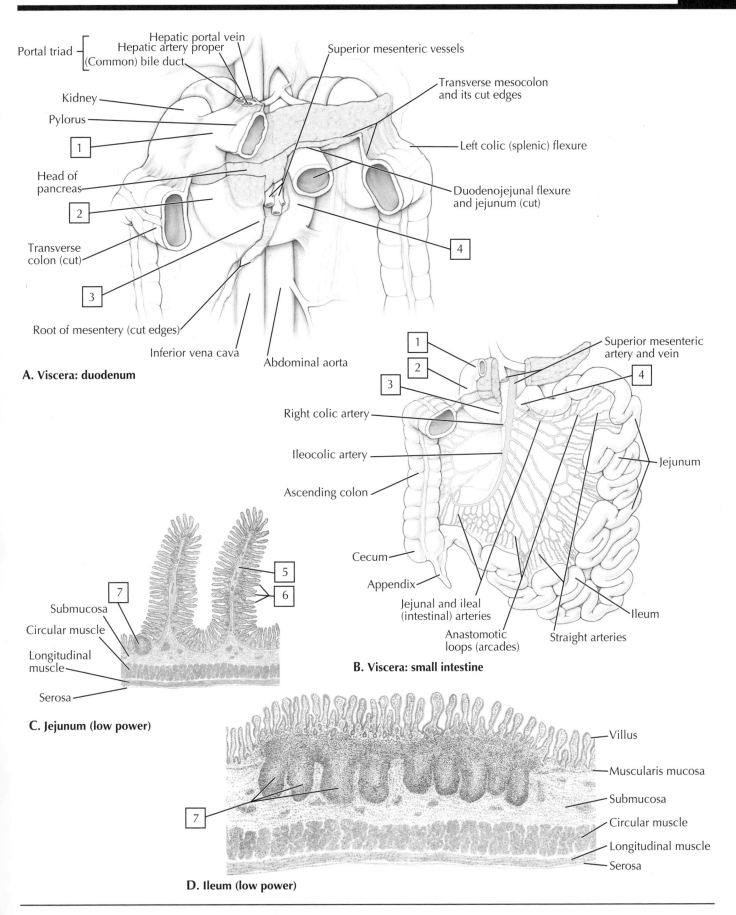

Portal triad
Hepatic portal vein
Hepatic artery proper
(Common) bile duct
Superior mesenteric vessels
Transverse mesocolon and its cut edges
Kidney
Pylorus
1
Left colic (splenic) flexure
Head of pancreas
Duodenojejunal flexure and jejunum (cut)
2
4
Transverse colon (cut)
3
Root of mesentery (cut edges)
Inferior vena cava
Abdominal aorta

A. Viscera: duodenum

1
2
3
Superior mesenteric artery and vein
4
Right colic artery
Ileocolic artery
Ascending colon
Jejunum
Cecum
Appendix
Ileum
Jejunal and ileal (intestinal) arteries
Anastomotic loops (arcades)
Straight arteries

B. Viscera: small intestine

Submucosa
Circular muscle
Longitudinal muscle
Serosa
5
6
7

C. Jejunum (low power)

Villus
Muscularis mucosa
Submucosa
Circular muscle
Longitudinal muscle
Serosa
7

D. Ileum (low power)

The large intestine is supplied by both the **superior** and **inferior mesenteric arteries**, because the proximal portion of the large bowel is derived from the embryonic midgut and the distal portion from the hindgut (distal transverse colon to rectum). The large intestine includes the:

- Cecum (and its vermiform appendix)
- Ascending colon (retroperitoneal)
- Transverse colon (has a transverse mesocolon)
- Descending colon (retroperitoneal)
- Sigmoid colon (has a sigmoid mesocolon)
- Rectum (retroperitoneal)
- Anal canal (lies below the pelvic diaphragm and ends as the anus)

The large intestine serves primarily to reabsorb water and electrolytes from the feces and to store feces until they are eliminated from the body. The large intestine has the same layers as the small intestine, but the mucosa does not have villi or circular folds; **lymphatic nodules** are common. **Goblet cells** also are common and secrete mucus, which lubricates the bowel lumen and facilitates the passage of feces. The mucosa has partial folds called **plicae semilunares**, and the outer longitudinal smooth muscle layer is organized into three thickened bands (**taeniae coli**) that run from the cecum to the rectum and help propel the feces along the length of the bowel. Contraction of the muscle layers produces sacculations called **haustrae** that give the colon its typical appearance. Additionally, the colon is studded with small sacs of fat (**appendices epiploicae**).

The terminal end of the large intestine is the rectum and anal canal. Normally, the anal canal is closed because of the tonic contraction of the **internal** (smooth muscle) and **external** (skeletal muscle) **anal sphincters**. When the rectum is distended by fecal material, the internal sphincter relaxes but defecation does not occur until the voluntary external sphincter is relaxed and the smooth muscles of the distal colon and rectum contract.

COLOR the following features of the large intestine, using a different color for each feature:

- [ ] 1. Cecum and appendix
- [ ] 2. Ascending colon
- [ ] 3. Transverse colon
- [ ] 4. Descending colon
- [ ] 5. Sigmoid colon
- [ ] 6. Rectum
- [ ] 7. Anal canal
- [ ] 8. Internal anal sphincter (involuntary, smooth muscle; parasympathetic innervation)
- [ ] 9. External anal sphincter (voluntary, skeletal muscle; somatic innervation)

Clinical Note:

Colonic diverticulosis usually is an acquired herniation of colonic mucosa through the muscular wall, creating a diverticulum or little saccule that may contain a fecal deposit or concretion. This condition is most common in the distal colon and sigmoid colon and may be caused by exaggerated peristaltic contractions, increased intraluminal pressure, and/or an intrinsic weakness in the muscular wall.

Colorectal cancer is second only to lung cancer in site-specific mortality and accounts for about 15% of cancer-related deaths in the United States. Risk factors include heredity, diet high in fat, increasing age, inflammatory bowel disease, and the presence of polyps.

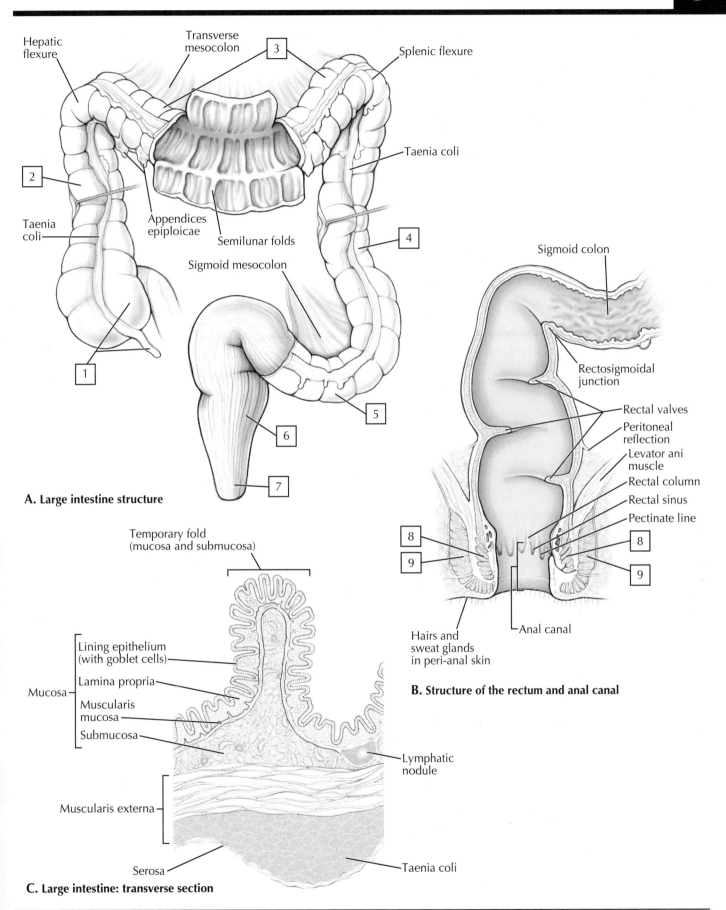

A. Large intestine structure

Hepatic flexure

Transverse mesocolon

[3]

Splenic flexure

[2]

Taenia coli

Taenia coli

Appendices epiploicae

Semilunar folds

Sigmoid mesocolon

[4]

[1]

[5]

[6]

[7]

Sigmoid colon

Rectosigmoidal junction

Rectal valves

Peritoneal reflection

Levator ani muscle

Rectal column

Rectal sinus

Pectinate line

[8]   [8]

[9]   [9]

Hairs and sweat glands in peri-anal skin

Anal canal

B. Structure of the rectum and anal canal

Temporary fold (mucosa and submucosa)

Lining epithelium (with goblet cells)

Lamina propria

Mucosa

Muscularis mucosa

Submucosa

Muscularis externa

Lymphatic nodule

Serosa

Taenia coli

C. Large intestine: transverse section

The liver is the largest solid organ in the body and anatomically is divided into four lobes:
- Right lobe (largest lobe)
- Left lobe
- Quadrate lobe (lies between the gallbladder and the round ligament of the liver)
- Caudate lobe (lies between the IVC, ligamentum venosum, and porta hepatis)

Functionally, the liver is divided into right and left lobes based upon its vasculature, with each lobe receiving a major branch of the hepatic artery, portal vein, hepatic vein (drains the liver's blood into the IVC), and biliary drainage.

FEATURE	DESCRIPTION
Lobes	Divisions, in functional terms, into right and left lobes, with anatomical subdivisions of right lobe into quadrate and caudate lobes
Round ligament	Ligament that contains obliterated umbilical vein
Falciform ligament	Peritoneal reflection off anterior abdominal wall with round ligament in its margin
Ligamentum venosum	Ligamentous remnant of fetal ductus venosus, allowing fetal blood from placenta to bypass liver
Coronary ligaments	Reflections of peritoneum from liver to diaphragm
Bare area	Area of liver pressed against diaphragm that lacks visceral peritoneum
Porta hepatis	Site at which vessels, ducts, lymphatics, and nerves enter or leave liver

The liver is important because it receives the venous drainage from the GI tract, its accessory organs, and the spleen via the portal vein (see Plate 5-18). The liver serves a number of important functions:
- Storage of energy sources (glycogen, fat, protein, and vitamins)
- Production of cellular fuels (glucose, fatty acids, and keto acids)
- Production of plasma proteins and clotting factors
- Metabolism of toxins and drugs
- Modification of many hormones
- Production of bile acids
- Excretion of substances (bilirubin)
- Storage of iron and many vitamins
- Phagocytosis of foreign materials that enter the portal circulation from the bowel

Liver cells receive blood from the **portal vein** (about 75%) and from the **hepatic artery proper** (about 25%). Hepatocytes (liver cells) are arranged in plates of cells that are separated from each other by **hepatic sinusoids**. The blood moves from the portal vein and hepatic arteriole branches through the sinusoid to the **central vein**. This arrangement forms **hepatic lobules** composed of hexagonal units of cells around the central vein. At the margin of the lobule is the **portal triad**, made up of a branch of the hepatic artery, a branch of the portal vein, and a bile duct. From the central vein, blood flows into the hepatic veins and IVC. The sinusoids contain **phagocytic cells** (Kupffer cells) that clear damaged red blood cells and foreign antigens. Bile is produced by the hepatocytes (about 900 ml/day) and drains into intralobular bile ductules and then the larger bile ducts (right and left). Ultimately, bile is collected into the **gallbladder**, where it is stored and concentrated.

COLOR the following features of the liver, using the suggested colors for each feature:
- [ ] 1. IVC (blue)
- [ ] 2. Gallbladder (green)
- [ ] 3. Round ligament of the liver (yellow)
- [ ] 4. Hepatic artery branch (at portal triad) (red)
- [ ] 5. Portal vein branch (at portal triad) (blue)
- [ ] 6. Bile duct (at portal triad) (green)
- [ ] 7. Several hepatocytes (brown)

Clinical Note:
Cirrhosis of the liver is largely an irreversible disease, characterized by diffuse fibrosis, parenchymal nodular regeneration, and disturbed hepatic architecture. Progressive fibrosis disrupts portal blood flow (leading to portal hypertension), beginning at the level of the sinusoids and central veins. Common causes of cirrhosis include:
- Alcoholic liver disease (60%-70%)
- Viral hepatitis (10%)
- Biliary diseases (5%-10%)
- Genetic causes (5%)
- Other (10%-15%)

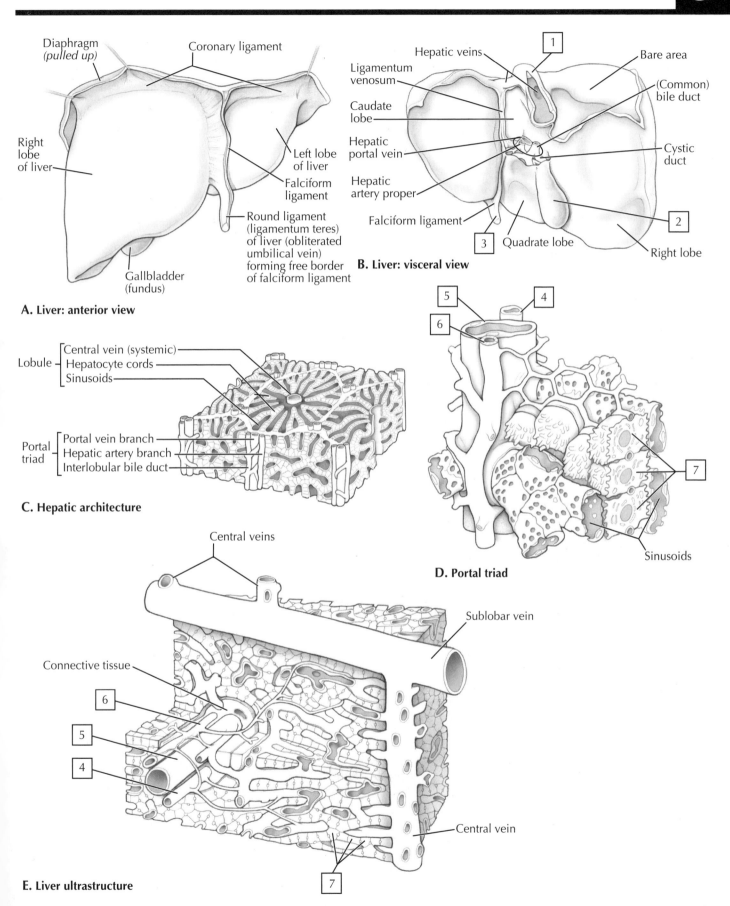

A. Liver: anterior view

Diaphragm (*pulled up*)

Coronary ligament

Right lobe of liver

Left lobe of liver

Falciform ligament

Round ligament (ligamentum teres) of liver (obliterated umbilical vein) forming free border of falciform ligament

Gallbladder (fundus)

B. Liver: visceral view

Hepatic veins

Ligamentum venosum

Caudate lobe

Hepatic portal vein

Hepatic artery proper

Falciform ligament

Bare area

(Common) bile duct

Cystic duct

Quadrate lobe

Right lobe

C. Hepatic architecture

Lobule
- Central vein (systemic)
- Hepatocyte cords
- Sinusoids

Portal triad
- Portal vein branch
- Hepatic artery branch
- Interlobular bile duct

D. Portal triad

Sinusoids

E. Liver ultrastructure

Central veins

Connective tissue

Sublobar vein

Central vein

Gallbladder

The gallbladder stores and concentrates bile, which is secreted by the hepatocytes in the liver. The bile, once secreted by the hepatocyte, takes the following journey:

- Passes into a bile canaliculus (capillary)
- Passes from canaliculi into intralobular ductules
- Passes from intralobular ductules to bile ducts
- Collects in the right and left hepatic ducts
- Enters the common hepatic duct
- Enters the cystic duct and is stored and concentrated in the gallbladder
- Upon stimulation (largely by vagal efferents and cholecystokinin [CCK]), bile leaves the gallbladder and enters the cystic duct
- Passes inferiorly down the common bile duct
- Enters the hepatopancreatic ampulla (of Vater)
- Empties into the second part of the duodenum

The liver produces about 900 ml of bile per day, and between meals it is stored in the gallbladder (capacity of about 30-50 ml), where it is also concentrated. Consequently, bile that reaches the duodenum is a mixture of the more dilute bile directly flowing from the liver and the concentrated bile from the gallbladder. The mucosa of the gallbladder is specialized for electrolyte and water absorption, which allows the gallbladder to concentrate the bile.

Exocrine Pancreas

The pancreas is both an **exocrine** and **endocrine** organ (see Plate 11-6). The pancreas lies posterior to the stomach in the floor of the **lesser sac** (omental bursa) and is a retroperitoneal organ except for the distal tail, which is in contact with the spleen. The pancreatic head is nestled within the C-shaped curve of the duodenum, with its uncinate process lying posterior to the superior mesenteric vessels.

The acinar cells of the exocrine pancreas (a compound tubuloacinar gland) secrete a number of enzymes that are necessary for digestion of proteins, starches, and fats. The pancreatic ductal cells secrete fluid with a high bicarbonate content that neutralizes the acid entering the duodenum from the stomach. Pancreatic secretion is under neural (vagus nerve) and hormonal control (secretin and CCK), and the pancreatic exocrine secretions empty primarily into the main pancreatic duct, which joins the common bile duct at the hepatopancreatic ampulla (of Vater).

COLOR the following features of the gallbladder and pancreas, using a different color for each feature:

- [ ] 1. **Gallbladder**
- [ ] 2. **Common hepatic duct**
- [ ] 3. **Cystic duct**
- [ ] 4. **Common bile duct**
- [ ] 5. **Pancreas**
- [ ] 6. **Hepatopancreatic ampulla**
- [ ] 7. **Main pancreatic duct**

Clinical Note:

Gallstones occur in 10% to 20% of the population in developed countries and usually are precipitates of cholesterol (crystalline cholesterol monohydrate, 80%) or pigment stones (bilirubin calcium salts, 20%). Risk factors include increasing age, obesity, female gender, rapid weight loss, estrogenic factors, and gallbladder stasis. The stone may pass through the duct system, collect in the gallbladder, or block the cystic or common bile ducts, causing inflammation and obstruction to the flow of bile. **Pancreatic cancer** is the fifth leading cause of cancer deaths in the United States. Most of these cancers arise from the exocrine pancreas, and about 60% are found in the head of the pancreas (can cause obstructive jaundice). Metastases are common.

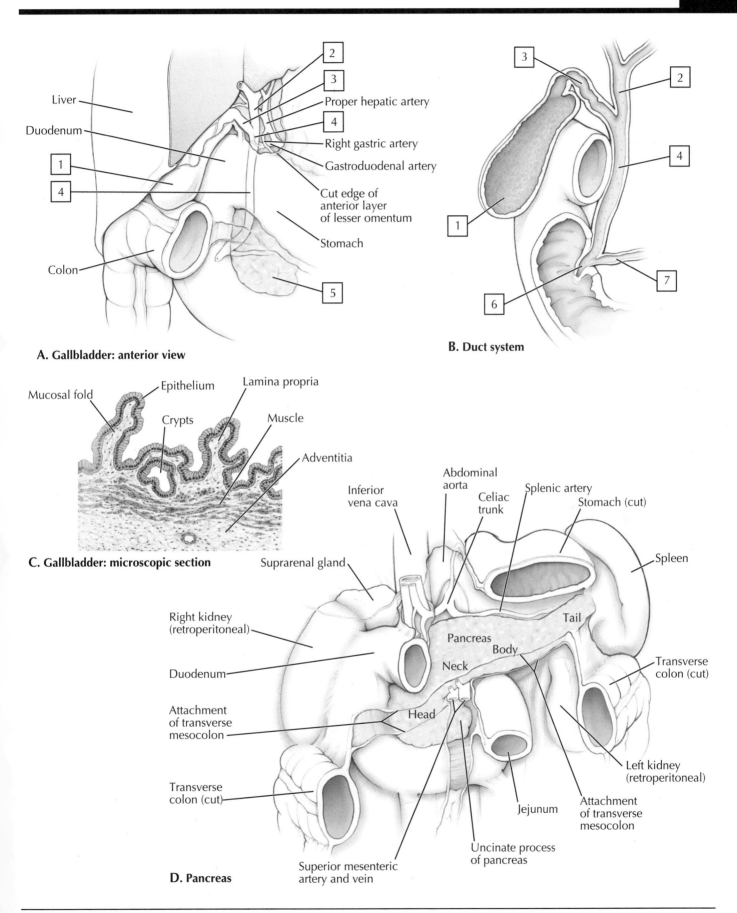

A. Gallbladder: anterior view

Liver
Duodenum
$\boxed{1}$
$\boxed{4}$
Colon

$\boxed{2}$
$\boxed{3}$
Proper hepatic artery
$\boxed{4}$
Right gastric artery
Gastroduodenal artery
Cut edge of anterior layer of lesser omentum
Stomach
$\boxed{5}$

B. Duct system

$\boxed{3}$
$\boxed{2}$
$\boxed{4}$
$\boxed{1}$
$\boxed{6}$
$\boxed{7}$

C. Gallbladder: microscopic section

Mucosal fold
Epithelium
Lamina propria
Crypts
Muscle
Adventitia

D. Pancreas

Inferior vena cava
Abdominal aorta
Celiac trunk
Splenic artery
Stomach (cut)
Spleen
Suprarenal gland
Right kidney (retroperitoneal)
Duodenum
Attachment of transverse mesocolon
Transverse colon (cut)
Pancreas
Neck
Body
Tail
Head
Transverse colon (cut)
Left kidney (retroperitoneal)
Attachment of transverse mesocolon
Jejunum
Uncinate process of pancreas
Superior mesenteric artery and vein

For each description below (1-4), color or highlight the relevant structure on the image

1. This is the most extensive mesentery in the abdominopelvic cavity.

2. This organ is suspended from the liver by the hepatogastric ligament.

3. This portion of the small bowel is retroperitoneal.

4. This retroperitoneal structure is both an endocrine and exocrine organ.

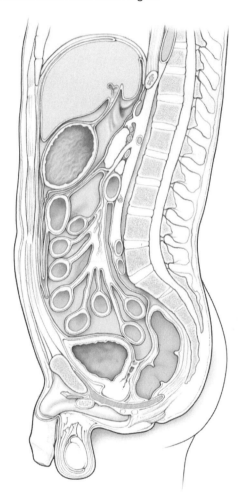

5. Which of the following structures is involved in a hiatal hernia?
   A. Duodenum
   B. Gallbladder
   C. Jejunum
   D. Sigmoid colon
   E. Stomach

6. Which of the following features is unique to the colon?
   A. Haustra
   B. Lymphatic nodules
   C. Mesentery
   D. Simple columnar epithelium
   E. Visceral peritoneum

7. Histologically, the portal triad refers to the presence of a branch of the portal vein and hepatic artery, and which of the following structures?
   A. Bile duct
   B. Central vein
   C. Hepatic sinusoid
   D. Hepatocyte cords
   E. Kupffer cells

8. The cul-de-sac posterior to the stomach and anterior to the pancreas is known by this term. _____

9. Bile leaving the gallbladder passes down the common bile duct and enters which portion of the gastrointestinal tract?
   _____

10. As food enters the oral cavity and is mixed with saliva, what enzyme is secreted by the serous glands of the tongue that aids in digestion? _____

ANSWER KEY

1. Mesentery of the small intestine (jejunum and ileum)

2. Stomach

3. Duodenum

4. Pancreas

Stomach

Pancreas

Duodenum

Mesentery of the small intestine (jejunum and ileum)

5. E

6. A

7. A

8. Lesser sac (omental bursa)

9. Second part of the duodenum

10. Lingual lipase

Chapter 9 **Urinary System**

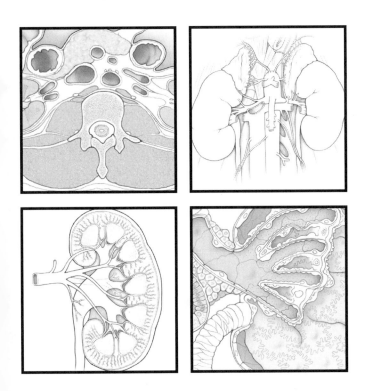

The urinary system includes the following components:
- **Kidneys:** paired retroperitoneal organs that filter the plasma and produce urine; they are located high in the posterior abdominal wall just anterior to the muscles of the posterior wall
- **Ureters:** course retroperitoneally from the kidney to the pelvis and convey urine from the kidneys to the urinary bladder
- **Urinary bladder:** lies subperitoneally in the anterior pelvis, stores urine, and, when appropriate, discharges the urine via the urethra
- **Urethra:** courses from the urinary bladder to the exterior

The kidneys function to:
- Filter plasma and begin the process of urine formation
- Reabsorb important electrolytes, organic molecules, vitamins, and water from the filtrate
- Excrete metabolic wastes, metabolites, and foreign chemicals, such as drugs
- Regulate fluid volume, composition, and pH
- Secrete hormones that regulate blood pressure, erythropoiesis, and calcium metabolism
- Convey urine to the ureters, which then conduct the urine to the bladder

The kidneys filter about 180 L of fluid each day through a tuft of capillaries known as the **glomerulus**, which then delivers the filtrate to a tubule and collecting duct system that, together with the glomerulus, is called the **nephron**. Each kidney has about 1.25 million nephrons, which are the functional units of the kidney. Grossly, each kidney measures about 12 cm long × 6 cm wide × 3 cm thick and weighs about 150 g, although variability is common. Approximately 20% of the blood pumped by the heart passes to the kidney each minute for plasma filtration, although most of the fluid and important plasma constituents are returned to the blood as the filtrate courses down the tubules of the nephron.

Each ureter is about 24 to 34 cm long, lies in a retroperitoneal position and contains a thick smooth muscle wall. The urinary bladder serves as a reservoir for the urine and is a muscular "bag" that expels the urine, when appropriate. The urethra in the female is short (3-5 cm) and in the male is long (about 20 cm). The male urethra runs through the prostate gland, the external urethral sphincter, and the corpus spongiosum of the penis (see Plate 10-8).

COLOR each of the following structures, using a different color for each structure:
- ☐ 1. **Kidney**
- ☐ 2. **Ureter**
- ☐ 3. **Urinary bladder**
- ☐ 4. **Urethra**

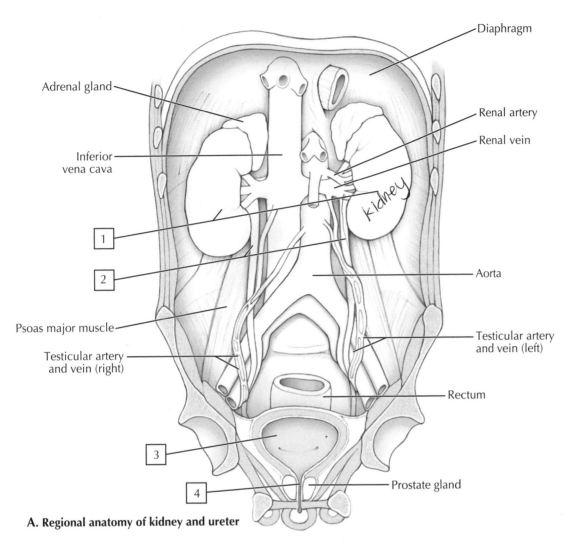

Diaphragm

Adrenal gland

Renal artery

Renal vein

Inferior vena cava

kidney

1

2

Aorta

Psoas major muscle

Testicular artery and vein (left)

Testicular artery and vein (right)

Rectum

3

Prostate gland

4

A. Regional anatomy of kidney and ureter

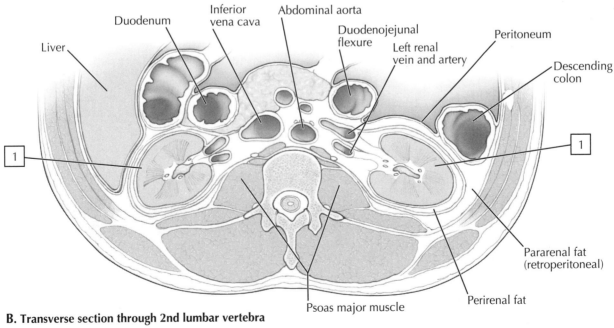

Liver

Duodenum

Inferior vena cava

Abdominal aorta

Duodenojejunal flexure

Left renal vein and artery

Peritoneum

Descending colon

1

1

Pararenal fat (retroperitoneal)

Perirenal fat

Psoas major muscle

B. Transverse section through 2nd lumbar vertebra

Each kidney is enclosed in a **capsule** and, when viewed internally, displays a distinct **cortex** (outer layer) and **medulla** (inner layer). Nephrons are located in the outer cortex and in a juxtamedullary region, or the deepest part of the cortex. The **tubules** of the cortical nephrons extend only a short distance into the medulla, whereas the tubules of the juxtamedullary nephrons extend deep within the medulla. The renal medulla is characterized by the presence of 8 to 15 **pyramids** (collections of tubules), which taper down at their apex to form the papilla, where the urine drips into a **minor calyx**. Several minor calices form a **major calyx**, and several major calices empty into a single **renal pelvis** and the proximal **ureter**.

Each kidney is supplied by a large renal artery, which then divides into the following branches:
- **Segmental arteries:** one artery for each of about five segments
- **Interlobar arteries:** several arise from each segmental artery and course between the renal pyramids, ascending to the cortex and arching over the base of each pyramid
- **Arcuate arteries:** the arching terminal portions of the interlobar arteries at the base of each renal pyramid
- **Interlobular arteries:** arise from the arcuate arteries and ascend into the renal cortex (90% of the blood flow to the kidney perfuses the renal cortex)
- **Afferent arterioles:** arise from the interlobular arteries and pass (one each) to the nephron's glomerulus to form the glomerular capillary tuft
- **Efferent arterioles:** glomerular capillaries of the juxtamedullary nephrons reunite to form efferent arterioles that descend into the medulla and form the **vasa recta** countercurrent system and peritubular capillary network (maintains an osmotic gradient for tubular function; see Plate 9-3)

COLOR each of the following features of the kidney, using a different color for each feature:

☐ 1. Kidney
☐ 2. Renal vein
☐ 3. Proximal ureter
☐ 4. Renal artery
☐ 5. Renal cortex
☐ 6. Renal pyramids (medulla)
☐ 7. Minor calices
☐ 8. Major calices
☐ 9. Renal pelvis

Clinical Note:

Precipitates within the kidney can form **renal stones** (nephrolithiasis) that can enter the urinary collecting system and cause renal colic (loin to groin pain) and potentially obstruct the flow of urine. About 12% of the U.S. population will have renal stones, which are two to three times more common in males and relatively uncommon in African Americans and Asian Americans. The types of stones include:
- Calcium oxalate (phosphate): about 75% of stones
- Magnesium ammonium phosphate: about 15% of stones
- Uric acid or cystine: about 10% of stones

As the renal stone passes through the major calyx and renal pelvis to the ureter, it is more likely than not to obstruct flow in one of these three locations (or all three):
- Junction between the renal pelvis and proximal ureter
- In the ureter, where it crosses the common iliac vessels (mid ureter)
- At the ureterovesical junction, where the ureter passes through the muscular wall of the urinary bladder

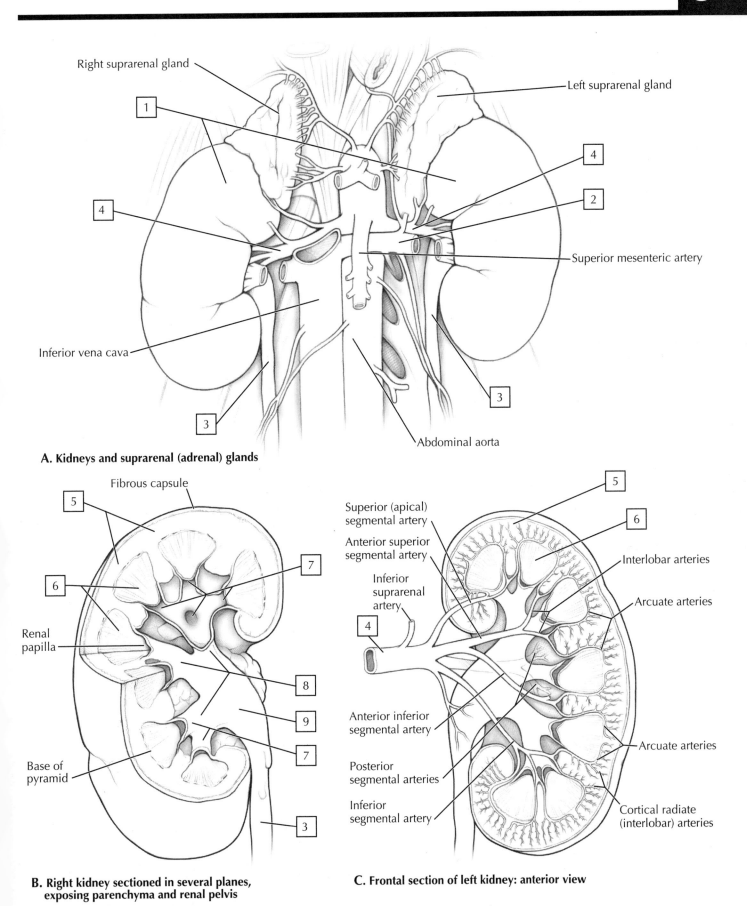

Right suprarenal gland

Left suprarenal gland

1

4

4

2

Superior mesenteric artery

Inferior vena cava

3

3

3

Abdominal aorta

A. Kidneys and suprarenal (adrenal) glands

Fibrous capsule

5

5

6

6

Superior (apical) segmental artery

Anterior superior segmental artery

Interlobar arteries

Inferior suprarenal artery

Arcuate arteries

7

6

4

Renal papilla

8

9

Anterior inferior segmental artery

7

Base of pyramid

Posterior segmental arteries

Arcuate arteries

3

Inferior segmental artery

Cortical radiate (interlobar) arteries

B. Right kidney sectioned in several planes, exposing parenchyma and renal pelvis

C. Frontal section of left kidney: anterior view

The nephrons differ somewhat in structure depending on their location; **cortical nephrons** have their glomeruli in the upper or midcortex and generally have short **loops of Henle** (tubules that dilute the urine but do not concentrate it), as opposed to **juxtamedullary nephrons**, which have long loops of Henle that extend deep into the inner medulla. Juxtamedullary nephrons account for only about 10% to 15% of the total nephrons in the kidney and are important for concentrating the urine.

Each nephron, which is the functional unit of the kidney that produces the ultrafiltrate of blood plasma and eventually forms the urine, consists of the following elements:
- **Glomerulus:** a capillary tuft formed by the afferent arteriole, which is encased in **Bowman's capsule** and is responsible for filtering the plasma
- **Proximal convoluted tubule (PCT):** connected to the glomerulus, it receives the plasma ultrafiltrate and conveys it down the loop of Henle
- **Loop of Henle:** consists of a single long tubule of varying thickness and lined with epithelial cells that are involved in reabsorption and secretion along the tubule's length
- **Distal convoluted tubule (DCT):** receives the remaining tubular fluid from the loop of Henle, monitors its osmolarity and conveys the fluid to the collecting duct
- **Collecting duct:** terminal end of the nephron where the final concentration of the urine is "fine tuned" before it is conveyed to the minor calices

The glomerulus filters the plasma. This ultrafiltrate is devoid of cells and virtually all proteins (unless they are smaller in size than albumin). The endothelium of the glomerulus is fenestrated but prevents the passage of blood cells. **Podocytes** envelop the fenestrated endothelium and keep proteins from being filtered.

Adjacent to the afferent arteriole that delivers blood to the glomerulus is a specialization of the DCT wall called the **macula densa**, which monitors the NaCl in the fluid of the DCT and, if low, stimulates the release of **renin** from juxtaglomerular cells that ultimately causes an increase in angiotensin II and aldosterone (renin-angiotensin-aldosterone [RAA] system). These hormones stimulate NaCl and water reabsorption by the nephron (angiotensin II acts on the proximal tubule and aldosterone acts on the collecting duct). The juxtaglomerular cells adjacent to the macula densa of the DCT also monitor blood pressure in the afferent arteriole and, if low, release renin to elevate blood pressure via the RAA system and sympathetic activity.

COLOR the following features of the nephron, using the colors suggested for each feature:

- [ ] 1. **Proximal tubule: convoluted and straight segments (blue)**
- [ ] 2. **Juxtamedullary glomerulus (purple)**
- [ ] 3. **Distal ascending loop of Henle (thick limb and DCT) (orange)**
- [ ] 4. **Thin descending and ascending loop of Henle (green)**
- [ ] 5. **Collecting duct (gray)**
- [ ] 6. **Cells lining the DCT (orange)**
- [ ] 7. **Afferent arteriole (red)**
- [ ] 8. **Juxtaglomerular cells (purple)**
- [ ] 9. **Endothelium of glomerular capillaries (yellow)**
- [ ] 10. **Podocytes (brown)**
- [ ] 11. **Bowman's capsule (green)**
- [ ] 12. **Epithelium of PCT (blue)**

Plate 9-3　　　　　　　　　　　　　　　　　　**Urinary System**

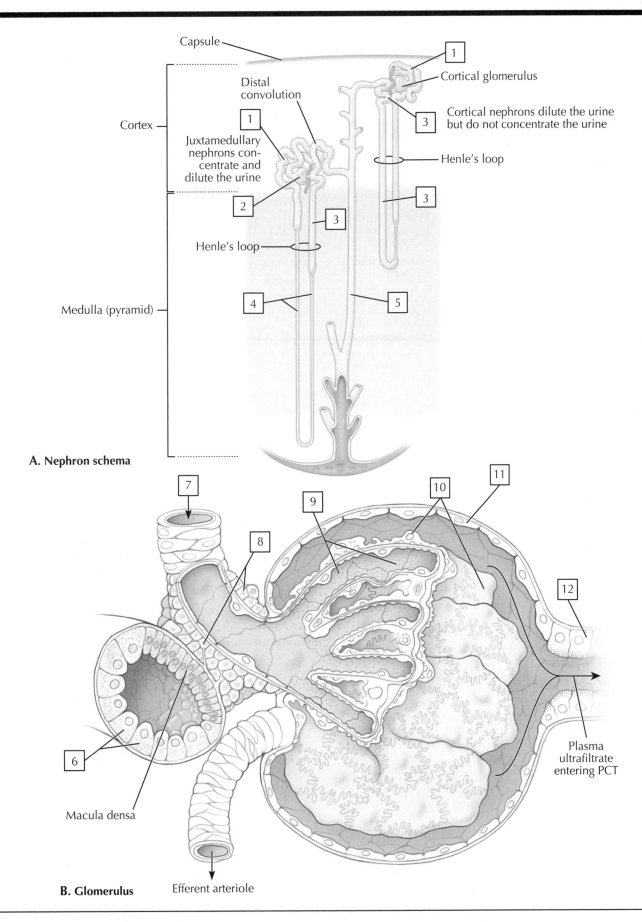

Capsule

Distal convolution

1

Cortex

Juxtamedullary nephrons concentrate and dilute the urine

2

Henle's loop

3

Medulla (pyramid)

4

5

A. Nephron schema

1

Cortical glomerulus

3

Cortical nephrons dilute the urine but do not concentrate the urine

Henle's loop

3

7

10

11

9

8

12

6

Macula densa

Plasma ultrafiltrate entering PCT

B. Glomerulus   Efferent arteriole

Glomerular Filtration

The volume of fluid filtered by the renal glomeruli per unit time is called the **glomerular filtration rate (GFR)**. Remember that in the average person, about 180 L of fluid is filtered per day (125 ml/min) and, since plasma accounts for about 3 L of our total blood volume, that means that the kidneys filter the blood plasma about 60 times per day! The amount of blood delivered to the glomerulus or leaving it is controlled by neural and hormonal mechanisms acting on the afferent and efferent arterioles.

Tubular Reabsorption

Once the ultrafiltrate of the plasma enters the PCT, it is modified by the renal tubules, as summarized in the following table.

REABSORPTION OF SEVERAL COMPONENTS FROM THE ULTRAFILTRATE

SUBSTANCE	AMOUNT FILTERED/DAY	PERCENT REABSORBED
Water	180 L	99
Sodium	630 g	99.5
Glucose	180 g	100
Urea	54 g	44

Reabsorption occurs both by diffusion and by mediated transport. For example, many substances are reabsorbed in combination with sodium (cotransported). Except in the descending limb of the loop of Henle, sodium is actively reabsorbed in all tubular regions, and water reabsorption is by diffusion and is dependent upon sodium reabsorption. About two thirds of the sodium and water is reabsorbed in the proximal tubule; in fact, tubular reabsorption is generally high for nutrients, ions, and water, but lower for waste products such as urea (see table above: 44% reabsorption).

Tubular Secretion

Tubular secretion involves a process whereby substances in the capillaries that parallel the renal tubules diffuse or are actively transported into the tubular lumen. Important substances secreted include:
- Hydrogen ions
- Potassium
- Organic anions such as choline and creatinine (waste product of muscle)
- Foreign chemicals

Renal Sodium and Water Regulation

Sodium filtration is regulated at the level of the glomerulus by the **baroreceptor reflex**, and its reabsorption is regulated at the tubular level by **aldosterone** (secreted by the adrenal cortex), which stimulates reabsorption. Other factors also play a role but water reabsorption is linked to sodium movement until it reaches the collecting duct system, where water then comes under the control of **vasopressin** (antidiuretic hormone, ADH). Low ADH levels result in a dilute urine (water excretion), whereas high ADH levels activate water channels (called **aquaporins**) that reabsorb water and create a concentrated urine.

The kidneys also play an important role in regulating the following:
- Water retention is facilitated by ADH and the countercurrent multiplier system (renal vasa recta), which creates a medullary interstitial fluid that is hyperosmotic
- Potassium levels, by both tubular reabsorption and secretion
- Calcium and vitamin D homeostasis, in concert with parathyroid hormone
- Homeostatic regulation of plasma hydrogen ion concentration (acid-base balance) in concert with the respiratory system
- Regulation of bicarbonate concentration and generation of new bicarbonate by the production and excretion of ammonium

COLOR each of the following dynamic features of tubular function, using the colors suggested for each feature:
- 1. **Water movement (blue)**
- 2. **Solute movement (yellow)**
- 3. **Filtrate (green)**
- 4. **PCT tubule cells (brown) (possess a high surface area for reabsorption)**
- 5. **Thin descending segment cells of the loop of Henle**
- 6. **DCT cells**
- 7. **Collecting duct cells**

Plate 9-4   **Urinary System**

A. Nephron and collecting ducts

PCT
Reabsorption of organic nutrients, inorganic ions and H_2O

DCT
Secretion of ions and waste products and reabsorption of Na^+, CL^-, and H_2O (hormonally regulated)

Glomerulus

Efferent arteriole

Afferent arteriole

Renal glomerulus
Produces ultrafiltrate

Descending limb

Collecting duct
Reabsorption of ions and H_2O (ADH regulated) and secretion of ions; fine tunes urine

Ascending limb

Loop of Henle
Reabsorption of H_2O (descending) and NaCl (ascending)

Toward renal calyx

B. Tubule epithelium

Proximal convoluted tubule

Distal convoluted tubule

Cortex
Medulla

Loop of Henle
Descending limb
Ascending limb

Collecting duct

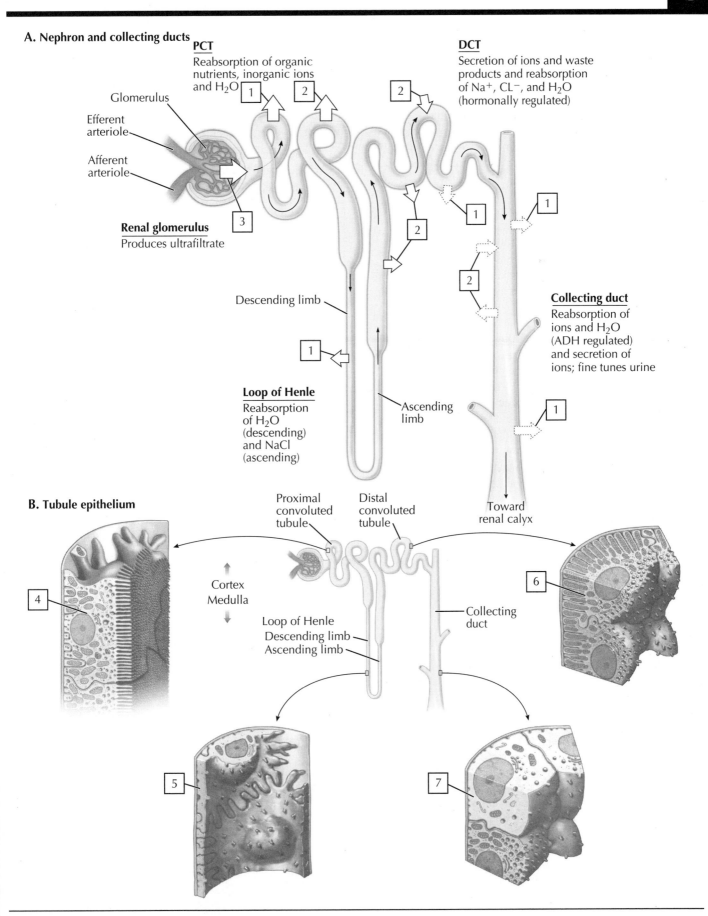

The renal calices, pelvis, ureters, bladder and proximal urethra are lined by **transitional epithelium** (urothelium) that has the unique ability to "unfold" or expand as the passageways or bladder become distended. The ureters are enveloped in smooth muscle arranged in 3 layers, but the bladder is enveloped with smooth muscle that is randomly mixed in its orientation and is known as the **detrusor** ("drive away") **muscle**. The proximal urethra in both sexes is lined with transitional epithelium, which then gives way to pseudostratified columnar and stratified squamous epithelium as the urethra opens to the exterior.

The urinary bladder lies **subperitoneally** behind the pubic symphysis. The bladder stores the urine until it is appropriate to void (urination) and can hold up to 800 to 1000 ml of urine. The interior, posteroinferior wall of the bladder demonstrates a smooth area called the **trigone**, demarcated by the two ureteric openings superiorly and the single urethral opening at the base of the bladder.

Micturition (voiding or urination) involves several important steps:
- Normally sympathetic nerve fibers relax the bladder wall, allowing for distension, and constrict the internal urethral sphincter (smooth muscle) located at the neck of the bladder (females do not have this internal urethral sphincter)
- Micturition is initiated by the stimulation of stretch receptors in the detrusor muscle, sending afferent signals to the spinal cord levels S2-S4 via the pelvic splanchnic nerves
- Parasympathetic efferents (via pelvic splanchnics) induce a reflex contraction of the detrusor muscle, relaxation of the internal sphincter in males, and enhance the "urge" to void
- When convenient (and sometimes not!), somatic efferents via the pudendal nerve (S2-S4) cause voluntary relaxation of the external urethral sphincter (both sexes) and micturition occurs
- When empty, the external sphincter contracts (in males the bulbospongiosus muscle expels that last few drops of urine from the urethra), and the detrusor muscle once again relaxes under sympathetic control

The female urethra is short (3-5 cm), is encircled by the urethral sphincter (blends with another skeletal muscle called the sphincter urethrovaginalis; see Plate 3-16), and opens into the vestibule. The male urethra is longer (about 20 cm) and descriptively is divided into three parts:
- **Prostatic urethra**: proximal portion of the male urethra that runs through the prostate gland
- **Membranous urethra**: short, middle portion that is enveloped by the external urethral sphincter (skeletal muscle)
- **Spongy (penile, cavernous) urethra**: courses through the bulb of the penis, the pendulous portion of the penis, and the glans penis to open at the external urethral orifice

In both sexes, urethral glands open into the lumen and lubricate the urethral mucosa (see Plate 3-16, bulbo-urethral glands in males and greater vestibular glands in females).

COLOR the following features of the urinary bladder and urethra, using a different color for each feature:

- [ ] 1. Detrusor muscle of the female bladder wall
- [ ] 2. Trigone in the female and male bladder
- [ ] 3. Female urethra
- [ ] 4. Sphincter urethrae muscle in the female
- [ ] 5. Internal urethral sphincter in the male
- [ ] 6. Membranous urethra
- [ ] 7. External urethral sphincter in the male
- [ ] 8. Spongy urethra
- [ ] 9. Prostatic urethra

Clinical Note:
Stress incontinence (involuntary release of urine) usually occurs with an increase in intra-abdominal pressure caused by coughing, sneezing, defecation, or lifting. Normally, the sphincter mechanism (urethral sphincter) is strong enough to keep the urine from leaving the bladder. However, weakening of the sphincter mechanism of the bladder, vagina, and other support structures of the pelvic floor can lead to stress incontinence; predisposing factors include multiparity (multiple childbirths, leading to stretching of the sphincter during vaginal delivery), obesity, chronic cough, and heavy lifting.

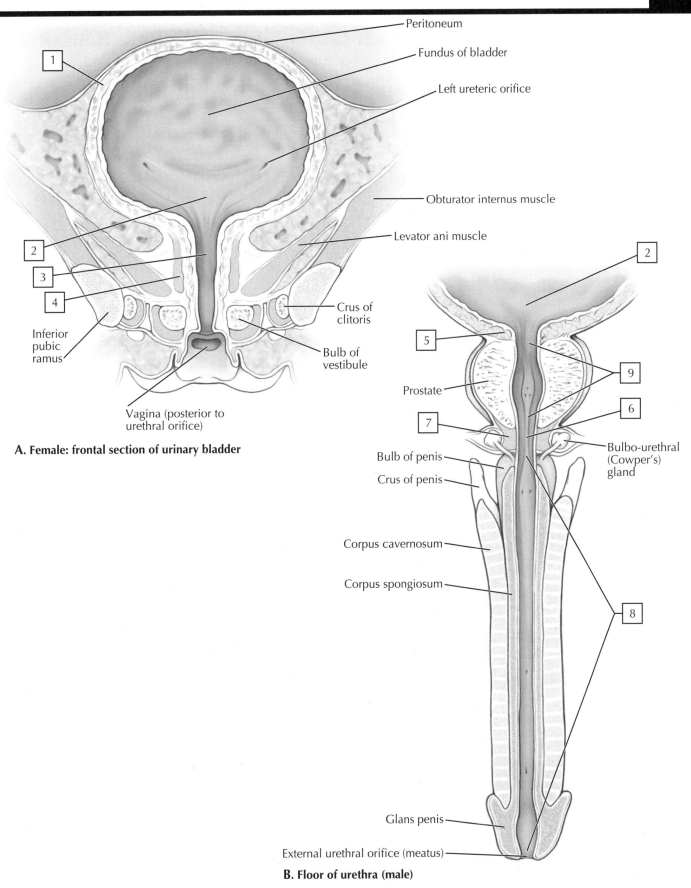

Peritoneum

Fundus of bladder

Left ureteric orifice

Obturator internus muscle

Levator ani muscle

Crus of clitoris

Bulb of vestibule

Inferior pubic ramus

Vagina (posterior to urethral orifice)

A. Female: frontal section of urinary bladder

Prostate

Bulb of penis

Crus of penis

Bulbo-urethral (Cowper's) gland

Corpus cavernosum

Corpus spongiosum

Glans penis

External urethral orifice (meatus)

B. Floor of urethra (male)

For each description below (1-4), color the relevant structure or feature on the image

1. This region of the kidney contains the most nephrons and their glomeruli.

2. Most of the renal tubules and the vasa recta are found in this area.

3. These structures collect urine from each pyramid.

4. This structure conveys urine to the urinary bladder.

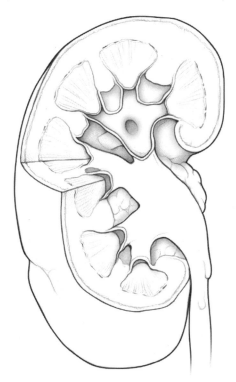

5. Descriptively, the kidneys do not reside within the abdominal peritoneal cavity nor are they suspended in a mesentery. What terminology would a clinician use to describe the location of the kidneys? _____

6. Renal stones may be passed down the ureter to the bladder but can become lodged at three primary points along their journey to the bladder. Where are these three points? _____

7. At the level of the renal glomerulus, cells envelop the glomerulus to prevent the passage of cells and proteins from being filtered. What are these cells called? _____

8. High levels of this hormone result in the retention (reabsorption) of water in the collecting ducts. _____

9. Which of the following nerves is critical for maintaining the voluntary urethral sphincter (external sphincter) in males and must be spared, if possible, during pelvic or perineal surgery?
   A. Femoral
   B. Inferior gluteal
   C. Obturator
   D. Pelvic splanchnics
   E. Pudendal

10. Which portion of the nephron is critical for monitoring the osmolarity of the tubular fluid?
    A. Bowman's capsule
    B. Collecting duct
    C. Distal convoluted tubule
    D. Loop of Henle
    E. Proximal convoluted tubule

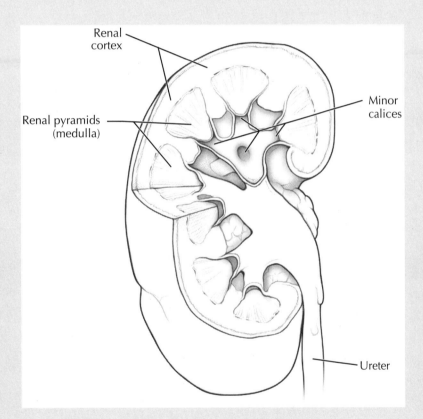

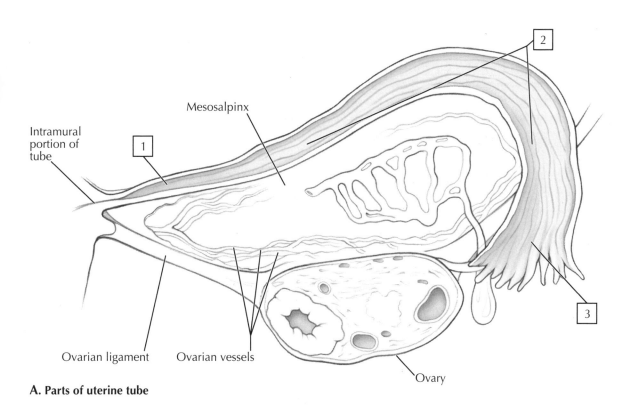

Intramural portion of tube

Mesosalpinx

1

2

3

Ovarian ligament

Ovarian vessels

Ovary

A. Parts of uterine tube

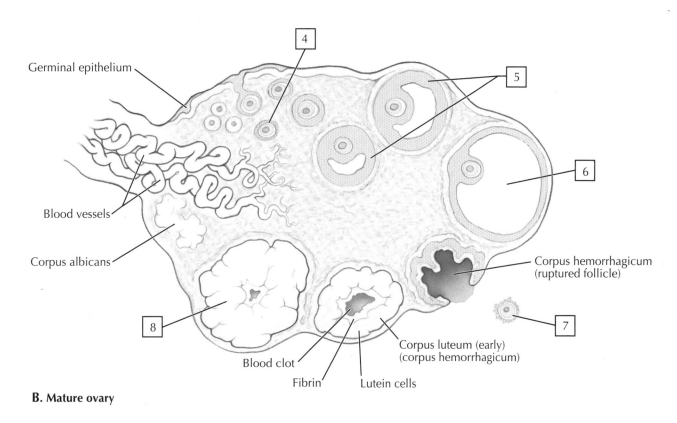

Germinal epithelium

4

5

6

Blood vessels

Corpus albicans

8

7

Corpus hemorrhagicum (ruptured follicle)

Blood clot

Fibrin

Lutein cells

Corpus luteum (early) (corpus hemorrhagicum)

B. Mature ovary

Uterus

The uterus (womb) is a pear-shaped organ suspended in the **broad ligament** (mesometrium) and tethered laterally by its connections to the uterine tubes and by the ovarian ligament and its attachment to the ovary. Additionally, reflecting from its anterolateral aspect is the **round ligament of the uterus,** a distal remnant of the female gubernaculum (the proximal remnant is the ovarian ligament attached to the ovary), which pulls the ovary down from its developmental site in the posterior abdominal wall into the pelvis. The round ligament of the uterus passes through the inguinal canal and ends as a fibrous fatty band in the labia majora (homologue to the male scrotum).

The uterus has several parts:

- **Fundus**: that part lying superior to the attachments of the two uterine tubes
- **Body**: the middle portion of the uterus that tapers inferiorly into the cervix
- **Cervix**: the "neck" of the uterus, it lies subperitoneally, has a narrow endocervical canal, and opens into the superior part of the vagina

The uterine wall is lined internally by the **endometrium**, which proliferates significantly during the first half of the menstrual cycle in preparation for the possible implantation of a conceptus and, if fertilization doesn't occur, degenerates and is sloughed off during the 3 to 5 days of **menstruation** that mark the beginning of the next menstrual cycle. The middle layer of the uterine wall is the **myometrium**, a thick smooth muscle layer, and the outer layer is the **perimetrium**, a serous layer (visceral peritoneal covering).

Vagina

The vagina is a musculoelastic tube extending from the cervix to its opening in the vestibule. The lumen is lined by a stratified, squamous, nonkeratinized epithelium that is lubricated by mucus from cervical glands.

COLOR the following features of the uterus and vagina, using a different color for each feature:

- [ ] 1. **Fundus of the uterus**
- [ ] 2. **Body of the uterus**
- [ ] 3. **Cervix of the uterus**
- [ ] 4. **Vagina**
- [ ] 5. **Stratum basale (regenerates a new stratum functionale after menstruation) of the endometrium**
- [ ] 6. **Stratum functionale (thick surface layer that proliferates and is sloughed off during menstruation) of the endometrium**
- [ ] 7. **Uterine glands**

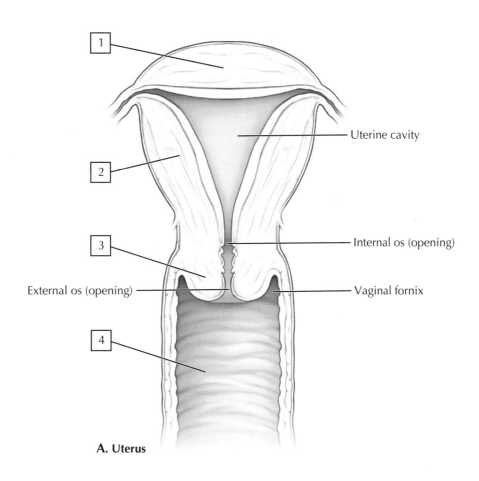

Uterine cavity

Internal os (opening)

External os (opening)

Vaginal fornix

A. Uterus

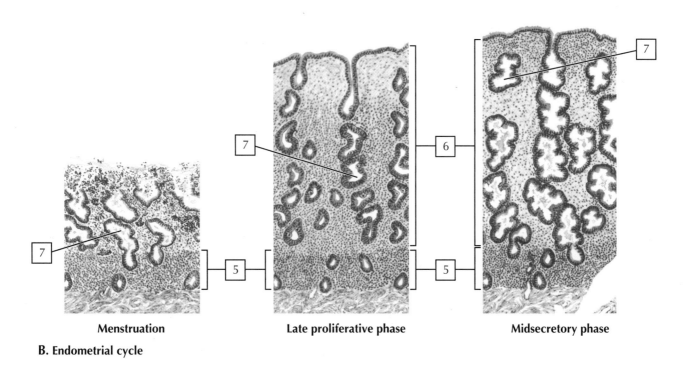

Menstruation

Late proliferative phase

Midsecretory phase

B. Endometrial cycle

The menstrual cycle is divided into three phases:

- **Follicular**: begins with menses on day 1 of the cycle and coincides with the proliferation of the granulosa cells in a selected follicle
- **Ovulatory**: happens midcycle around day 14 and coincides with ovulation of the oocyte by the mature graafian follicle, induced by the LH and FSH surges
- **Luteal**: following ovulation, the follicular cells transform into the corpus luteum and produce large amounts of progesterone, estrogen, and inhibin (negative feedback on the hypothalamus to inhibit GnRH; LH and FSH also participate in this feedback)

During the follicular phase, the rising levels of estrogen feed back onto the hypothalamus and pituitary to increase the surge of GnRH that is followed by the LH and FSH peaks during the ovulatory phase. If fertilization does not occur, the corpus luteum degenerates beginning around the 25th day of the cycle and menses commence after the 28th day, as the new menstrual cycle begins again.

If fertilization and implantation occur, then the plasma levels of estrogen and progesterone continually increase, with estrogen stimulating the myometrium growth and progesterone inhibiting uterine contractility so the fetus can reach term (9 months) before birth. The **corpus luteum** is responsible for the secretion of these hormones during the first 2 months, under the stimulation of **human chorionic gonadotropin (hCG)** secreted by the trophoblast cells of the implant. After about 60 to 80 days, the placenta takes over and secretes the estrogen and progesterone necessary to maintain the pregnancy.

The menstrual cycle also results in changes in the uterine endometrium and includes the following phases:

- **Menstrual**: lasts about 3 to 5 days and marks the beginning of the cycle when the endometrium degenerates (because no implantation has occurred) and is sloughed off as the menstrual flow
- **Proliferative**: from about day 5 to 14, when the endometrium thickens tremendously; this growth is stimulated by estrogen
- **Secretory**: after ovulation, the endometrium increases its secretory activity (nutrient-rich mucus) under the influence of progesterone ("promotes gestation"), becomes edematous and thickens in anticipation of a possible implantation

COLOR the following features of the menstrual cycle, using the colors suggested for each feature:

1. **Corpus luteum (yellow with a red center)**
2. **Veins and venous lakes of the endometrium (blue)**
3. **Spiral arteries of the endometrium during the cycle (red)**
4. **LH levels (line in table) (orange)**
5. **FSH levels (brown)**
6. **Progesterone levels (blue)**
7. **Estrogen levels (green)**
8. **Inhibin levels (purple)**

Clinical Note:
Approximately 10% to 15% of infertile couples may benefit from various **assisted reproductive strategies,** including:
- Artificial insemination: use of a donor's sperm
- GIFT: gamete intrafallopian transfer
- IUI: intrauterine insemination (with a partner's sperm or a donor's sperm)
- IVF/ET: in vitro fertilization with embryo transfer into the uterine cavity
- ZIFT: in vitro fertilization with zygote transfer into the fallopian tube

Plate 10-4 **Reproductive System**

Menstrual Cycle

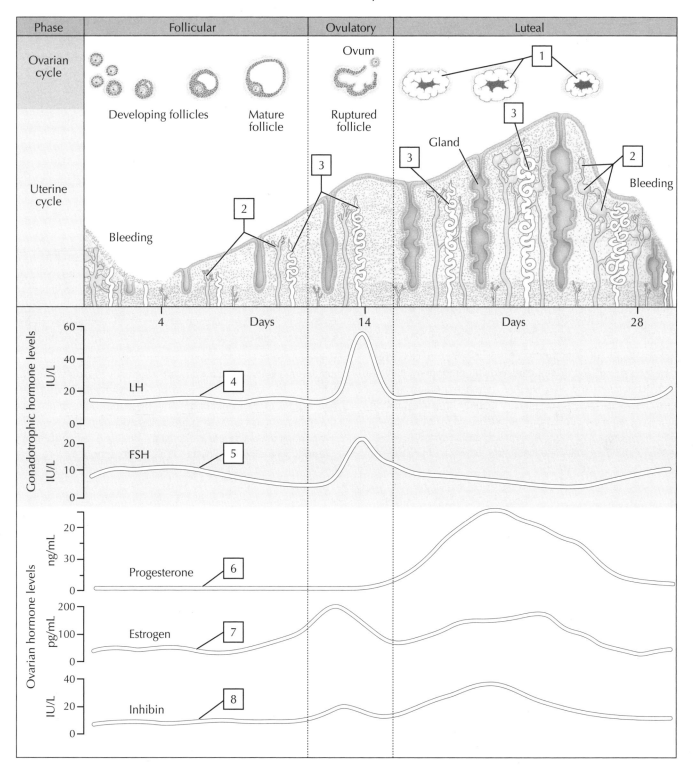

Phase	Follicular	Ovulatory	Luteal

Ovarian cycle

Ovum

Developing follicles Mature follicle Ruptured follicle

1

3

Gland

3

2

Bleeding

Uterine cycle

2

3

Bleeding

4 Days 14 Days 28

Gonadotrophic hormone levels

60
40
IU/L 20
0

LH 4

20
IU/L 10
0

FSH 5

Ovarian hormone levels

20
ng/mL 30
0

Progesterone 6

200
pg/mL 100
0

Estrogen 7

40
IU/L 20
0

Inhibin 8

The female breast extends from approximately the 2nd to the 6th ribs and from the sternum medially to the midaxillary line laterally. The mammary gland tissue lies in the **superficial fascia**, histologically is really a modified sweat gland that develops under hormonal influence, and is supported by strands of fibrous tissue called the **suspensory ligaments** (of Cooper). The nipple usually lies at approximately the 4th intercostal space and is surrounded by the pigmented **areola**. The glandular architecture includes the following features:

- **Secretory alveoli**: cells in the lobules of tubuloalveolar glands release "milk" via merocrine (exocytotic release of the protein secretory product) and apocrine (fatty component of the secretion released in membrane-enclosed droplets) mechanisms
- **Intralobular ducts**: collect the alveolar secretions and convey them along to interlobular ducts
- **Interlobular ducts**: coalesce into about 15 to 25 lactiferous ducts
- **Lactiferous ducts**: drain the milk toward the nipple and exhibit dilated segments just deep to the nipple called lactiferous sinuses, before opening on the nipple surface.

The **areola** contains sebaceous glands, sweat glands, and modified mammary glands (of Montgomery), along with numerous sensory nerve endings. These glands moisten the nipple and keep it supple.

Breast development is under the control of prolactin, GH, estrogen, progesterone, and adrenocorticoids. In pregnancy, elevated prolactin, estrogen, and progesterone increase development of the tubuloalveolar glands but inhibit milk production. **Lactation** occurs when estrogen and progesterone levels fall dramatically at birth while prolactin levels remain high and oxytocin levels increase to stimulate milk release. In the absence of pregnancy or suckling (active nursing), the tubuloalveolar glands regress and become inactive. After menopause, the glandular tissue largely atrophies and is replaced by fat, although some of the lactiferous ducts may remain.

COLOR the following features of the female breast, using a different color for each feature:

- [ ] 1. Areola
- [ ] 2. Nipple
- [ ] 3. Lactiferous ducts
- [ ] 4. Lactiferous sinuses
- [ ] 5. Fatty subcutaneous tissue
- [ ] 6. Gland lobules

Clinical Note:

Fibrocystic changes (disease) is a general term covering a large group of benign conditions that occur in about 80% of women and are often related to cyclic changes in the maturation and involution of the glandular tissue. Fibroadenoma, the second most common tumor of the breast after carcinoma, is a benign neoplasm of the glandular epithelium. Both conditions can present with palpable masses and warrant follow-up evaluation.

Breast cancer (usually ductal carcinoma or invasive lobular carcinoma) is the most common malignancy in women. Approximately two thirds of all cases occur in postmenopausal women. About 50% of the cancers occur in the upper outer quadrant of the breast (region closest to the axilla) and metastases via the lymphatics usually occur in the axilla, because about 75% of the lymph from the breast drains to these lymph nodes.

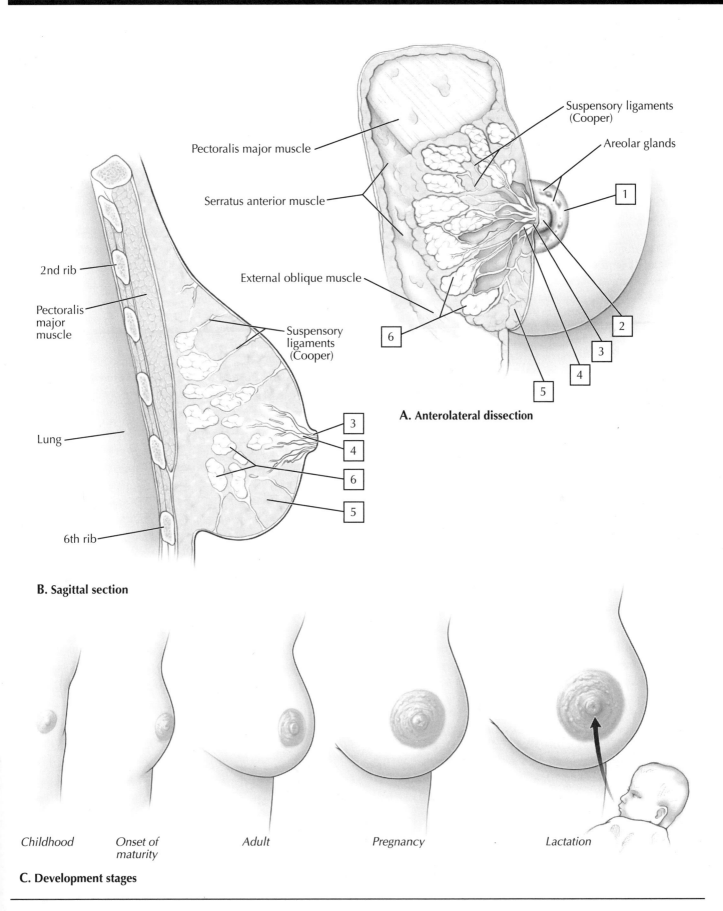

Suspensory ligaments (Cooper)

Areolar glands

Pectoralis major muscle

Serratus anterior muscle

External oblique muscle

1

2

3

4

5

6

A. Anterolateral dissection

2nd rib

Pectoralis major muscle

Lung

6th rib

Suspensory ligaments (Cooper)

3

4

6

5

B. Sagittal section

Childhood

Onset of maturity

Adult

Pregnancy

Lactation

C. Development stages

The male reproductive system is composed of the following structures:
- **Testes**: the paired gonads of the male reproductive system, they are egg shaped and about the size of a chestnut, produce the male germ cells called **spermatozoa**, and reside in the scrotum (externalized from the abdominopelvic cavity)
- **Epididymis**: a convoluted tubule that receives the spermatozoa and stores them as they mature (stretched out, it is almost 23 feet long!)
- **Ductus (vas) deferens**: a muscular (smooth muscle) tube about 40 to 45 cm long that conveys sperm from the epididymis to the ejaculatory duct (seminal vesicle)
- **Seminal vesicles**: paired tubular glands that lie posterior to the prostate, are about 15 cm long, produce seminal fluid, and join the ductus deferens at the **ejaculatory duct**
- **Prostate gland**: a walnut-sized gland that surrounds the urethra as it leaves the urinary bladder and produces prostatic fluid that is added to semen (sperm suspended in glandular secretions)
- **Urethra**: a canal that passes through the prostate gland, enters the penis, and conveys the semen for expulsion from the body during ejaculation

The male reproductive viscera are summarized in the following table.

FEATURE	CHARACTERISTICS
Testes	Develop in retroperitoneal abdominal wall and descend into scrotum
Epididymis	Consists of head, body, and tail; functions in maturation and storage of sperm
Ductus (vas) deferens	Passes in spermatic cord through inguinal canal to join duct of seminal vesicle (ejaculatory duct)
Seminal vesicles	Secrete alkaline seminal fluid
Prostate gland	Surrounds prostatic urethra and secretes prostatic fluid

The pelvic extent of the ductus deferens, the seminal vesicles, and prostate gland lie deep to the peritoneum of the male pelvis. The peritoneum reflects off of the pelvic walls, passes over the superior aspect of the bladder and onto the anterior and lateral aspects of the lower rectum. The trough formed by this peritoneal reflection between the bladder anteriorly and the rectum posteriorly is called the **rectovesical pouch**, and is the lowest extent of the abdominopelvic peritoneal cavity in the male (in the sitting or standing position).

The seminal vesicles produce a viscous, alkaline fluid (about 70% of the seminal fluid in semen) that helps to both nourish the spermatozoa and protect them from the acidic environment of the female vagina. The prostate produces about 20% of the semen (spermatozoa plus the glandular secretions) and consists of a thin, milky, slightly alkaline secretion that helps to liquefy the rather coagulated semen after it is deposited in the female vagina. The prostatic secretion also contains citric acid, proteolytic enzymes, sugars, phosphate, and various ions (calcium, sodium, potassium, etc.). Each ejaculation contains about 2 to 6 ml of semen, has a pH of about 7 to 8, and normally contains from 150 to 600 million spermatozoa.

COLOR the following features of the male reproductive system, using a different color for each feature:
- ☐ **1. Ductus deferens**
- ☐ **2. Testis**
- ☐ **3. Epididymis**
- ☐ **4. Prostate gland**
- ☐ **5. Seminal vesicle**

Clinical Note:

Benign prostatic hypertrophy (BPH) is fairly common and usually occurs in aging males (90% of men over the age of 80 will have some BPH). This growth can lead to symptoms that may include urinary urgency, decreased stream force, frequency of urination, and nocturia (frequent nighttime urges to urinate).

Prostate cancer is the second most common visceral cancer in males (lung cancer is first) and the second leading cause of death in men older than 50 years. Seventy percent of the cancers arise in the outer gland (adenocarcinomas) and are palpable by digital rectal examination.

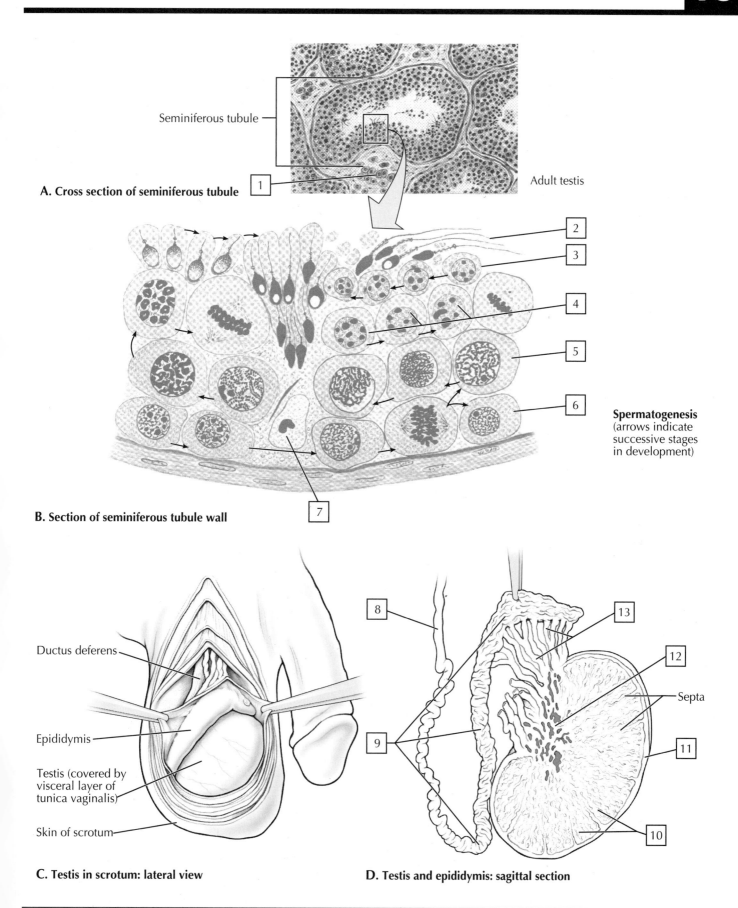

A. Cross section of seminiferous tubule

Seminiferous tubule

1

Adult testis

Spermatogenesis
(arrows indicate
successive stages
in development)

B. Section of seminiferous tubule wall

Ductus deferens

Epididymis

Testis (covered by
visceral layer of
tunica vaginalis)

Skin of scrotum

C. Testis in scrotum: lateral view

Septa

D. Testis and epididymis: sagittal section

Urethra

The male urethra is about 20 cm long and descriptively is divided into three parts:

- **Prostatic urethra**: proximal portion of the male urethra that runs through the prostate gland
- **Membranous urethra**: short, middle portion that is enveloped by the external urethral sphincter (skeletal muscle)
- **Spongy (penile, cavernous) urethra**: courses through the bulb of the penis, the pendulous portion of the penis and the glans penis to open at the external urethral orifice

As the prostatic urethra leaves the urinary bladder, it is surrounded by a sphincter of smooth muscle, the **internal urethral sphincter**. This sphincter is under sympathetic control and closes off the urethra during ejaculation so that semen cannot pass into the bladder and urine into the urethra. The membranous urethra also is surrounded by a sphincter, the **external urethral sphincter**, which is skeletal muscle and innervated by branches of the **pudendal nerve** (somatic control). We have voluntary control of this sphincter.

The proximal portion of the spongy urethra receives the openings of two small glands, the **bulbo-urethral (Cowper's) glands**, which reside in the external urethral sphincter (deep transverse perineal muscle). These pea-sized glands secrete a clear, viscous alkaline mucus. Before ejaculation, these glands lubricate the lumen of the spongy urethra and neutralize its acidic environment, thus preparing the way for the semen.

Penis

The penis provides a common outlet for urine and semen and is the copulatory organ in the male. It is composed of three bodies of erectile tissue:

- **Corpora cavernosa**: two lateral erectile bodies that begin along the ischiopubic ramus and meet at about the level of the pubic symphysis to form the dorsal columns of the pendulous portion of the penis
- **Corpus spongiosum**: a single erectile body of tissue the begins in the midline of the perineum (bulb of the penis) and joins with the corpora cavernosa to form the ventral aspect of the pendulous portion of the penis (contains the spongy urethra)

The proximal portion of each of these cavernous bodies (the parts residing in the perineum) is covered by a thin layer of skeletal muscle (ischiocavernosus and bulbospongiosus muscle; see Plate 3-16), but the distal two thirds of the three erectile bodies are wrapped in a dense connective tissue fascial sleeve **(Buck's fascia)**. The corpus spongiosum contains the spongy urethra and possesses less erectile tissue, so as not to obstruct the flow of semen during ejaculation by compressing the urethral lumen. Erection is achieved by parasympathetic stimulation, which relaxes the smooth muscle of the arterial walls supplying the erectile tissue and allows the flow of blood to engorge the erectile tissue sinuses. The erection compresses the veins, thus keeping the blood in the cavernous sinuses to maintain erection.

The spongy urethra passes into a dilated region called the navicular fossa within the glans penis and then terminates at the external urethral orifice. Along its length, the spongy urethra has openings for small urethral mucous glands (of Littre) that lubricate the urethral lumen.

COLOR the following features of the male urethra and penis, using a different color for each feature:

- [ ] 1. **Prostatic urethra**
- [ ] 2. **Membranous urethra**
- [ ] 3. **Bulbo-urethral glands**
- [ ] 4. **Spongy urethra**
- [ ] 5. **Corpora cavernosa**
- [ ] 6. **Corpus spongiosum**
- [ ] 7. **Deep (Buck's) fascia of the penis (in cross section)**

Clinical Note:

Erectile dysfunction (ED) is an inability to achieve and/or maintain penile erection sufficient for sexual intercourse. Its occurrence increases with age and may be caused by a variety of factors, including:

- Depression, anxiety, and stress disorders
- Spinal cord lesions, MS, or prior pelvic surgery
- Vascular factors such as atherosclerosis, high cholesterol, hypertension, diabetes, smoking, and medications used to control these factors
- Hormonal factors

Available drugs to treat ED target the smooth muscle of the penile arteries, causing then to relax so that blood may pass easily into the cavernous sinuses.

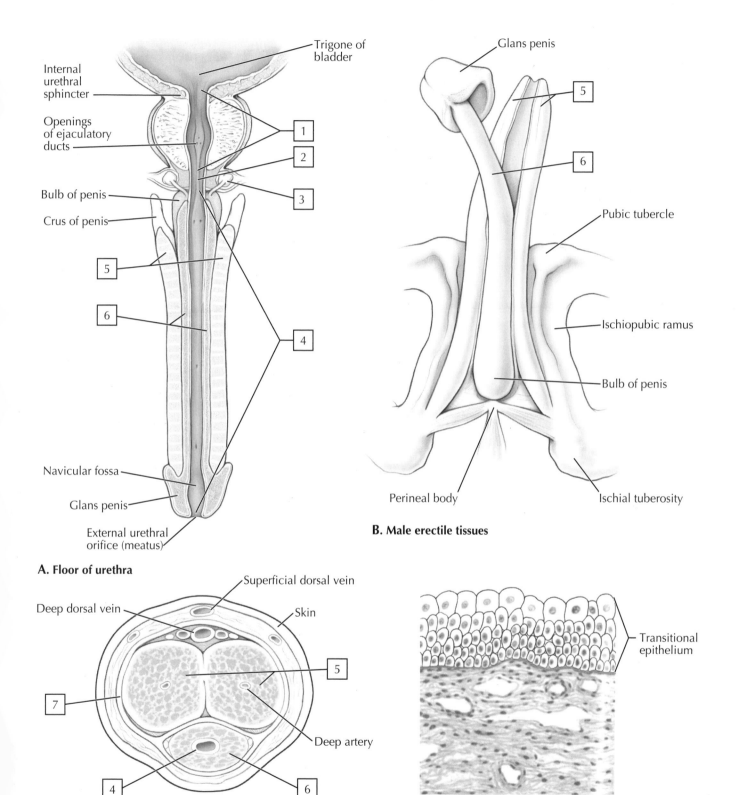

Trigone of bladder

Internal urethral sphincter

Openings of ejaculatory ducts

Bulb of penis

Crus of penis

[1]

[2]

[3]

[5]

[6]

[4]

Navicular fossa

Glans penis

External urethral orifice (meatus)

A. Floor of urethra

Glans penis

[5]

[6]

Pubic tubercle

Ischiopubic ramus

Bulb of penis

Perineal body

Ischial tuberosity

B. Male erectile tissues

Superficial dorsal vein

Deep dorsal vein

Skin

[5]

[7]

Deep artery

[4]

[6]

C. Section through body of penis

Transitional epithelium

D. Transitional epithelium in prostatic and membranous urethra

REVIEW QUESTIONS

1. Fertilization of the human ovum normally occurs in which of the following sites?
   A. Ampulla of the uterine tube
   B. Fimbriated portion of the uterine tube
   C. Fundus of the uterus
   D. Intramural portion of the uterine tube
   E. Isthmus of the uterine tube

2. While the interplay of all essential hormones is important in reproduction, which of the following is most important in maintaining a pregnancy?
   A. Estrogen
   B. FSH
   C. Inhibin
   D. LH
   E. Progesterone

3. Infertility in a 23 year-old man appears to be related to a lack of testosterone. Which of the following cells may be responsible for this condition?
   A. Leydig cells
   B. Seminiferous tubule cells
   C. Sertoli cells
   D. Spermatids
   E. Spermatogonial cells

For each statement below (4-6), color the relevant feature or structure in the image

4. The ovaries are tethered to the uterus by this structure.

5. The vulva is demarcated by this hairless fold of tissue.

6. This portion of the uterus is often involved in cancer, and its epithelium can be easily assessed and monitored clinically by a routine PAP smear.

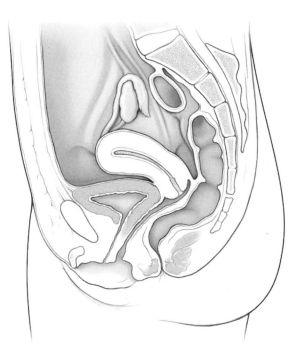

7. If the ovum is fertilized and implants in the uterine wall, it is maintained hormonally during the first 2 or 3 months by this structure. _____

8. Sperm undergo their final maturation in this structure. _____

9. Which male structure accounts for about 70% of the volume of the ejaculate?_____

10. The penile urethra is found in this erectile body of tissue ._____

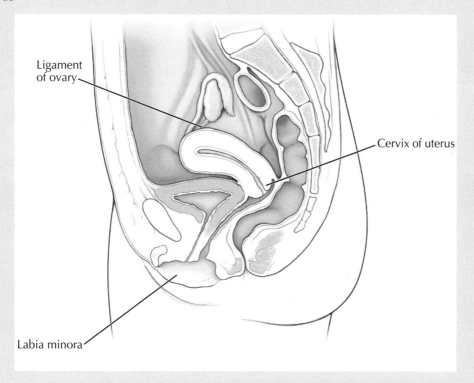

Chapter 11 Endocrine System

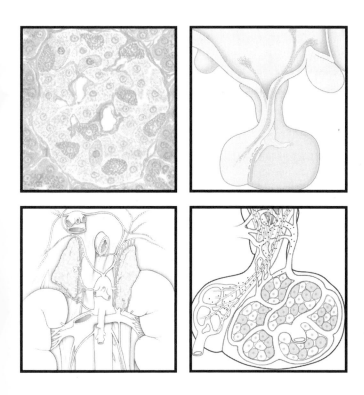

The endocrine system, along with the nervous and immune systems, facilitates communication, integration, and regulation of many of the body's functions. Specifically, the endocrine system interacts with target sites (cells and tissues), many a great distance away, by releasing hormones into the blood stream. Generally speaking, the endocrine glands and hormones share several additional features:

- Secretion is controlled by **feedback mechanisms**
- Hormones bind target receptors on cell membranes or within cells (cytoplasmic or nuclear)
- Hormone action may be slow to appear but may have long-lasting effects
- Hormones are chemically diverse molecules (amines, peptides and proteins, steroids)

Hormones can communicate via a variety of cell-to-cell interactions, including:

- **Autocrine**: on another cell as well as upon itself
- **Paracrine**: directly upon an adjacent or nearby cell
- **Endocrine**: at a great distance by the bloodstream
- **Neurocrine**: like a neurotransmitter except released into the bloodstream

Major hormones and the tissues responsible for their release are summarized in the table below.

Additionally, the **placenta** releases human chorionic gonadotropin (hCG), estrogens, progesterone, and human placental lactogen (hPL), whereas other cells release a variety of growth factors. The endocrinology of the reproductive system will be covered separately in that section.

Actually, there are many other hormones but the listing below covers only the major ones! As you can appreciate, the endocrine system is widespread and critically important in regulating bodily functions.

COLOR the major endocrine organs listed in the table, using a different color for each organ/tissue and noting the major hormone(s) secreted by each organ or tissue. Also note the pathway of a hormone in cell-to-cell communication, by tracing the arrows in red in the bottom diagram.

SUMMARY OF THE MAJOR HORMONES

TISSUE/ORGAN	HORMONE
1 Hypothalamus	Antidiuretic hormone (ADH), oxytocin, thyrotropin-releasing hormone (TRH), corticotropin-releasing hormone (CRH), growth hormone–releasing hormone (GHRH), gonadotropin-releasing hormone (GnRH), somatostatin (SS), dopamine (DA)
2 Pineal gland	Melatonin
3 Anterior pituitary	Adrenocorticotropic hormone (ACTH), thyroid-stimulating hormone (TSH), growth hormone (GH), prolactin, follicle-stimulating hormone (FSH), luteinizing hormone (LH)
3 Posterior pituitary	Oxytocin, vasopressin (antidiuretic hormone, ADH)
4 Thyroid gland	Thyroxine (T_4), triiodothyronine (T_3), calcitonin
5 Parathyroid glands	Parathyroid hormone (PTH)
6 Thymus gland	Thymopoietin, thymulin, thymosin, thymic humeral factor
7 Heart	Atrial natriuretic peptide (ANP)
8 Digestive tract	Gastrin, secretin, cholecystokinin (CCK), motilin, gastric inhibitory peptide (GIP), glucagon, SS, vasoactive intestinal peptide (VIP), ghrelin
Liver	Insulin-like growth factors (IGF)
9 Adrenal glands	Cortisol, aldosterone, androgens, epinephrine (E), norepinephrine (NE)
10 Pancreatic islets	Insulin, glucagon, SS, VIP, pancreatic polypeptide
11 Kidneys	Erythropoietin (EPO), calcitriol, renin, urodilatin
12 Fat	Leptin
13 Ovaries	Estrogens, progestins, inhibin, relaxin
14 Testes	Testosterone, inhibin
White cells and some connective tissue cells	Various cytokines (interleukins, colony-stimulating factors, interferons, tumor necrosis factor [TNF])

Plate 11-1   **Endocrine System**

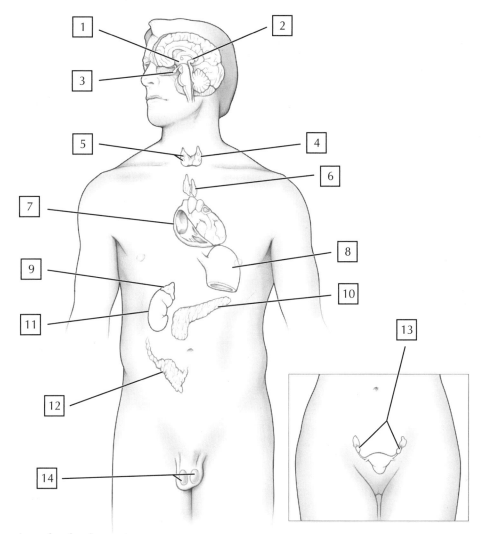

A. Overview of endocrine system

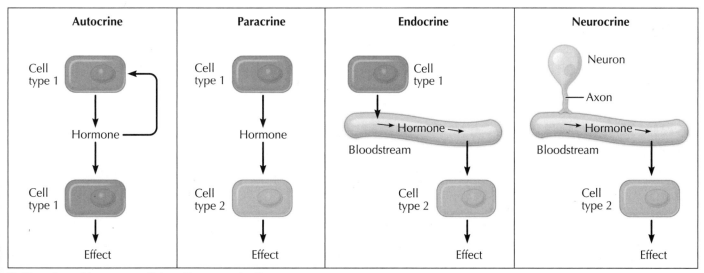

B. Overview of hormone cell-to-cell communication

Netter's Anatomy Coloring Book

Plate 11-1

Hypothalamus

The hypothalamus was reviewed previously (see Plate 4-11) and comprises a portion of the diencephalon along with the thalamus and epithalamus (pineal gland). Functionally, the hypothalamus is very important in visceral control and homeostasis. Its neuroendocrine cells release hormones into the hypothalamic-hypophyseal portal system that stimulate or inhibit the secretory cells of the anterior pituitary gland. Neuroendocrine cells in the hypothalamus (paraventricular and supra-optic nucleus) also send axons into the posterior pituitary gland and median eminence, which really is a downgrowth of the brain's diencephalon. These axons release hormones into the systemic vasculature of the posterior pituitary, although it should be remembered that they are synthesized and initially released from the hypothalamus.

Pituitary Gland

The pituitary gland (hypophysis) lies within a bony seat or "saddle" called the sella turcica of the sphenoid bone and is connected to the overlying hypothalamus by a stalk called the **infundibulum**. This pituitary stalk contains blood vessels and axons originating from several nuclei in the hypothalamus. The pituitary gland has three parts:

- **Anterior lobe**: also called the **adenohypophysis**, it is derived from an upward growth of the ectodermal tissue of the oropharynx (Rathke's pouch) and secretes six different hormones
- **Posterior lobe**: also called the **neurohypophysis**, it is a neural extension of the hypothalamus that contains blood vessels and axonal terminals arising from the paraventricular and supra-optic nuclei of the hypothalamus; releases two hormones
- **Intermediate lobe**: an intervening lobe between the anterior and posterior lobes that is poorly developed in humans, displaying a small cleft or space and intervening connective tissue; has no endocrine function

COLOR the following features of the hypothalamus and pituitary gland, using a different color for each feature:

- [ ] 1. Cells and axons of the paraventricular nucleus of the hypothalamus
- [ ] 2. Cells and axons of the supra-optic nucleus of the hypothalamus
- [ ] 3. Cleft and connective tissue of the intermediate lobe
- [ ] 4. Anterior pituitary
- [ ] 5. Posterior pituitary

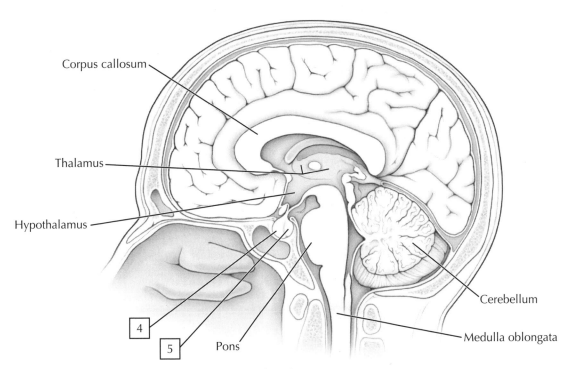

A. Hypothalamus and pituitary gland: midsagittal section

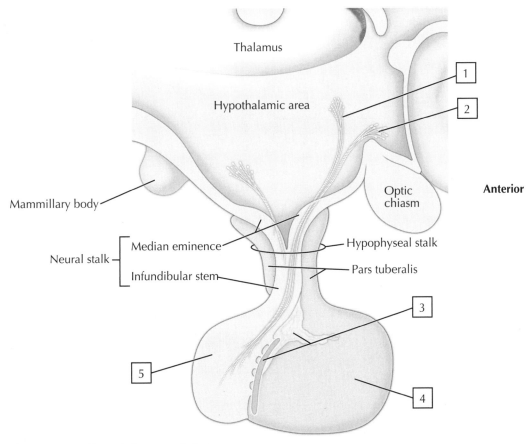

B. Structure of hypothalamus and pituitary

The neuroendocrine cells of the hypothalamus release hormones into the hypothalamic-hypophyseal portal system that stimulate or inhibit the secretory cells of the anterior pituitary. These hormones include (abbreviations from table on Plate 11-1):

- **TRH**: stimulates the release of TSH
- **CRH**: stimulates the release of ACTH
- **GHRH**: stimulates the release of GH
- **SS**: inhibits the release of GH
- **GnRH**: stimulates the release of LH and FSH
- **DA**: inhibits the release of prolactin

The cells of the anterior pituitary are of two primary types (based upon their histological staining characteristics) and release the following hormones:

- **Thyrotropes (somatotropes)**: acidophilic cells (stain red) that secrete **GH**, which stimulates overall body growth, organ growth, increased lean body mass, and bone growth
- **Lactotropes (mammotropes)**: acidophilic cells (stain red) that secrete prolactin, which stimulates breast development and promotes milk production
- **Thyrotropes**: basophilic cells (stain blue) that secrete **TSH**, which stimulates the development and release of thyroxine from the thyroid gland
- **Corticotropes**: basophilic cells (stain blue) that secrete **ACTH**, which stimulates the adrenal cortex to release cortisol
- **Gonadotropes**: basophilic cells (stain blue) that secretes **LH** and **FSH**, which promote gamete production and hormone synthesis in the gonads

The axons that course from the hypothalamus to the posterior pituitary (neurohypophysis) can either store the hormones in the axon terminals until stimulated to release them or can release them immediately into the capillary system of the gland. Their release is controlled by neuronal and hormonal input on the hypothalamus. These hormones include:

- **Oxytocin**: stimulates milk ejection from the breast and uterine contractions during labor
- **ADH**: causes vasoconstriction and an increase in blood pressure (that is why ADH also is called **vasopressin**), and acts on the kidney to reabsorb water and help the body retain fluids

COLOR the following features of hormonal release from the pituitary gland, using the suggested colors for each feature:

- [ ] 1. **Supra-optic and paraventricular neurons and their axons (purple)**
- [ ] 2. **Acidophils of the anterior pituitary (red)**
- [ ] 3. **Basophils of the anterior pituitary (blue)**
- [ ] 4. **GH (arrow) targeting the liver (orange)**
- [ ] 5. **TSH (arrow) targeting the thyroid gland (brown)**
- [ ] 6. **ACTH (arrow) targeting the adrenal cortex (yellow)**
- [ ] 7. **FSH (arrows) targeting the testis and ovary (blue)**
- [ ] 8. **LH (arrows) targeting the testis and ovary (red)**
- [ ] 9. **Prolactin (arrow) targeting the breast (green)**
- [ ] 10. **Liver's release of insulin-like growth factors (IGFs) (pink)**

Plate 11-3   **Endocrine System**

Pituitary Function

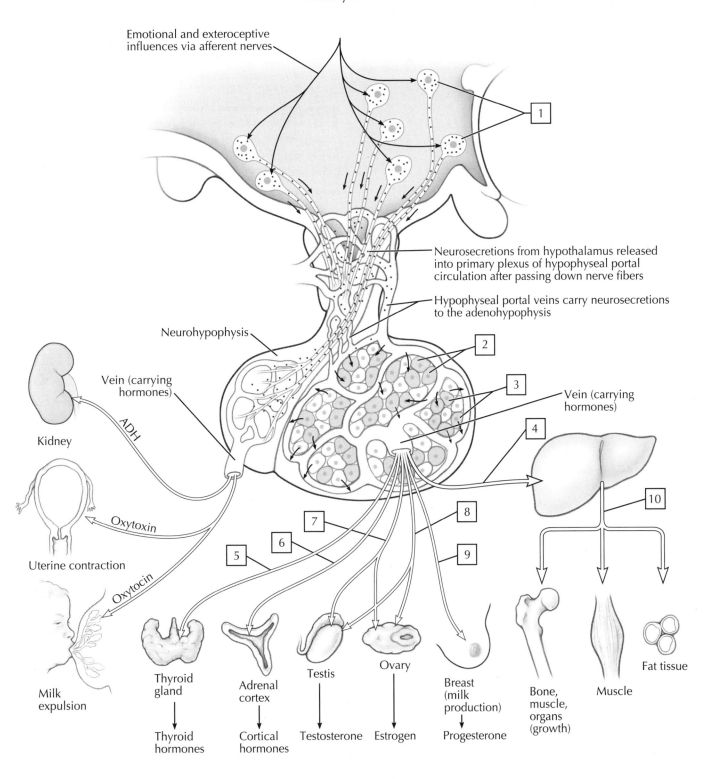

Emotional and exteroceptive
influences via afferent nerves

1

Neurosecretions from hypothalamus released
into primary plexus of hypophyseal portal
circulation after passing down nerve fibers

Hypophyseal portal veins carry neurosecretions
to the adenohypophysis

Neurohypophysis

2

Vein (carrying
hormones)

3

Vein (carrying
hormones)

Kidney

ADH

4

10

Vein (carrying
hormones)

Uterine contraction

Oxytoxin

5

6

7

8

9

Oxytocin

Milk
expulsion

Thyroid
gland

Adrenal
cortex

Testis

Ovary

Breast
(milk
production)

Bone,
muscle,
organs
(growth)

Muscle

Fat tissue

Thyroid
hormones

Cortical
hormones

Testosterone

Estrogen

Progesterone

Thyroid

The thyroid gland is a **ductless endocrine gland** that weighs about 20 g and consists of a right and left lobe joined by an isthmus. In about 50% of the population there is a small pyramidal lobe extending cranially from the gland. The thyroid lies anterior to the trachea and just inferior to the cricoid cartilage and, like most endocrine organs, has a rich vascular supply.

FEATURE	CHARACTERISTICS
Lobes	Right and left, with a thin isthmus joining them
Blood supply	Superior and inferior thyroid arteries
Venous drainage	Superior, middle, and inferior thyroid veins
Pyramidal lobe	Variable (50% of time) superior extension of thyroid tissue

The thyroid is composed of follicles formed by surrounding epithelial cells that synthesize, store, and secrete thyroxine (T_4, 90% of its secretion) and triiodothyronine (T_3). The follicular cells actively take up iodine to iodinate tyrosine molecules, forming T_3 and T_4, and storing them linked to thyroglobulin in the thyroid follicle (the only endocrine gland that stores its hormone to any significant degree). When stimulated by TSH, the thyroglobulin is endocytosed and T_3 and T_4 are released into the bloodstream. T_4 is really a prehormone that is converted to the more active T_3 by the target tissues. These hormones:

- Increase the metabolic rate of tissues
- Increase the consumption of oxygen
- Increases heart rate, ventilation, and renal function
- Is needed for GH production and is especially important for CNS growth

COLOR the following features of the thyroid gland, using a different color for each feature:

- [ ] **1. Superior thyroid arteries, from the external carotid artery, supplying the gland and inferior thyroid arteries from the subclavian artery**
- [ ] **2. Internal jugular veins and their branches draining the thyroid gland**
- [ ] **3. Internal carotid arteries**
- [ ] **4. Thyroid gland, the isthmus and pyramidal lobe**
- [ ] **5. Follicular cells surrounding a thyroglobulin-filled follicle**

Parathyroids

The parathyroid glands are paired superior and inferior glands located on the posterior aspect of the thyroid gland. Although there are usually four glands, their number and location can vary. The parathyroid glands secrete **PTH** in response to a decrease of calcium in the bloodstream. PTH acts on bone to cause resorption and release of calcium, and acts on the kidney to reabsorb calcium. PTH also alters vitamin D metabolism, which is critical for calcium absorption from the GI tract.

COLOR the following features of the parathyroid glands, using a different color for each feature:

- [ ] **6. Parathyroids (superior and inferior pairs)**
- [ ] **7. Target tissue sites (bone, kidney, small intestine)**

Clinical Note:

Graves' disease, an autoimmune disease, is the most common cause of hyperthyroidism in patients younger than 40 years, and affects women seven times more frequently than men. Excess synthesis and release of thyroid hormone results in thyrotoxicosis, which upregulates tissue metabolism and leads to sweating, nervousness, excitability, insomnia, goiter (enlarged thyroid gland), warm and velvety skin, an increase in appetite, weight loss, shortness of breath, muscular weakness, and exophthalmos (bulging eyes).

Hypothyroidism is a disease in which the thyroid gland produces inadequate amounts of thyroid hormone to meet the body's needs. It is more common in women than men and leads to dry, brittle hair; lethargy; memory impairment; slow speech; edema of the face; sensations of coldness; diminished sweating; slow pulse; enlarged heart; course, dry skin; and muscle weakness.

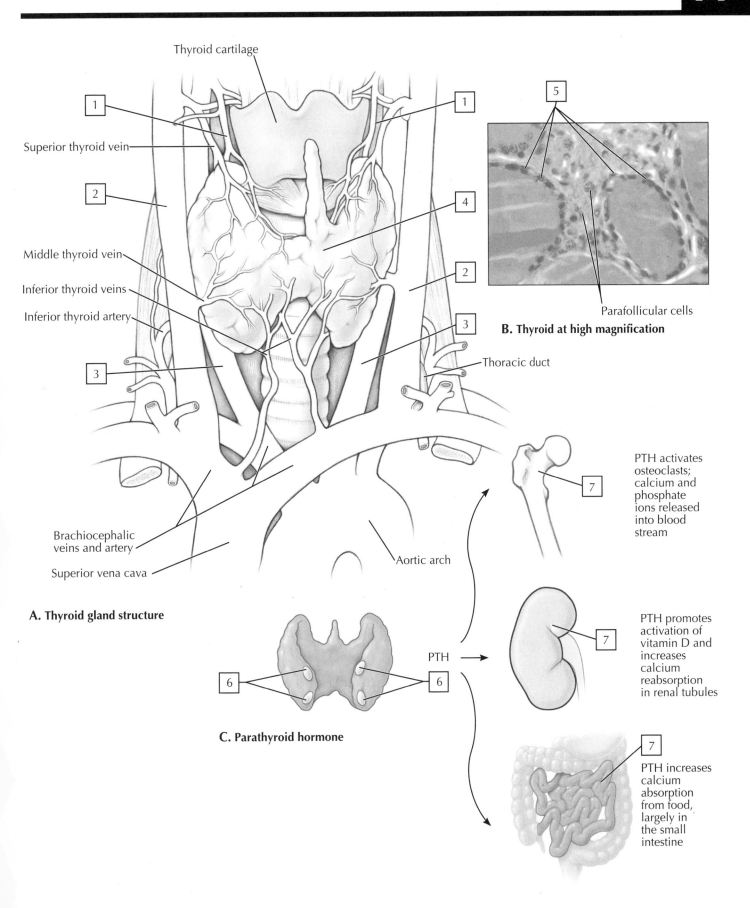

Thyroid cartilage

1

1

Superior thyroid vein

2

Middle thyroid vein

Inferior thyroid veins

Inferior thyroid artery

4

2

3

3

3

Thoracic duct

Brachiocephalic veins and artery

Superior vena cava

Aortic arch

A. Thyroid gland structure

5

Parafollicular cells

B. Thyroid at high magnification

7

PTH activates osteoclasts; calcium and phosphate ions released into blood stream

7

PTH promotes activation of vitamin D and increases calcium reabsorption in renal tubules

PTH

6

6

C. Parathyroid hormone

7

PTH increases calcium absorption from food, largely in the small intestine

The paired adrenal (suprarenal) glands are **retroperitoneal ductless endocrine glands** that are nestled above the superior pole of each kidney, below the overlying diaphragm. Each gland normally weighs about 7 to 8 g, is highly vascularized, and consists of an outer **cortex** and an inner **medulla**. The right adrenal gland is often pyramidal in shape and the left gland is semilunar in shape.

Adrenal Cortex

Both the adrenal cortex and medulla are richly vascularized by a radially oriented plexus of vessels. The cortex produces more than two dozen steroid hormones and structurally is divided into three distinct histologic regions:

- **Zona glomerulosa**: the outer cortical region that lies just beneath the gland's capsule and produces mineralocorticoids, principally aldosterone
- **Zona fasciculata**: a middle region that produces glucocorticoids, principally cortisol (most important in humans), corticosterone, and cortisone
- **Zona reticularis**: the innermost cortical region that produces androgens

Aldosterone plays a critical role in regulating the extracellular fluid compartment (ECF) and blood volumes and in maintaining potassium balance. When the ECF compartment and blood volumes are reduced (e.g., from diarrhea or hemorrhage), renin is released from the kidney, which increases angiotensin II levels. Angiotensin II is a potent stimulator of aldosterone secretion, which then acts on sweat glands, salivary glands, the intestines, and kidneys to retain sodium and water in an effort to increase ECF and blood volume.

Cortisol has both direct and indirect actions on a number of tissues, and is considered a hormone that is released during stress:

- Causes muscle wasting
- Fat deposition
- Hyperglycemia
- Insulin resistance
- Osteoporosis
- Immune suppression (anti-inflammatory) and anti-allergic actions
- Decreased connective tissue production leading to poor wound healing
- Increased neural excitability
- Increased glomerular filtration rate (water diuresis), sodium retention, and potassium loss

Adrenal androgens play a role in puberty in both sexes and in females are the primary source of circulating androgens. They are responsible for the growth of pubic and axillary hair in women, whereas testicular testosterone does this in males. In general, the effects of androgens are anabolic, leading to increased muscle mass and bone formation. They also cause sebaceous gland hypertrophy (leading to acne), hairline recession, and growth of facial hair (think of the effects of anabolic steroid abuse by athletes).

Adrenal Medulla

The medulla produces two hormones, which classically have been thought of as neurotransmitters, but in this instance are true hormones, because they are released into the bloodstream. The cells of the adrenal medulla are actually the **postganglionic elements of the sympathetic division of the autonomic nervous system** (ANS) and produce the "fight or flight" response. The two hormones are:

- Epinephrine (E): accounts for about 80% of the medullary secretions
- Norepinephrine (NE): 20% of the medullary secretions, but plays a larger role as a neurotransmitter in the ANS

COLOR the following features of the adrenal gland, using a different color for each feature:

- [ ] **1. Adrenal glands**
- [ ] **2. Capsule of the gland (inset)**
- [ ] **3. Zona glomerulosa (aldosterone) (inset)**
- [ ] **4. Zona fasciculata (cortisol) and its cells (inset)**
- [ ] **5. Zona reticularis (androgens) and its cells (inset)**
- [ ] **6. Medulla (E and NE) and its cells (inset)**

Clinical Note:

Addison's disease is also referred to as chronic adrenal cortical insufficiency, and this disease usually does not manifest itself until about 90% of the adrenal cortex is destroyed. Manifestations include:

- Darkening of the hair
- Freckling of the skin; skin pigmentation
- Hypotension
- Loss of weight, anorexia, vomiting, and diarrhea
- Muscular weakness

Cushing's syndrome is caused by any condition that results in an increase in glucocorticoid levels. Clinical features include:

- Red cheeks and a "moon" face
- Shoulder fat pads ("buffalo hump") and thin arms and legs
- Bruises and thin skin
- Osteoporosis
- Pendulous abdomen with red skin striae
- Poor wound healing

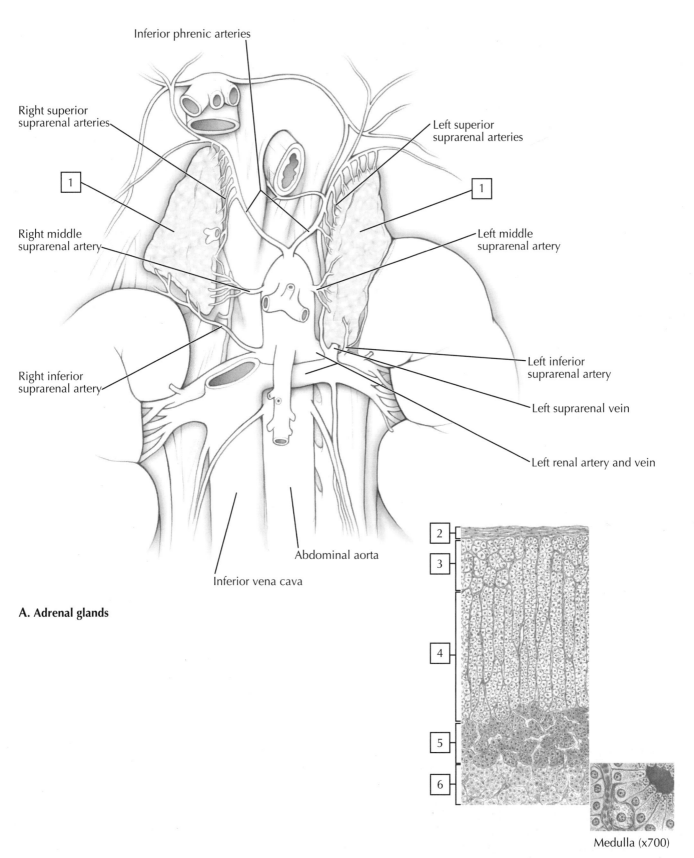

Inferior phrenic arteries

Right superior
suprarenal arteries

Left superior
suprarenal arteries

1

1

Right middle
suprarenal artery

Left middle
suprarenal artery

Left inferior
suprarenal artery

Right inferior
suprarenal artery

Left suprarenal vein

Left renal artery and vein

Abdominal aorta

Inferior vena cava

A. Adrenal glands

2

3

4

5

6

Medulla (x700)

B. Normal human suprarenal gland

The endocrine pancreas is represented by clusters of islet cells (of Langerhans), a heterogeneous population of cells responsible for the elaboration and secretion primarily of (several other hormones also are elaborated by the islets to a lesser extent):

- **Glucagon**: secreted by the alpha cells
- **Insulin**: secreted by the beta cells
- **Somatostatin (SS)**: secreted by the delta cells

Glucagon is a **fuel-mobilization hormone** that acts on the liver to break down glycogen and stimulates hepatic gluconeogenesis from amino acids. This results in an **increase in blood glucose concentration**. Glucagon also acts on adipose tissue to stimulate lipolysis and the release of fatty acids. The net effect of glucagon is that glucose, fatty acid, and keto acid levels in the bloodstream increase.

Insulin is a **fuel-storage hormone**. Insulin secretion increases in the presence of an increase in plasma glucose levels, especially after a meal. The major fuels of the body are glucose, fatty acids, and keto acids (derived from fatty acid metabolism). Insulin **stimulates the uptake of glucose** into cells, where it is stored in the form of glycogen (especially in the liver and muscle). Insulin also stimulates fat synthesis and inhibits lipolysis. Finally, insulin stimulates the uptake of amino acids into cells and their storage as protein. The net effect is that blood levels of glucose and keto acids are decreased.

Little is known about the role of SS from the pancreas. It may inhibit the release of many of the GI and pancreatic exocrine and endocrine secretions, and it is already known to inhibit GH release.

COLOR the following features of the endocrine pancreas, using the colors suggested for each feature:

- ☐ 1. **Pancreas (head, uncinate process, body, and tail) (green; see Plate 8-10)**
- ☐ 2. **Delta cells (light blue) (SS)**
- ☐ 3. **Alpha cells (orange) (glucagon)**
- ☐ 4. **Acini of the exocrine pancreas outside the islets (red)**
- ☐ 5. **Beta cells (yellow) (insulin)**

Clinical Note:

Diabetes mellitus (DM) affects about 15 million people in the United States, and that percentage is probably an underestimate. There are two types of DM:

- **Type I:** insulin-dependent DM, in which insulin is absent or almost absent in the pancreatic islets because of the destruction of the islets by the body's immune system (autoimmune disease), thus requiring exogenous insulin administration
- **Type II:** non–insulin-dependent DM, in which insulin is present in the plasma at normal or above normal levels but the target cells are hyporesponsive to the insulin; about 90% of DM is of the type II variety

Vascular complications account for about 80% of all deaths related to DM, and can include:

- **Retinopathy:** vascular microaneurysms and hemorrhages in vessels supplying the retina
- **Ischemic stroke:** cerebrovascular thrombosis, often from plaques that rupture in the carotid or cerebral vessels
- **Myocardial infarct:** occlusion of the coronary arterial branches supplying the heart
- **Kidney disease:** glomerulosclerosis of the renal glomerular vessels
- **Atherosclerosis:** plaque formation in the aorta and its major branches

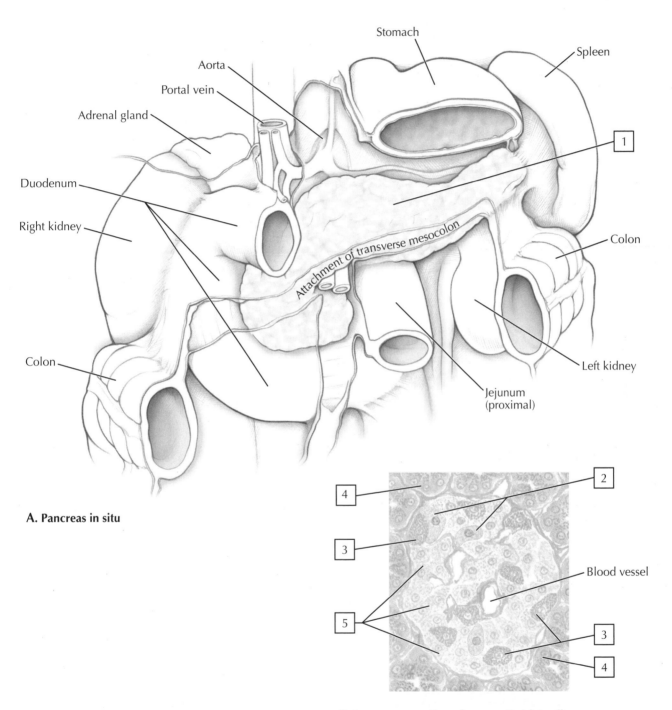

Stomach

Spleen

Aorta

Portal vein

Adrenal gland

1

Duodenum

Colon

Right kidney

Attachment of transverse mesocolon

Left kidney

Colon

Jejunum
(proximal)

A. Pancreas in situ

4

2

3

5

Blood vessel

3

4

B. Low-power section of pancreatic islet cells

Puberty usually occurs between the ages of 10 and 14 years and marks the maturation of the reproductive organs in both sexes, as well as the development of the secondary sex characteristics. One to two years before puberty, adrenal androgen levels increase (adrenarche) and are responsible in both sexes for the early development of pubic and axillary hair and an increase in growth.

At puberty, the following events occur:
• Hypothalamus increases the release of GnRH
• GnRH stimulates the release of LH and FSH by the anterior pituitary
• In females, LH targets the ovary to produce androgens that are then converted to estrogens (E), LH also stimulates the production of progesterone (P), and FSH stimulates the production of E from androgens
• E then induces the changes in the accessory sex organs and secondary sex characteristics seen in puberty
• In males, LH acts on the testes to stimulate the production of testosterone (T), and T and FSH together act on the testes to promote development of the spermatozoa
• T induces the changes in the accessory sex organs and secondary sex characteristics seen in puberty

The secondary sex characteristics commonly associated with puberty are illustrated and listed in the facing page.

COLOR the features of puberty summarized in the illustration, using the colors suggested for each feature:

- [ ] 1. ACTH arrow (targeting the adrenal glands) (green)
- [ ] 2. FSH arrow (targeting the ovaries and testes) (orange)
- [ ] 3. LH arrow (targeting the ovaries and testes) (brown)
- [ ] 4. Adrenal androgens (pink)
- [ ] 5. Adrenal cortex (yellow)
- [ ] 6. Ovaries (pink/light red)
- [ ] 7. Testes (gray)
- [ ] 8. Estrogen arrow (targets female sex characteristics) (red)
- [ ] 9. Estrogen arrow (targets male sex characteristics) (blue)
- [ ] 10. Progesterone arrow (targets female sex characteristics) (gold)
- [ ] 11. Testosterone arrow (targets male sex characteristics) (purple)

Plate 11-7   **Endocrine System**

Onset of Puberty

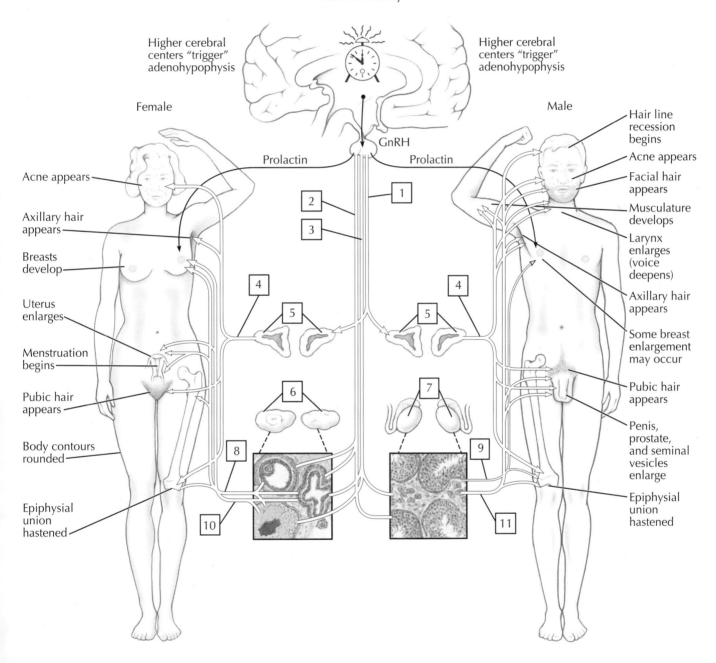

Higher cerebral
centers "trigger"
adenohypophysis

Higher cerebral
centers "trigger"
adenohypophysis

Female

Male

GnRH

Prolactin

Prolactin

Acne appears

Hair line
recession
begins

Acne appears

Facial hair
appears

Axillary hair
appears

Musculature
develops

Breasts
develop

Larynx
enlarges
(voice
deepens)

Uterus
enlarges

Axillary hair
appears

Menstruation
begins

Some breast
enlargement
may occur

Pubic hair
appears

Pubic hair
appears

Body contours
rounded

Penis,
prostate,
and seminal
vesicles
enlarge

Epiphysial
union
hastened

Epiphysial
union
hastened

1
2
3
4
4
5
5
6
7
8
9
10
11

Digestive System Hormones

It probably is fair to say that the largest endocrine organ in the human body is the gastrointestinal (GI) tract. The complex physiology of the GI tract involving digestion, absorption, peristalsis, metabolism, and storage is regulated by the complex and integrated actions of the endocrine, neuroendocrine, nervous, and immune systems. The sheer number of different hormones involved is beyond the scope of this book, but some of the "major players" deserve to be introduced.

The composition of **saliva** is modified by the actions of ADH and aldosterone, whereas major GI hormones regulate the **secretory activity** of the stomach, pancreas, and liver. Likewise, **hormones** such as insulin, glucagon, cortisol, epinephrine, norepinephrine, and growth hormone play key roles in organic metabolism. The regulation of the body's energy stores, eating and fasting, obesity control, and thermoregulation all involve the integrated mechanisms of the endocrine and neuroendocrine systems.

However, when focusing principally on the abdominal GI tract, five major hormones play key roles. Dozens of other minor hormones and neuroendocrine molecules are necessary for optimal functioning, but these five are primary and are summarized in the following table.

Universal among these hormones is the fact that they participate in a **feedback mechanism** that regulates the internal environment of the GI tract and they act on multiple target cells. Even between meals, hormones like motilin initiate the "**migrating myoelectric complex**" (MMC), which consists of waves of peristalsis that clean the GI tract of residual food particles and move them into the colon. This essentially flushes the stomach and small intestine of bacteria that might otherwise flourish, multiply there, and cause disease.

COLOR the following arrows demonstrating the target sites of major GI hormones, using the suggested color for each hormone's arrow:

- [ ] **1. Gastrin (red)**
- [ ] **2. Secretin (blue)**
- [ ] **3. CCK (green)**
- [ ] **4. GIP (yellow)**
- [ ] **5. Motilin (orange)**

HORMONE	NEUROENDOCRINE CELL TYPE AND LOCATION	STIMULUS FOR SECRETION	PRIMARY ACTION	OTHER ACTIONS
Gastrin	**G cell** Stomach, duodenum	Vagus, organ distention, amino acids	Stimulate HCl secretion	Inhibit gastric emptying
Secretin	**S cell** Duodenum	Acid	Stimulate pancreatic ductal cell H_2O and HCO_3^- secretion	Inhibit gastric secretion, inhibit gastric motility, and stimulate bile duct secretion of H_2O and HCO_3^-
Cholecystokinin	**I cell** Duodenum, jejunum	Fat, vagus	Stimulate enzyme secretion by pancreatic acinar cells and contract the gallbladder	Inhibit gastric motility
GIP	**K cell** Duodenum, jejunum	Fat	Inhibit gastric secretion and motility	Stimulate insulin secretion
Motilin	**M cell** Duodenum, jejunum		Increased motility and initiates the MMC	

Plate 11-8   **Endocrine System**

Major GI Hormones

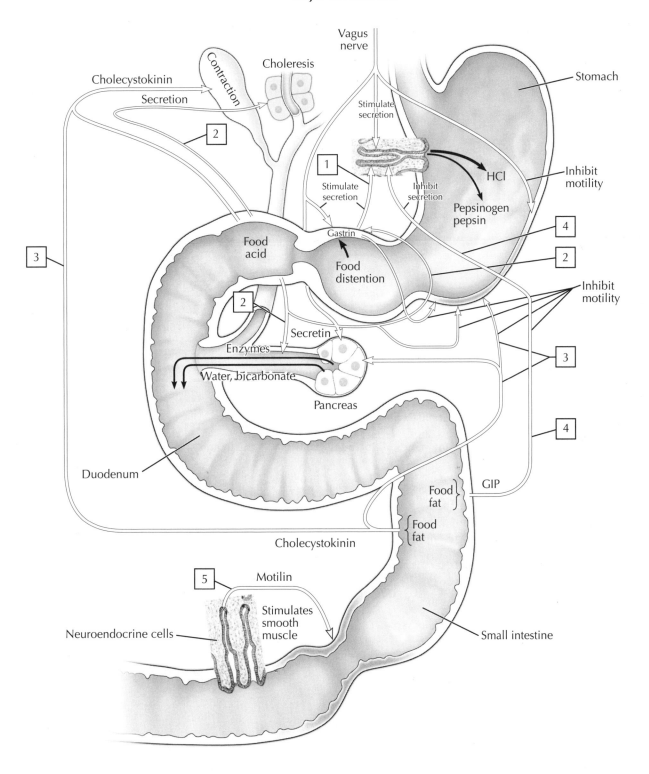

Cholecystokinin

Contraction

Choleresis

Secretion

2

Vagus nerve

Stomach

Stimulate secretion

1

Stimulate secretion

Inhibit secretion

HCl

Inhibit motility

Pepsinogen pepsin

4

3

Food acid

Gastrin

Food distention

2

2

Inhibit motility

Secretin

Enzymes

3

Water, bicarbonate

Pancreas

Duodenum

4

Food fat

GIP

Food fat

Cholecystokinin

5

Motilin

Stimulates smooth muscle

Neuroendocrine cells

Small intestine

1. Which of the following endocrine organs is responsible for uterine contraction, milk expulsion, and concentration of the urine?
   A. Adrenal cortex
   B. Kidney
   C. Ovary
   D. Parathyroids
   E. Posterior pituitary

2. When a hormone is released into the bloodstream by an axon, which of the following types of cell-cell communication is occurring?
   A. Autocrine
   B. Endocrine
   C. Holocrine
   D. Neurocrine
   E. Paracrine

3. Graves' disease is an autoimmune disease caused by the excess synthesis and release of thyroid hormone. Which of the following symptoms is most likely to be observed in this condition?
   A. Coldness
   B. Dry skin
   C. Edema of the face
   D. Excitability
   E. Slow pulse

4. Cushing's syndrome is characterized by an increase secretion of what hormone from which gland (be specific)? _____
   _____

5. One hormone in particular is known to be a "fuel-mobilization" hormone and another a "fuel-storage" hormone. Name these two hormones. _____

6. Which endocrine organ (fat excluded) is probably the largest of the endocrine organs? _____

For each description below (7-10), color the appropriate endocrine organ in the image

7. This endocrine organ regulates the circulating amounts of calcium (an increase) in the bloodstream.

8. Somatostatin (SS), released from this structure, inhibits the release of growth hormone (GH).

9. This endocrine gland releases cortisol, aldosterone, androgens, epinephrine, and norepinephrine.

10. Gonadotropes are released by basophilic cells in this endocrine organ.

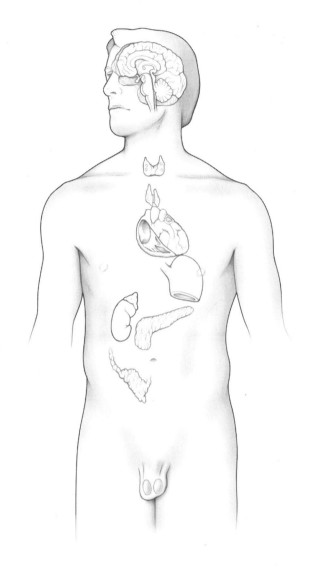

1. E

2. D

3. D

4. Glucocorticoids (principally cortisol) from the adrenal cortex (zona fasciculata)

5. Glucagon and insulin (from the pancreas)

6. Gastrointestinal tract

7. Parathyroid gland (PTH)

8. Hypothalamus

9. Adrenal gland

10. Anterior pituitary gland

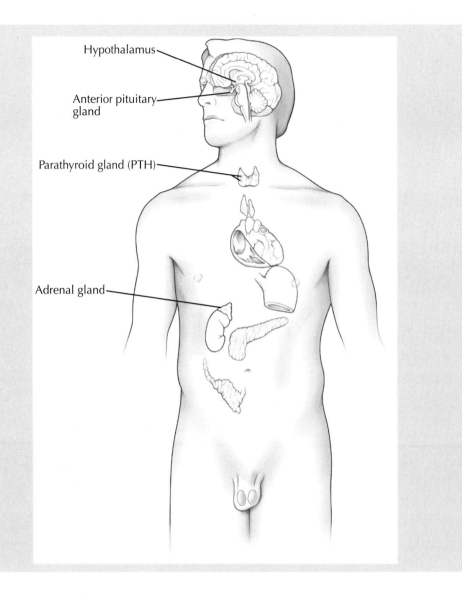

Hypothalamus

Anterior pituitary gland

Parathyroid gland (PTH)

Adrenal gland

Index

Note: Locators cited are plate numbers. Numbers in regular type indicate the discussion; **boldface** numbers indicate the art in the plate.

Brachial plexus (Continued)
  terminal branches, 4-29, **4-29**
  trunks, 4-29, **4-29**
Brachial vein, 5-20, **5-20**
Brachialis muscle, 3-19, **3-19**, 3-24, **3-24**
Brachiocephalic trunk, **5-12**, 5-14, **5-14**, **8-4**
Brachiocephalic veins, **5-20**, **6-7**
Brachioradialis muscle, **3-21**, 3-22, **3-22**, 3-24, **3-24**
Brachium (arm), **1-1**
Brain, 1-11, **1-11**
  dural lining, 1-13, **1-13**
  midsagittal and basal anatomy, 4-6, **4-6**
  oxygen consumption, **5-2**
  parts of, 4-4, **4-4**
Brain ventricles, **4-5**, **4-6**
  fourth, 4-17, **4-17**
  lateral, **4-7**, **4-9**, 4-17, **4-17**
  third, 4-17, **4-17**
Brainstem, 1-11, **4-21**
Branches of abdominal aorta, 5-14
Branches of inferior mesenteric artery, 5-15, **5-15**
Branches of superior mesenteric artery, 5-15, **5-15**
Breast, **1-1**, 10-5, **10-5**
Broad ligament of uterus, 10-1, **10-1**
Bronchi
  main, **7-1**, 7-5, **7-5**
  secondary, 7-5, **7-5**
  tertiary, 7-5, **7-5**
Bronchial artery, **5-14**
Bronchioles, 7-5
  terminal, **7-6**
Bronchus-associated lymphatic tissue, 6-6, **6-6**
Buccal (cheek), **1-1**
Buccal artery, **5-9**
Buccal surface, **8-3**
Buccinator muscle, 3-1, **3-1**, **3-2**, **3-5**, **8-2**
Buck's fascia, 10-8, **10-8**
Buffy coat, 5-1, **5-1**
Bulb of penis, **9-5**, **10-8**
Bulb of vestibule, **3-16**, **5-16**, **9-5**, 10-1, **10-1**
Bulbocavernosus muscle, 3-16, **3-16**
Bulbospongiosus muscle, **5-16**, **10-1**
Bulbourethral gland, **3-16**, **9-5**, **10-6**, 10-8, **10-8**
Bundle branches, ventricular, 5-5, **5-5**
Bursa, 1-9
  iliopectineal, **2-16**
  omental, 8-5, **8-5**, **8-6**
  shoulder joint, 2-11, **2-11**
  suprapatellar, **2-18**

C

Calcaneocuboid joint, 2-20
Calcaneofibular ligament, 2-20, **2-20**
Calcaneus (heel of foot), **1-1**, 2-19, **2-19**
Calcarine fissure, **4-24**
Calcium deficiency, 2-1
Calf, **1-1**
Calices, renal, 9-2, **9-2**
Calvaria, 2-2
Cancer
  breast, 10-5
  colorectal, 8-8
  lung, 7-5
  pancreatic, 8-10

Cancer (Continued)
  prostate, 10-6
  testicular, 10-7
Canines, 2-4, **2-4**, 8-3, **8-3**
Capillaries, **4-2**, 5-7, **5-7**
  alveolar, 7-6
  glomerular, endothelium of, 9-3, **9-3**
Capillary endothelial cell, 7-6, **7-6**
Capillary loops of dermal papillae, **1-12**
Capillary lumen, **7-6**
Capillary plexus of alveoli, **7-6**
Capitate, 2-13, **2-13**, **2-14**, **3-23**
Capsular ligaments of shoulder, 2-11, **2-11**
Capsule
  of adrenal gland, 11-5, **11-5**
  Bowman's, 9-3, **9-3**
  fibrous
    renal, **9-2**
    of synovial joint, **1-8**
  of lymph node, **6-1**
  splenic, 6-5, **6-5**
Carbon dioxide diffusion pathways, **7-6**
Carcinomas, 1-5
Cardiac muscle, 1-10
Cardiac notch, **7-5**
Cardiac part of stomach, 8-6, **8-6**
Cardiac plexus, **4-19**
Cardiac tamponade, 5-3
Cardiac veins, 5-6, **5-6**
Cardiovascular system
  general organization, 5-2, **5-2**
  prenatal and postnatal circulation, 5-22, **5-22**
Carotid canal, **2-3**
Carotid sheath, 3-7, **3-7**
Carotid triangle of neck, 3-7, **3-7**
Carpal bones, **1-7**, 2-13, **2-13**
Carpal tunnel, 2-13
Carpometacarpal joints, 2-14
Carpus (wrist), **1-1**
Cartilage, **1-6**
  articular, **1-8**, 2-1, **2-1**, **2-12**, 2-16
  contributing to nose, 7-2, **7-2**
  costal, 2-8, **2-8**
  elastic, 1-7
  hyaline, 1-7
  laryngeal, 3-6, **3-6**, **7-4**
  septal, 2-3, 7-2, **7-2**
  thyroid, **3-5**, **7-1**
  tracheal, 7-5
Cartilaginous joints, 1-8, **1-8**
  primary, 2-8
Cataract, 4-23
Catheterization of chest wall, 3-11
Cauda equina, 4-13, **4-13**, **4-18**
Caudal (inferior), 1-2, **1-2**
Caudate nucleus, **4-5**, 4-7, **4-7**, **4-9**
Cavernous venous sinus, 5-11, **5-11**
Cecum, 8-1, **8-1**, **8-7**, 8-8, **8-8**
Celiac trunk, 5-14, **5-14**, 5-15, **5-15**, 5-22, **8-5**, **8-10**
Cell body, **4-1**
Cell-mediated response, 6-3
Cell nucleus, 1-4, **1-4**
Cell-to-cell communication, hormonal, 11-1, **11-1**
Cells lining distal convoluted tubule, 9-3, **9-3**
Cementum, 8-3, **8-3**
Central artery, 6-5, **6-5**

Central band, **3-23**
Central lobule, **4-12**
Central nervous system, 1-11, **1-11**
Central sulcus, **4-4**
Central tendon of perineum, 3-16
Central veins, hepatic, **8-9**
Central venous sinus of bone, **2-1**
Centrioles, 1-4, **1-4**
Centromedian thalamic nucleus, **4-10**
Cephalic vein, 5-20, **5-20**
Cephalon (head), 1-1, **1-1**
Cerebellar cortex, **4-12**
Cerebellar peduncles, 4-6, **4-6**
Cerebellum, 1-11, 4-4, **4-5**, **4-10**, 4-12, **4-12**, **11-2**
  Purkinje cell of, **4-1**
Cerebral aqueduct (of Sylvius), **4-12**, **4-17**
Cerebral cortex, 1-11, **1-11**
  cortical connections, 4-5, **4-5**
  lobes of, 4-4, **4-4**
  pyramidal cell of, **4-1**
Cerebral longitudinal fissure, **4-5**, **4-6**
Cerebrospinal fluid (CSF), 4-17, **4-17**, 4-18, **4-18**
Cerebrum
  lobes, 4-4, **4-4**
  pia mater covering, 4-18, **4-18**
Cervical curvature, 2-5, **2-5**
Cervical dermatomes (C2-C8), 4-16, **4-16**
Cervical lymph nodes, **6-1**
Cervical plexus, 1-11, **1-11**, 4-28, **4-28**
Cervical vertebrae, 2-5, **2-5**. See also Atlas (C1); Axis (C2)
  bifid spine, 2-6, **2-6**
  body of, 2-6, **2-6**, **3-8**
  foramen transversarium, 2-6, **2-6**
  intervertebral discs, 2-6, **2-6**
  lamina, 2-6, **2-6**
  transverse process, 2-6, **2-6**
  vertebral canal, 2-6, **2-6**
Cervicis (neck), 1-1, **1-1**
Cervix of uterus, **10-1**, 10-3, **10-3**
Chambers of eye, **4-23**
Cheek, **1-1**
Chest, 1-1
Chief cells, 8-6, **8-6**
Choanae, **3-4**, **3-5**, **7-2**, **8-4**
Cholecystokinin, 11-8, **11-8**
Chondrocytes, **1-6**
Choroid, 4-23, **4-23**, **4-24**
Choroid plexus, **4-9**
  in lateral ventricles, 4-17, **4-17**
Chronic obstructive pulmonary disease, 7-5
Ciliary body, 4-20, 4-23, **4-23**, **4-24**
Ciliary process, 4-23, **4-23**
Cingulate cortex, limbic, **4-10**
Cingulate gyrus, **4-6**, 4-8, **4-8**
Circular folds, 8-7, **8-7**
Circular muscle, 1-10, **1-10**, **6-6**, **8-7**
Circulation
  intrapulmonary, 7-6, **7-6**
  prenatal and postnatal, 5-22, **5-22**
Circumduction, 1-3, **1-3**
Circumflex subscapular artery, **5-12**
Circumvallate papillae, 3-4, **3-4**
Cirrhosis of liver, 5-19, 8-9
Cisterna chyli, **6-1**, **6-7**

Gluteal muscles, 3-25, **3-25**
Gluteus (buttocks), **1-1**
Gluteus maximus muscle, **3-15**, 3-25, **3-25**, **3-26**, **4-31**
Gluteus medius muscle, 3-25, **3-25**, **3-26**, **4-31**
Gluteus minimus muscle, 3-25, **3-25**, **3-26**
Goblet cells, 8-8, **8-8**
Golgi apparatus, 1-4, **1-4**, **4-1**
Gonadal arteries, 5-14, **5-14**
Gonadotropes, 11-3
Gonadotrophic hormone levels, **10-4**
Gonadotropin-releasing hormone (GnRH), 11-7, **11-7**
Graafian follicle, mature, 10-2, **10-2**
Gracilis muscle, **3-26**, 3-28, **3-28**, 3-32, **3-32**
Graves disease, 11-4
Gray matter, 4-5, **4-5**, **4-14**
  spinal cord, 4-13, **4-13**, 4-14
Gray ramus communicans, **4-15**
Great auricular nerve, 4-28, **4-28**
Great cardiac vein, 5-6, **5-6**
Great cerebral vein (of Galen), **5-11**
Great saphenous vein, 5-21, **5-21**
Great toe, **1-1**
  distal phalanx of, **2-20**
  lumbar dermatome related to, 4-16, **4-16**
Greater curvature of stomach, 8-6
Greater omentum, 8-5, **8-5**, **8-6**
Greater sciatic foramen, **2-15**
Greater sciatic notch, **2-15**
Greater trochanter, **2-16**, **2-17**, **3-25**
Groin, **1-1**, **8-1**
  pull injury, 3-28
  thoracic dermatome related to, 4-16, **4-16**
Ground substance, **1-6**
Growth hormone (GH), 11-3, **11-3**
Gubernaculum, **3-13**
Gustatory cortex, **4-4**
Gut-associated lymphatic tissue, 6-6, **6-6**

H

Hair cells, otic, 4-25, **4-25**, 4-26, **4-26**
Hair follicles, 1-12, **1-12**
Hallux (great toe), **1-1**
Hamate, 2-13, **2-13**, **2-14**
Hamstrings, 3-26
Hand, **1-1**
  bones, 2-13, **2-13**
  intrinsic muscles, 3-23, **3-23**
Hard palate, **3-4**, **7-4**, 8-2, **8-2**
Haversian system, 2-1
Head, 1-1, **1-1**
  arteries, 5-8, **5-8**, 5-9, **5-9**
  veins, 5-11, **5-11**
Healing, 6-2
Hearing loss, 4-25
Heart, 1-13, **1-13**
  atria and ventricles, 5-4, **5-4**
  coronary arteries and cardiac veins, 5-6, **5-6**
  hormone, 11-1, **11-1**
  intrinsic conduction pathway, 5-5, **5-5**
  mediastinum, 5-3, **5-3**
  parasympathetic system effects, 4-20, **4-20**
  pericardium, 5-3, **5-3**
  sympathetic system effects, 4-19, **4-19**

Heart sounds, 5-4
Heel of foot, **1-1**
  pain from plantar fasciitis, 3-31
Helper T cells, 6-3
Hematoma, epidural, 5-10
Hemiazygos vein, 5-17, **5-17**
Hemispheres
  cerebellar, 4-12, **4-12**
  cerebral, 4-4, **4-4**, 4-5, **4-5**
Hemopericardium, 5-3
Hemorrhage, subarachnoid, 5-10
Henle's loop, 9-3, **9-3**, 9-4
Hepatic artery branch, 8-9, **8-9**
Hepatic artery proper, **8-10**
Hepatic flexure, **8-6**, **8-8**
Hepatic portal system, **5-19**
Hepatic portal vein, **5-17**
Hepatic veins, 5-18, **5-18**, **5-22**
Hepatocytes, 8-9, **8-9**
Hepatopancreatic ampulla, 8-10, **8-10**
Hernias
  hiatal, 8-6
  incisional, 3-12
  inguinal, 3-12, 3-13
  lineal alba, 3-12
  umbilical, 3-12
Herniation of nucleus pulposus, 2-7, **2-7**
Hiatal hernia, 8-6
Hilum, **7-5**
Hindgut, 5-15
Hinge (ginglymus) joints, 1-9, **1-9**
  humeroulnar, 2-12, **2-12**
  interphalangeal, 2-14
  talocrural, 2-20
  TMJ, 2-4, **2-4**
Hip bone, 2-15
Hip joint, 2-16, **2-16**
  muscles acting on, 3-32
  sacral plexus, **4-31**
Hippocampus, 4-8, **4-8**, 4-9, **4-9**
Hirschsprung's disease, 4-21
Hoarseness, 3-6, 7-4
Homunculus, 4-4, **4-4**
Hook of hamate, **2-14**
Hormones, 11-1, **11-1**
  of digestive system, 11-8, **11-8**
  fuel-mobilization and fuel-storage, 11-6
  of pituitary gland, 11-3, **11-3**
Humeroradial joint, 2-12, **2-12**
Humeroulnar joint, 2-12, **2-12**
Humerus, **1-7**, **1-9**, 2-10, **2-10**, **3-19**, **3-24**
Humoral response, 6-3
Huntington's disease, 4-7
Hyaline cartilage, 1-7, 2-1, **2-1**
Hydrocephalus, 4-17, **4-17**
Hydrochloric acid, **11-8**
Hyoglossus muscle, 3-4, **3-4**, 3-5
Hyoid bone, **3-4–3-6**, **7-1**, **7-4**
Hyperextension injury of neck, 2-9
Hyperopia, 4-24
Hypersensitivity, 6-7
Hypertension, 5-2
  portal, 5-19
Hypochondriac region, **8-1**
Hypodermis, 1-12, **1-12**
Hypoglossal canal, **2-3**
Hypoglossal nerve (XII), **2-3**, 4-22, **4-22**, **4-28**
Hypophyseal stalk, **11-2**

Hypophysis, **4-11**
Hypothalamic artery, **5-10**
Hypothalamic nuclei
  arcuate, 4-11, **4-11**
  dorsomedial, 4-11, **4-11**
  mammillary, 4-11, **4-11**
  paraventricular, 4-11, **4-11**
  posterior, 4-11, **4-11**
  supraoptic, 4-11, **4-11**
  ventromedial, 4-11, **4-11**
Hypothalamohypophyseal tract, **4-11**
Hypothalamus, 4-6, **4-6**, 4-8, **4-8**, 4-11, **4-11**, 11-1, **11-1**, 11-2, **11-2**
Hypothenar eminence, 3-23
Hypothenar muscles, **3-24**
Hypothyroidism, 11-4

I

Ileocolic artery, 5-15, **5-15**, **8-7**
Ileocolic vein, **5-19**
Ileum, 8-1, **8-1**, 8-7, **8-7**
Iliac crest, **3-25**
Iliac lymph nodes, **6-1**, **6-6**, 6-7, **6-7**
Iliac tuberosity, **2-15**
Iliacus muscle, 3-14, **3-14**, 3-27, **3-27**
Iliocostalis muscle, 3-10, **3-10**
Iliofemoral ligament, 2-16, **2-16**
Iliohypogastric nerve, 4-30, **4-30**
Ilioinguinal nerve, 4-30, **4-30**
Iliolumbar ligament, **2-15**
Iliopectineal bursa, **2-16**
Iliopsoas muscle, 3-27, **3-27**, 3-28
Iliotibial tract, **3-26**
Ilium, 2-15, **2-15**, **6-6**
Immature lymphocytes, 6-4, **6-4**
Immunity
  adaptive, 6-3, **6-3**
  innate, 6-2, **6-2**
Immunodeficiencies, 6-7
Immunological surveillance, 6-2
Incisional hernias, 3-12
Incisors, 2-4, **2-4**, 8-3, **8-3**
Inclusions, 1-4
Incontinence, stress, 9-5
Incus, **4-25**
Indirect inguinal hernias, 3-13
Infarction, myocardial, 5-6
Infected cell
  displaying antigen, 6-3, **6-3**
  dying, 6-3, **6-3**
Inferior (caudal), 1-2, **1-2**
Inferior alveolar artery, 5-9, **5-9**
Inferior colliculus, **4-12**
Inferior concha, 7-2, **7-2**
Inferior gluteal artery, 5-16, **5-16**
Inferior gluteal nerve, 4-31, **4-31**
Inferior mesenteric artery, 5-14, **5-14**, 5-15, **5-15**
Inferior mesenteric vein, **5-17**, **5-18**, 5-19, **5-19**
Inferior nasal concha, 2-2, **2-2**, 2-3, **2-3**, **4-23**
Inferior oblique muscle, 3-3, **3-3**
Inferior part of duodenum, 8-7, **8-7**
Inferior petrosal sinus, **5-11**
Inferior pharyngeal constrictor muscle, 3-5, **3-5**
Inferior phrenic artery, **5-14**, **11-5**
Inferior phrenic vein, **5-18**
Inferior pubic ramus, **9-5**
Inferior rectal artery, 5-16, **5-16**

Neck (Continued)
  veins, 5-11, **5-11**
  whiplash, 2-9
Nephrons, 9-3, **9-3**
Nerve plexuses
  deep dermal, **1-12**
  of enteric nervous system, 4-21, **4-21**
  spinal, 1-11, **1-11**, 4-28, **4-28**, 4-29, **4-29**,
    4-30, **4-30**, 4-31, **4-31**
Nervous system, 1-11, **1-11**
Neural stalk, **11-2**
Neurocranium, 2-2
Neurocrine cell-to-cell interaction, 11-1, **11-1**
Neuroeffector junctions, **4-15**
Neuroendocrine cells, **11-8**
Neurohypophysis, **4-11**, 11-2, **11-3**
Neurons
  in gut, 4-21
  postganglionic parasympathetic, 4-20, **4-20**
  postganglionic sympathetic, 4-19, **4-19**
  preganglionic parasympathetic, 4-20, **4-20**
  preganglionic sympathetic, 4-19, **4-19**
  structure of, 4-1, **4-1**
  supraoptic and paraventricular, 11-3, **11-3**
Neurotubules, **4-1**, 4-3
Neurovascular bundle, intercostal, **3-11**
Neutrophils, 1-6, **1-6**, 5-1, **5-1**, 6-2, **6-2**
Nipple, 10-5, **10-5**
  thoracic dermatome related to, 4-16, **4-16**
Nissl substance, **4-1**
Norepinephrine, 4-19, 11-5
Normal pressure hydrocephalus, 4-17
Nose, **1-1**, 7-2, **7-2**
Nucleolus, 1-4, **1-4**
Nucleus (pl. nuclei), **4-1**
  of cell, 1-4, **1-4**
  hypothalamic, 4-11, **4-11**
  of muscie, **1-10**
  thalamic, 4-10, **4-10**
Nucleus pulposus, 2-5, **2-5**
  herniating, 2-7, **2-7**

O

Oblique sinus, 5-3
Obliquus capitis inferior muscle, 3-10, **3-10**
Obliquus capitis superior muscle, 3-10, **3-10**
Obstructive hydrocephalus, 4-17
Obturator artery, **5-13**, 5-16, **5-16**
Obturator externus muscle, 3-28, **3-28**
Obturator internus muscle, 3-15, **3-15**, **3-16**,
  3-25, **3-25**
Obturator nerve, 4-30, **4-30**
Occipital artery, 5-8, **5-8**
Occipital bone, 2-2, **2-2**, 2-3
  basilar part, **3-4**, **3-5**, **3-8**, 7-2
Occipital condyle, **2-3**, 2-6
Occipital lobe, 1-11, **1-11**, 4-4, **4-4**
Occipital pole, **4-6**
Occipital sinus, **5-11**
Occipitalis muscle, 3-1, **3-1**
Occipitomastoid suture, 2-2, **2-2**
Oculomotor nerve (III), **2-3**, 4-22, **4-22**
Olecranon (back of elbow), **1-1**, **2-12**, **3-19**,
  3-22
Olecranon fossa, **2-10**
Olfaction, 4-27, **4-27**
Olfactory cell, **4-1**

Olfactory cortex, **4-4**
Olfactory epithelium, 4-27, **4-27**
Olfactory nerve (I), 4-22, **4-22**
Olfactory nerve bundles, **2-3**
Olfactory receptors, 4-27, **4-27**
Olfactory stria, **4-27**
Olfactory tract, 4-8, **4-8**
Oligodendrocytes, 4-1, 4-2, **4-2**
Omental bursa, 8-5, **8-5**, **8-6**
Omohyoid muscle, 3-7, **3-7**, **4-28**
Oocytes, 10-2
Ophthalmic artery, 5-10
Ophthalmic nerve (V₁), branches of, **2-3**
Opponens digiti minimi muscle, 3-23, **3-23**,
  3-32
Opponens pollicis muscle, 3-23, **3-23**
Opposition, thumb, 2-14
Optic canal, **2-3**
Optic chiasm, **4-6**, **4-11**, **4-12**, 4-24, **11-2**
Optic disc, 4-23
Optic nerve (II), **2-3**, 3-3, 4-22, **4-22**, 4-24
Oral cavity, **7-1**, 8-1, 8-2, **8-2**
Orbicularis oculi muscle, 3-1, **3-1**
Orbicularis oris muscle, **1-10**, 3-1, **3-1**
Orbit, **7-3**
Organ of Corti, 4-25, **4-25**
Organelles, 1-4
Oris (mouth), **1-1**
Oropharynx, 3-5, **3-5**, 7-1, **7-1**, 7-4, **7-4**, **8-4**
Osteoarthritis, 1-8
Osteoblasts, 2-1
Osteoclasts, 2-1, **11-4**
Osteocytes, 2-1, **2-1**
Osteon, 2-1, **2-1**
Osteoporosis, 1-7
Otic (ear), **1-1**
Otic ganglion, **4-20**
Otitis media, acute, 7-2
Otoliths, 4-26, **4-26**
Outer hair cells, 4-25, **4-25**
Outflow to pulmonary trunk, 5-4, **5-4**
Oval window, **4-25**
Ovarian hormone levels, **10-4**
Ovaries, 10-1, **10-1**, 10-2, **10-2**, 11-1, **11-1**,
  11-7, **11-7**
Ovulated ovum, 10-2, **10-2**
Oxygen diffusion pathways, **7-6**
Oxytocin, 11-3, **11-3**

P

Palate
  hard, **3-4**, **7-4**, 8-2, **8-2**
  muscles, 3-4, **3-4**
  soft, 3-5, **3-5**, **7-1**, **7-2**, **7-4**, 8-2, **8-2**, 8-4, **8-4**
Palatine bone, 2-2, **2-2**, 2-3, **2-3**, **7-2**
Palatine raphe, **8-2**
Palatine tonsil, **3-4**, 4-27, 8-2, **8-2**, **8-4**
Palatoglossus muscle, 3-4, **3-4**
Palatopharyngeus muscle, 3-4, **3-4**
Palm (palmar), **1-1**
  pronation, 1-3, **1-3**
  supination, 1-3, **1-3**
Palmar aponeurosis, **3-21**
Palmar interossei muscles, 3-23, **3-23**
Palmar ligament, 2-14, **2-14**
Palmar radiocarpal ligaments, 2-14, **2-14**
Palmar venous arches, **5-20**

Palmaris longus muscle, 3-21, **3-21**, **3-24**
Palmaris longus tendon, **3-21**
Pancreas, 8-1, 11-6, **11-6**
  exocrine, 8-10, **8-10**
Pancreatic islets, 11-1, **11-1**, **11-6**
Papillae of tongue, 3-4, 4-27, **4-27**
Papillary dermis, 1-12, **1-12**
Papillary muscles, 5-4, **5-4**, 5-5
Para-aortic (lumbar) nodes, 6-7, **6-7**
Paracrine cell-to-cell interaction, 11-1, **11-1**
Parahippocampal gyrus, 4-8, **4-8**, 4-9
Paranasal sinuses, 7-3, **7-3**
Pararenal fat, **9-1**
Parasagittal planes, 1-2
Parasympathetic division of ANS, 4-20, **4-20**,
  4-21, **4-21**
Parathyroid gland, 11-1, **11-1**, 11-4, **11-4**
Parathyroid hormone (PTH), target tissues,
  11-4, **11-4**
Paraumbilical veins, 5-19, **5-19**
Paraventricular nucleus of hypothalamus, cells
  and axons of, 11-2, **11-2**
Paravermis zone, 4-12, **4-12**
Parietal bones, **1-7**, 2-2, **2-2**, 2-3
Parietal cells, 8-6, **8-6**
Parietal layer of serous pericardium, 5-3, **5-3**
Parietal lobe, 1-11, **1-11**, 4-4, 4-4
Parietal peritoneum, 1-13, **1-13**, 8-5, **8-5**
Parietal pleura, 1-13, **1-13**, 7-5, **7-5**
Parietomastoid suture, 2-2, **2-2**
Parkinson's disease, 4-7
Parotid gland, 8-2, **8-2**, 8-4
Pars distalis, 4-11
Pars intermedia, 4-11
Pars tuberalis, 4-11, **11-2**
Passive immunity, 6-3, **6-3**
Patella (kneecap), **1-1**, **1-7**, 2-17, **2-17**, **2-18**,
  3-27, **3-28**
Patellar ligament, **3-27**, **3-28**
Patellar reflex, 3-27
Patellofemoral joint, 2-18
Pathogens, 6-2, **6-2**
Pectinate line, **8-8**
Pectineus muscle, 3-28, **3-28**
Pectoral girdle, 2-10, **2-10**
Pectoralis major muscle, **3-17**, 3-18, **3-18**,
  10-5
Pectoralis minor muscle, **3-17**, 3-18, **3-18**
Peduncles, cerebellar, 4-6, **4-6**, 4-12, **4-12**
Pelvic bone, 2-15
Pelvic girdle, 1-7, **1-7**, 2-15, **2-15**
Pelvic splanchnic nerves, **4-20**, 4-21, **4-21**
Pelvis, 1-1, **1-1**
  acetabulum, 1-9, **1-9**
  arteries, 5-16, **5-16**
  muscles, 3-15, **3-15**
  weakened, 3-25
Penis, **3-16**, **9-5**, **10-6**, 10-8, **10-8**
Pennate muscle, 1-10, **1-10**
Pepsinogen, **11-8**
Peptic ulcers, 8-6
Periarterial lymphatic sheath, 6-5, **6-5**
Pericardium, 1-13, **1-13**, 5-3, **5-3**, **7-1**, 7-5
Pericyte, **5-7**
Perikaryon, 4-1
Perimysium, 1-10, **1-10**
Perineal artery, 5-16, **5-16**
Perineal body, **3-16**, **10-1**

Pulse points
   lower limb, 5-13
   upper limb, 5-12
Pulvinar, **4-7**, 4-10, **4-10**
Purkinje cell of cerebellum, **4-1**
Purkinje system, 5-5, **5-5**
Putamen, **4-5**, 4-7, **4-7**
Pyloric antrum, 8-6, **8-6**
Pyloric canal, 8-6, **8-6**
Pyramidal cell of cerebral cortex, **4-1**
Pyramidal lobe of thyroid gland, 11-4, **11-4**
Pyramidalis muscle, 3-12, **3-12**
Pyramids, renal, 9-2, **9-2**

Q

Quadrate muscle, 1-10, **1-10**
Quadratus femoris muscle, 3-25, **3-25**
Quadratus lumborum muscle, 3-14, **3-14**
Quadratus plantae muscle, 3-31, **3-31**
Quadriceps femoris tendon, **2-18**, **3-27**

R

Radial artery, 5-12, **5-12**
Radial collateral ligament, 2-12, **2-12**, **2-14**
Radial nerve, 4-29, **4-29**
Radial tuberosity, **2-12**
Radial vein, 5-20, **5-20**
Radiate ligaments, **2-8**, 2-9, **2-9**
Radiocarpal joint, 2-14
Radioulnar joints
   muscles acting on, 3-24
   pronation and supination, 3-20, **3-20**
Radius, **1-8**, 2-12, **2-12**, **2-13**, **3-19**
Ramus of ischium, **2-15**
Reabsorption from ultrafiltrate, 9-4, **9-4**
Reciprocal synapse, 4-3, **4-3**
Rectal valves, **8-8**
Rectosigmoidal junction, **8-8**
Rectouterine pouch, **10-1**
Rectovesical pouch, 8-5, 10-6, **10-6**
Rectum, **3-15**, 8-1, **8-1**, **8-5**, 8-8, **8-8**, **9-1**, 10-6
   veins, **5-18**
Rectus abdominis muscle, 3-12, **3-12**
Rectus capitis anterior muscle, 3-8
Rectus capitis lateralis muscle, 3-8
Rectus capitis posterior major muscle, 3-10, **3-10**
Rectus capitis posterior minor muscle, 3-10
Rectus femoris muscle, **1-10**, 3-27, **3-27**, 3-32, **3-32**
Rectus sheath, 3-12, **3-12**
Red blood cells, **1-6**, 5-1, **5-1**, **6-5**, 7-6, **7-6**
Red pulp, 6-5
Referred pain, of angina pectoris, 5-6
Reflexes, patellar, 3-27
Regulatory proteins, plasma, **5-1**
Renal arteries, 5-14, **5-14**, **9-1**, 9-2, **9-2**, **11-5**
Renal cortex, 9-2, **9-2**
Renal medulla, **9-3**
Renal papilla, **9-2**
Renal pelvis, 9-2, **9-2**
Renal pyramids, 9-2, **9-2**
Renal stones, 9-2
Renal veins, 5-18, **5-18**, **9-1**, 9-2, **9-2**, **11-5**
Renin-angiotensin-aldosterone system, 9-3
Reposition, thumb, **2-14**

Reproductive system
   female
      breast, 10-5, **10-5**
      features of, 10-1, **10-1**
      menstrual cycle, 10-4, **10-4**
      ovaries and uterine tubes, 10-2, **10-2**
      uterus and vagina, 10-3, **10-3**
   male
      features of, 10-6, **10-6**
      testis and epididymis, 10-7, **10-7**
      urethra and penis, 10-8, **10-8**
Respiratory system
   mechanics of ventilation, 7-6, **7-6**
   nasal cavity and nasopharynx, 7-2, **7-2**
   organization of, 7-1, **7-1**
   oropharynx, laryngopharynx, and larynx, 7-4, **7-4**
   paranasal sinuses, 7-3, **7-3**
   trachea and lungs, 7-5, **7-5**
Rete testis, 10-7, **10-7**
Reticular cells, 6-1
Reticular dermis, 1-12, **1-12**
Reticular fibers, 1-6, **1-6**
Retina, 4-23, **4-23**, 4-24, **4-24**
Retinal cell, **4-1**
Retino-geniculo-calcarine pathway, **4-24**
Retraction, 1-3, **1-3**
Retromandibular branches, 5-9
Retromandibular vein, 5-11, **5-11**
Retroperitoneal viscera, 8-5, **8-5**
Retropharyngeal space, **3-7**, 3-8
Rhinosinusitis, 7-3
Rhomboid major muscle, 3-9, **3-9**, 3-17, **3-17**
Rhomboid minor muscle, **3-9**, 3-17, **3-17**
Ribosomes, 1-4, **1-4**
Ribs, 1-7, **1-7**
   angle of, 2-8, **2-8**
   first, **1-11**, **3-8**, **3-11**, **4-29**, **5-3**
   head of, 2-8, **2-8**
   neck of, 2-8, **2-8**
   tubercle of, 2-8, **2-8**
   twelfth, 3-9
Rickets, 2-1
Right atrium, 5-4, **5-4**
Right brachiocephalic vein, 5-17, **5-17**
Right colic artery, 5-15, **5-15**, **8-7**
Right colic vein, **5-19**
Right common iliac artery, 5-16, **5-16**
Right coronary artery, 5-6, **5-6**
Right gastric artery, **8-10**
Right gastric vein, **5-19**
Right gonadal vein, 5-18, **5-18**
Right hepatic artery, **5-15**
Right lymphatic duct, 6-1, **6-1**, **6-7**
Right lymphatic trunk, **6-6**
Right superior rectal veins, 5-19, **5-19**
Right ventricle, 5-4, **5-4**
Rima glottidis, 7-4
Risorius muscle, 3-1, **3-1**
Rods, 4-24, **4-24**
Root of tongue, **3-5**, **8-4**
Roots of brachial plexus, 4-29, **4-29**
Roots of teeth, **7-3**, 8-3, **8-3**
Rotation
   lateral, 1-3
   medial, 1-3
Rotator cuff muscles, 2-11, 3-17, **3-17**
Rotator cuff tendons, 2-11

Rotatores cervicis muscles, **3-10**
Rotatores thoracis muscles, **3-10**
Rough endoplasmic reticulum, 1-4, **1-4**, **4-1**
Round ligament of liver, 8-9, **8-9**
Round ligament of uterus, **10-1**
Round window, 4-25, **4-25**
Rubrospinal tract, 4-14, **4-14**
Rupture
   of anterior cruciate ligament, 2-18
   of biceps brachii tendon, 3-19

S

Saccule, 4-25, **4-25**, **4-26**
Sacral curvature, 2-5, **2-5**
Sacral dermatomes (S1-S5), 4-16, **4-16**
Sacral hiatus, **2-7**
Sacral plexus, **4-13**, 4-31, **4-31**
Sacral spinal cord, **4-21**
Sacral vertebrae
   anterior sacral foramina, 2-7, **2-7**
   lumbosacral articular surface, 2-7, **2-7**
   median sacral crest, 2-7, **2-7**
Sacrococcygeal joint, 2-15
Sacroiliac joint, 2-15
Sacroiliac ligaments, 2-15, **2-15**
Sacrospinous ligament, 2-15, **2-15**
Sacrotuberous ligament, 2-15, **2-15**, **3-25**
Sacrum, **1-11**, 2-5, **2-5**, 2-7, **2-7**, 2-15, **3-15**
Saddle joints, 1-9, **1-9**
   patellofemoral, 2-18
   sternoclavicular, 2-8
   thumb, 2-14
Sagittal planes, 1-2
Sagittal suture, 2-2, **2-2**
Salivary glands, 8-1, 8-2, **8-2**
Salpingopharyngeus muscle, 3-5
Salty taste, 4-27
Saphenous nerve, **4-30**
Sarcolemma, **1-10**
Sarcomas, 1-6
Sarcoplasm, **1-10**
Sartorius muscle, 3-27, **3-27**, 3-32, **3-32**
Sartorius tendon, **3-27**
Scala tympani, **4-25**
Scala vestibuli, **4-25**
Scalene muscles, 3-8, **3-8**
Scalp, **3-1**
Scaphoid bone, 2-13, **2-13**, 2-14, **3-23**
Scapula, 1-9, **1-9**, 2-10, **2-10**, **3-17**
   muscles acting on, 3-24
   spine of, 2-10, **2-10**, **3-9**, **3-17**, **3-18**
Schwann cells, 4-1, 4-2, **4-27**
Sciatic nerve, 4-31, **4-31**
Sciatica, 4-31
Sclera, 4-23, **4-23**, **4-24**
Scoliosis, **2-5**
Scrotum, **10-6**, 10-7
Sebaceous glands, 1-12, **1-12**
Secondary bronchi, 7-5, **7-5**
Secondary cartilaginous joint, **1-8**, 2-9, **2-9**
Secondary follicles, 10-2, **10-2**
Secondary spermatocytes, 10-7, **10-7**
Secretin, 11-8, **11-8**
Segmental arteries, 9-2, **9-2**
Sella turcica, **2-3**
Semicircular canals, 4-25, **4-25**, 4-26, **4-26**
Semilunar folds, **8-8**

Netter's Anatomy Coloring Book

Veins (Continued)
  carrying hormones from pituitary, **11-3**
  of endometrium, 10-4, **10-4**
  general organization of, 5-2, **5-2**
  of head and neck, 5-11, **5-11**
  of lower limb, 5-21, **5-21**
  of lymph node, 6-1, **6-1**
  subcutaneous, **1-12**
  of thorax, 5-17, **5-17**
  types of, 5-7, **5-7**
  of upper limb, 5-20, **5-20**
Venae comitantes, 5-20
Venous lakes of endometrium, 10-4,
  10-4
Venous sinuses, 5-11, **5-11**
  splenic, 6-5, **6-5**
Venous valves, 5-21, **5-21**
Ventral (anterior), 1-2, **1-2**
Ventral body cavities, 1-13, **1-13**
Ventral ramus, 4-15, **4-15**
  of spinal nerves, **4-30**
Ventral root, 4-15, **4-15**
Ventral thalamic nuclei, 4-10, **4-10**
Ventricles
  cardiac, 5-4, **5-4**
  cerebral, **4-5**, **4-6**
    fourth, 4-17, **4-17**
    lateral, **4-7**, **4-9**, 4-17, **4-17**
    third, 4-17, **4-17**
  laryngeal, 7-4, **7-4**
Ventricular bundle branches (Purkinje system),
  5-5, **5-5**
Ventricular tachycardia, 5-5
Venules, 5-7, **5-7**
Vermiform appendix, 6-6, **6-6**
Vermis, 4-12, **4-12**
Vertebra (pl. vertebrae), **1-7**
  body of, **1-8**, 2-5, **2-5**, **4-18**
  cervical. See Cervical vertebrae

Vertebra (pl. vertebrae) (Continued)
  coccygeal, 2-7, **2-7**
  intervertebral disc, 2-5, **2-5**
  levels, and nerve plexuses, **1-11**
  lumbar. See Lumbar vertebrae
  sacral
    anterior sacral foramina, 2-7, **2-7**
    lumbosacral articular surface, 2-7, **2-7**
    median sacral crest, 2-7, **2-7**
  spine of, **4-15**
  thoracic. See Thoracic vertebrae
  typical, 2-5, **2-5**
Vertebral artery, 5-8, **5-8**, 5-10, **5-10**, **5-12**
Vertebral column, 1-7, 2-5, **2-5**
Vertebral foramen, 2-5, **2-5**
Vertebral notches, 2-5
Vertigo, 4-26
Vesicle exocytosis, 4-3, **4-3**
Vesicouterine pouch, **10-1**
Vestibular folds, 7-4, **7-4**
Vestibular ganglion, and afferent axons, 4-26,
  4-26
Vestibule
  laryngeal, 7-4, **7-4**
  nasal, **7-2**
  otic, **4-25**
Vestibulocochlear nerve (VIII), **2-3**, 4-22,
  4-22, **4-25**
Villus, **6-6**, 8-7, **8-7**
Visceral layer of serous pericardium, 5-3,
  5-3
Visceral peritoneum, 1-13, **1-13**
Visceral pleura, 1-13, **1-13**, **7-5**
Viscerocranium, 2-2
Visual cortex, primary, 4-4, **4-4**, **4-10**
Visual system, 4-23, **4-23**, 4-24, **4-24**
Vitamin D deficiency, 2-1
Vitreous body, 4-23, **4-23**
Vocal folds, 3-6, **7-1**, 7-4, **7-4**

Vocal ligament, **3-6**, **7-4**
Vomer, 2-2, **2-2**, 2-3, **2-3**, 7-2, **7-2**, **7-3**

W

Waldeyer's lymphatic ring, 7-4
Walls of nasal cavity, 7-2, **7-2**
Water regulation, renal, 9-4, **9-4**
Whiplash, 2-9
White blood cells, 5-1, **5-1**, 6-1
  hormones, 11-1, **11-1**
White matter
  cerebral cortical, 4-5, **4-5**
  spinal cord, 4-13, **4-13**, 4-14, **4-14**
White pulp, 6-5, **6-5**
White ramus communicans, **4-15**
Wing of ilium, **2-15**
Wrist, **1-1**
  bones, 2-13, **2-13**
  carpal bones, **1-7**
  flexion and extension at, 1-3, **1-3**
  joints, 2-14, **2-14**
  muscles acting on, 3-24

X

Xiphoid process, 2-8, **2-8**

Z

Zona fasciculata, 11-5, **11-5**
Zona glomerulosa, 11-5, **11-5**
Zona reticularis, 11-5, **11-5**
Zonular fibers, 4-23, **4-23**
Zygapophysial joints, 2-9, **2-9**
Zygomatic arch, **3-2**
Zygomatic bone, 2-2, **2-2**
Zygomaticus major muscle, **3-1**
Zygomaticus minor muscle, **3-1**